CRASH COURSE
Pharmacology
SECOND EDITION

Series editor
Daniel Horton-Szar
BSc (Hons) MBBS (Hons)
GP Registrar
Northgate Medical Practice
Canterbury
Kent

Faculty advisor
Professor Clive Page, BSc, PhD
Sackler Institute of Pulmonary
Pharmacology
King's College
London

Pharmacology

SECOND EDITION

James S Dawson

MBChB 2001
Leicester University

First Edition Authors
Magali NF Taylor
Peter JW Reide

 Mosby

Edinburgh • London • New York • Oxford • Philadelphia • St Louis • Sydney • Toronto 2002

MOSBY
An imprint of Elsevier Limited

Commissioning Editor Alex Stibbe
Project Manager Colin Arthur
Project Development Manager Ruth Swan
Designer Andy Chapman
Illustration Management Mick Ruddy

First edition 1999
Second edition 2002
Reprinted 2003, 2004

ISBN 0723432465

British Library Cataloguing in Publication Data
A catalogue record for this book is available from the British Library

Library of Congress Cataloging in Publication Data
A catalog record for this book is available from the Library of Congress

Note
Medical knowledge is constantly changing. As new information becomes available, changes in treatment, procedures, equipment and the use of drugs become necessary. The author, editors and the publisher have taken care to ensure that the information given in this text is accurate and up to date. However, readers are strongly advised to confirm that the information, especially with regard to drug usage, complies with the latest legislation and standards of practice.

ELSEVIER SCIENCE
your source for books, journals and multimedia in the health sciences
www.elsevierhealth.com

The publisher's policy is to use paper manufactured from sustainable forests

Typeset by Kolam, Pondicherry, India
Printed in Spain by Graphycems

Preface

Believe it or not, pharmacology is a fairly logical subject; most drugs have simple mechanisms of action, and predictable side effects.

For me, its author, the purpose of this book is to present the basic concepts of how drugs act alongside the important aspects of physiology and disease.

Used alone, or in conjunction with lectures, this text should be more than sufficient to give you a good grounding in the subject of pharmacology, and allow you to sail through your exams.

I hope you find it as useful and enjoyable to use, as I have to write it.

Good luck.

James Dawson

The Second Edition of this book has been thoroughly revised and updated as a new edition. The book continues to provide a comprehensive and approachable text on pharmacology for medical students. As part of the Crash Course Series, the overall style is user friendly, consisting of concise bulleted text with many informative illustrations. The content provides a comprehensive overview of the core material needed to pass the pharmacology component of the undergraduate medical curriculum. At the end of the book, there is a self-assessment section consisting of multiple-choice questions, short-answer questions and essay questions which test the reader's understanding of the topic.

In line with the new style of curriculum recommended by the General Medical Council, the pharmacology is organized logically into body systems and the clinical relevance of the pharmacology is stressed throughout.

I have no doubt that this Second Edition will be widely used and provide a very useful study and revision aid for students. It provides a refreshing means of bringing the medical student up to speed in pharmacology and will help make pharmacology easily understood.

Professor Clive Page
Faculty Advisor

In the six years since the First Editions were published, there have been many changes in medicine, and in the way it is taught. These Second Editions have been largely rewritten to take these changes into account, and keep Crash Course up to date for the twenty-first century. New material has been added to include recent research and all pharmacological and disease management information has been updated in line with current best practice. We have listened to feedback from hundreds of students who have been using Crash Course and have improved the structure and layout of the books accordingly: pathology material has been closely integrated with the relevant basic medical science; there are more multiple-choice questions and the clarity of text and figures is better than ever.

The principles on which we developed the series remain the same, however. Medicine is a huge subject, and the last thing a student needs when exams are looming is to waste time assembling information from different sources, and wading through pages of irrelevant detail. As before, Crash Course brings you all the information you need, in compact, manageable volumes that integrate basic medical science with clinical practice. We still tread the fine line between producing clear, concise text and providing enough detail for those aiming at distinction. The series is still written by medical students with recent exam experience, and checked for accuracy by senior faculty members from across the UK.

I wish you the best of luck in your future careers!

Dr Dan Horton-Szar
Series Editor

Acknowledgements

I would like to thank firstly and foremost Dan Horton-Szar for his constructive and enthusiastic e-mails, and his meticulous eye for detail.

My thanks go to Professor Clive Page, Division of Pharmacology and Therapeutics, King's College, London, and to Dr Iain Squire, Department of Medicine and Therapeutics, University of Leicester, for their help and assistance. Thanks particularly to Preet Panasar, Gillian Stead, Sarah Hobson, and the other pharmacists at the Leicester Royal Infirmary for the information and ideas they all provided me with.

I must also thank the team at Mosby's in London for their administrative role, and in particular Alex Stibbe, who offered me practical solutions to what seemed like insurmountable problems.

Finally I thank my friends and family.

Figure credits
Figures 1.1–3, 1.12, 1.13, 6.1, 6.4, 6.11, 7.1–4, 8.3, 9.1, 9.3–5, 10.2, 11.1–5, 11.7, 11.11, 11.16, 11.18, 12.1–3, 12.6–8 redrawn with kind permission from Integrated Pharmacology 2e, edited by Professor C Page, Dr M Curtis, Professor M Sutter, Professor M Walker and Professor B Hoffman, Mosby, 2002

Key to Icons

Dedication

This text is dedicated to my mum and dad for all the emotional and financial support they have given me, which has allowed me to study medicine, and achieve a goal I once thought unobtainable.

Contents

PRINCIPLES OF
PHARMACOLOGY

1. Introduction to Pharmacology

Molecular basis of pharmacology

What is pharmacology?

The word 'pharmacology' derives from the Greek word for drug, *pharmakon*.

Pharmacology is the study of the actions, mechanisms, uses, and adverse effects of drugs.

A drug is any natural or synthetic substance that alters the physiological state of a living organism. Drugs can be divided into two groups:

- Medicinal drugs are substances used for the prevention, treatment, and diagnosis of disease.
- Non-medicinal drugs, or social drugs, are substances used for recreational purposes. Non-medicinal drugs include illegal mood-altering substances such as cannabis, heroin, and cocaine as well as everyday substances such as caffeine, nicotine, and alcohol.

Although drugs are intended to have a selective action, this is rarely achieved.

There is always a risk of adverse effects associated with the use of any drug, and each time a drug is used the prescriber should be happy that the benefits of giving the drug outweigh potential drawbacks, or adverse effects.

Drug names and classification

A single drug can have a variety of names and belong to many classes.

Factors used for classifying drugs include their:

- Pharmacotherapeutic actions.
- Pharmacological actions.
- Molecular actions.
- Chemical nature.

The generic name of a drug is that which appears in official national pharmacopoeias. All drugs available on prescription or sold over the counter have a generic name that may vary from country to country. Newly-patented drugs usually have one generic name (e.g. salbutamol) and one brand or proprietary name (e.g. Ventolin®). However, once the patent expires, the marketing of the drug is open to any number of manufacturers and, although the generic name is retained, the variety of brand names inevitably increases.

How do drugs work?

Drugs cause a change in physiological function by interacting with the organism at the chemical level.

Certain drugs (e.g. general anaesthetics, antacids) work by means of their physicochemical properties, and these are said to have a non-specific mechanism of action. For this reason these drugs must be given in much higher doses (mg–g) than the more specific drugs.

Most drugs produce their effects by targeting specific cellular macromolecules. This may involve modification of DNA or RNA function, inhibition of transport systems or enzymes or, more commonly, action on receptors.

Detailed knowledge about the molecular structures of the cell are not required, though a simple understanding of them is useful in appreciating how drugs have their effects, and side effects.

Transport systems
Ion channels

Ion channels are pores located in the cell membrane that allow selective transfer of ions (charged species) in and out of the cell. Opening or closing of these channels, known as 'gating', occurs as a result of the channel proteins undergoing a change in shape. Gating is controlled either by transmitter substances or by the membrane potential (voltage-operated channels).

Some drugs modulate ion channel function directly by binding to a part of the channel protein itself, e.g. the blocking action of local anaesthetics on sodium channels. Other drugs interact with ion channels indirectly via a G-protein and other intermediates.

Carrier molecules

Transfer of ions and molecules against their concentration gradients is facilitated by carrier molecules located in the cell membrane. There are two types of carrier molecule:

- Energy-independent carriers are transporters (move one type of ion/molecule in one direction), symporters (move two or more ions/molecules), or antiporters (exchange one or more ions/molecules for one or more other ions/molecules).
- Energy-dependent carriers are termed pumps (e.g. the Na^+/K^+ ATPase pump).

Enzymes

Enzymes are protein catalysts that increase the rate of specific chemical reactions without undergoing any net change themselves during the reaction.

All enzymes are potential targets for drugs. Drugs either act as a false substrate for the enzyme, or they inhibit the enzyme's activity directly by binding to other sites on the enzyme protein.

Certain drugs may require enzymatic modification. This degradation converts a drug from its inactive form (prodrug) to its active form.

Receptors

Receptors are the means through which most drugs produce their effects.

A receptor is a specific protein molecule that is usually located in the cell membrane, though intracellular receptors and intranuclear receptors also exist. Agonist drugs mimic endogenous mediators and activate the receptor, while antagonist drugs bind to the receptor preventing receptor activation by endogenous mediators.

Synaptic transmitter substances and hormones, the body's chemical messengers, are natural ligands (i.e. molecules that bind with a molecular target) for receptors, and they have the following modes of action:

- Neurotransmitters are chemicals that are released from nerve terminals, diffuse across the synaptic cleft, and bind to pre- or postsynaptic receptors.
- Hormones are chemicals that, after being released into the bloodstream from specialized cells, act at neighbouring or distant cells.

Each cell expresses only certain receptors, depending on the function of the cell.

Receptor number and responsiveness to messengers can be modulated.

In many cases there is more than one receptor for each messenger, so that the messenger often has different pharmacological specificity and different functions according to where it binds (e.g. adrenaline). This may be a result of gene splicing and other processes that led to polypeptide diversity in evolution.

Using conventional molecular biology techniques, it is now possible to clone the genes encoding receptors and express them in cultured cells, so allowing their properties to be studied. In particular, substitutions of amino acid residues that may be caused by mutations can be reproduced, so that the relation between protein structure and function can be evaluated.

The four types of receptors for chemical messengers and growth factors are those:

- Linked directly to multimeric ion channels (ionotropic).
- Linked via G-proteins to membrane enzymes and intracellular processes (metabotropic).
- Linked directly to tyrosine kinases.
- Linked to DNA interactions (steroid receptors).

Receptors directly linked to ion channels

Receptors that are directly linked to ion channels (Fig. 1.1) are mainly involved in fast synaptic neurotransmission, where the delay between ligand binding and channel opening lasts only a matter of milliseconds. A classic example of a receptor linked directly to an ion channel is the nicotinic acetylcholine receptor (nicAChR). The nicAChR consists of five subunits—two α, one β, one γ, and one δ—each of molecular weight 40–58 kDa and of great sequence identity.

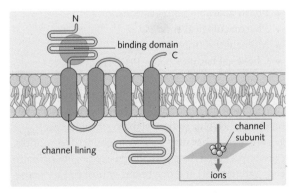

Fig. 1.1 General structure of the subunits of receptors directly linked to ion channels. (N, *N*-terminal; C, *C*-terminal.) (Redrawn from Page et al, 2002.)

The nicAChRs possess several characteristics:
- Acetylcholine (ACh) must bind to the *N*-termini of both α-subunits in order to activate the receptor.
- The whole receptor oligomer incorporates 20 transmembrane segments arranged around a central aqueous channel. One of the transmembrane helices (M_2) from each of the subunits is believed to form the lining of the channel.
- The receptor shows marked similarities with the two other receptors for fast transmission, namely the γ-aminobutyric acid ($GABA_A$) and glycine receptors.

G-protein-linked receptors

G-protein-linked receptors (Fig. 1.2) are involved in relatively rapid transduction, a response being generated in seconds. Muscarinic ACh, adrenergic, dopamine, serotonin, and opiate receptors are all examples of G-protein-linked receptors.

Molecular structure of the receptor

Most of the G-protein-linked receptors consist of a single polypeptide chain of 400–500 residues and have seven transmembrane α-helices. The third intracellular loop of the receptor is larger than the other loops, and this interacts with the G-protein.

The ligand-binding domain is buried within the membrane on one or more of the α-helical segments. This is unlike ion channel-coupled receptors, where the ligand binds to the extracellular *N*-terminal region—an area easily accessible to small hydrophobic molecules.

G-proteins

Fig. 1.3 describes the mechanism of G-protein-linked receptors:

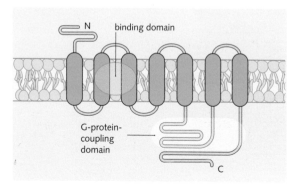

Fig. 1.2 General structure of the subunits of receptors linked to G-proteins. (N, *N*-terminal; C, *C*-terminal.) (Redrawn from Page et al, 2002.)

- In the resting state the G-protein exists as an unattached trimer consisting of α-, β-, and γ-subunits (Fig. 1.3A).
- The occupation of the receptor by an agonist produces a conformational change, causing its affinity for the trimer to increase. Subsequent association of the trimer with the receptor results in the dissociation of bound guanosine diphosphate (GDP) from the α-subunit. Guanosine triphosphate (GTP) replaces GDP in the cleft, thus activating the G-protein and causing the α-subunit to dissociate from the βγ-dimer (Fig. 1.3B).
- The α–GTP complex represents the active form of the G-protein (although this is not always the case: in the heart, potassium channels are activated by the βγ-dimer, and recent research has shown that the γ-subunit alone may play a role in activation). This component diffuses in the plane of the membrane, where it is free to interact with downstream effectors such as enzymes and ion channels. The βγ-dimer remains associated with the membrane owing to its hydrophobicity (Fig. 1.3C).
- The cycle is completed when the α-subunit, which has enzymic activity, hydrolyses the bound GTP to GDP. The GDP-bound α-subunit dissociates from the effector and recombines with the βγ-dimer (Fig. 1.3D).

This whole process results in an amplification effect because the binding of an agonist to the receptor can cause the activation of numerous G-proteins, which in turn can each, via their association with the effector, produce many molecules of product.

Targets for G-proteins

G-proteins interact with either ion channels or second messengers.

Ion channels

G-proteins may activate ion channels directly, e.g. muscarinic receptors in the heart are linked to potassium channels that open directly upon interaction with the G-protein, causing a slowing down of the heart rate.

Second messengers

Three second-messenger systems exist as targets of G-proteins (Fig. 1.4).

Adenylyl cyclase/cyclic AMP system

Many types of G-protein exist. This is probably attributable to the variability of the α-subunit. G_S

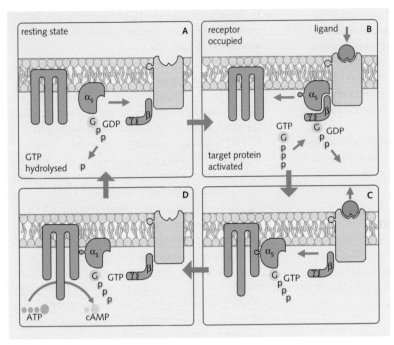

Fig. 1.3 Mechanism of G-protein-linked receptors. (α, β, γ, subunits of G-protein; cAMP, cyclic adenosine monophosphate; ATP, adenosine triphosphate; G, guanosine; GDP, GTP, guanosine di- and triphosphate; p, phosphate.) (Redrawn from Page et al, 2002.)

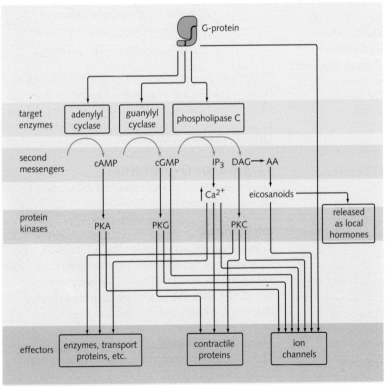

Fig. 1.4 Second-messenger targets of G-proteins and their effects. (cAMP, cyclic adenosine monophosphate; cGMP, cyclic guanosine monophosphate; DAG, diacylglycerol; IP_3, inositol (1,4,5) triphosphate; PK, protein kinase; AA, arachidonic acid.)

and G_i/G_o cause stimulation and inhibition, respectively, of the target enzyme adenylyl cyclase. This explains why muscarinic ACh receptors and β-adrenoreceptors located in the heart produce opposite effects.

The bacterial toxins cholera and pertussis can be used in order to determine which G-protein is involved in a particular situation. Each has enzymic action on a conjugation reaction with the α-subunit, such that:

- Cholera affects G_S causing continued activation of adenylyl cyclase. This explains why infection with cholera toxin results in uncontrolled fluid secretion from the gastrointestinal tract.
- Pertussis affects G_i and G_o causing continued inactivation of adenylyl cyclase. This explains why infection with *Bordetella pertussis* causes a 'whooping' cough, characteristic of this infection, as the airways are constricted, and the larynx experiences muscular spasms.

Adenylyl cyclase catalyses the conversion of adenosine triphosphate (ATP) to cyclic adenosine monophosphate (cAMP) within cells. The cAMP produced in turn causes activation of certain protein kinases, enzymes that phosphorylate serine and threonine residues in various proteins, thereby producing either activation or inactivation of these proteins. This can lead to:

- Increased lipolysis through activation of hormone-sensitive lipase.
- Reduced glycogen synthesis through inactivation of glycogen synthase.
- Increased glycogen breakdown through the activation of phosphorylase kinase and, therefore, conversion of inactive phosphorylase b to active phosphorylase a.

Activation of $β_1$-adrenergic receptors found in cardiac muscle results in activation of cAMP-dependent protein kinase A, which phosphorylates and opens voltage-operated calcium channels. This increases calcium levels in the cell and results in an increased rate and force of contraction.

In contrast, activation of $β_2$-adrenergic receptors found in smooth muscle causes activation of protein kinase and, therefore, phosphorylation, but inactivation of another enzyme (myosin light-chain kinase) needed for contraction.

Receptors linked to G_i inhibit adenylyl cyclase and reduce cAMP production. Examples of these receptors are the M_2 and M_4 muscarinic, the opioid, the 5-HT$_1$ (5-hydroxytryptamine) and the $α_2$-adrenoreceptors.

Phospholipase C/inositol phosphate system

Activation of M_1, M_3, 5-HT$_2$, peptide and $α_1$-adrenoreceptors, via G_q, cause activation of phospholipase C, a membrane-bound enzyme, which increases the rate of degradation of phosphatidylinositol (4,5) bisphosphate into diacylglycerol (DAG) and inositol (1,4,5) triphosphate (IP$_3$). DAG and IP$_3$ act as second messengers.

IP$_3$ binds to the membrane of the endoplasmic reticulum, opening calcium channels and increasing the concentration of calcium within the cell by 10–100 fold. Increased calcium levels may result in smooth muscle contraction, increased secretion from exocrine glands, increased hormone or transmitter release, or increased force and rate of contraction of the heart.

DAG, which remains associated with the membrane owing to its hydrophobicity, causes protein kinase C to move from the cytosol to the membrane where DAG can regulate its activity. There are at least six types of protein kinase C, with 50 or more targets having effects such as:

- Release of hormones and neurotransmitters.
- Smooth muscle contraction.
- Inflammation.
- Ion transport.
- Tumour promotion.

Guanylyl cyclase system

Guanylyl cyclase catalyses the conversion of GTP to cGMP. This cGMP goes on to cause activation of protein kinase G, which in turn phosphorylates contractile proteins and ion channels.

Transmembrane guanylyl cyclase activity is exhibited by the atrial natriuretic peptide receptor upon the binding of atrial natriuretic peptide.

Cytoplasmic guanylyl cyclase activity is exhibited when bradykinin activates receptors on the membrane of endothelial cells to generate nitric oxide, which then acts as a second messenger to activate guanylyl cyclase within the cell.

Sodium nitroprusside is a nitrovasodilator that relaxes the smooth muscle of arteries and veins by increasing cGMP production. Because both central venous pressure and arterial pressure drop, there is little change in cardiac output. Sodium nitroprusside is used for angina and hypertension.

Tyrosine-kinase-linked receptors

Tyrosine-kinase-linked receptors are involved in the regulation of growth and differentiation, and responses to metabolic signals.

The response time of enzyme-initiated transduction is slow (minutes). Examples include the receptors for insulin, platelet-derived growth factor, and epidermal growth factor.

Activation of tyrosine kinase receptors results in autophosphorylation of tyrosine residues leading to the activation of pathways involving protein kinases.

DNA-linked receptors

Corticosteroids, thyroid hormone, retinoic acid, and vitamin D are all molecules with receptors that are linked so as to interact with DNA. The receptors are intracellular and so agonists must pass through the cell membrane in order to reach the receptor. Receptor–agonist complexes are then transported to the nucleus. Once in the nucleus the complex can bind to specific DNA sequences and so alter the expression of specific genes. As a result, secondary transduction involving an increase or decrease in the synthesis of various proteins occurs. The process is much slower than for other receptor–ligand interactions, and the effects usually last longer.

Drugs, like naturally occurring chemical mediators, act on receptors located in the cell membrane, in the cytoplasm of the cell, or in the cell nucleus, to bring about a cellular, and eventually organ or tissue response.

Drugs and receptors

Drug–receptor interactions

Most drugs produce their effects by acting through specific protein molecules called receptors.

Receptors respond to endogenous chemicals in the body that are either synaptic transmitter substances (e.g. ACh, noradrenaline) or hormones (endocrine, e.g. insulin; or local mediators, e.g. histamine). These chemicals or drugs will do one of the following:

- Activate receptors and produce a subsequent response (agonists).
- Associate with receptors but not cause activation (antagonists). Antagonists reduce the chance of transmitters or agonists binding to the receptor and thereby oppose their action by effectively diluting or removing the receptors from the system.

Electrostatic forces initially attract a drug to a receptor. If the shape of the drug corresponds to that of the binding site of the receptor, then it will be held there temporarily by weak bonds or, in the case of irreversible antagonists, permanently by stronger covalent bonds. The number of bonds, and the level of perfection of fit, between drug and receptor determines the affinity of the drug for that receptor. The greater the number of bonds and the more perfect the fit, the higher the affinity.

The affinity is defined by the dissociation constant which is given the symbol K_d. The lower the K_d, the higher the affinity. K_d values in the nanomolar range represent drugs (D) with a high affinity for their receptor (R):

$$D + R \underset{k_{-1}}{\overset{k_{+1}}{\rightleftharpoons}} DR$$

The rate at which the forward reaction occurs is dependent upon the drug concentration [D] and the receptor concentration [R]:

Forward rate $= k_{+1} [D][R]$

The rate at which the backward reaction occurs is mainly dependent upon the interaction between the drug and the receptor [DR]:

Backward rate $= k_{-1} [DR]$

$$K_d = k_{-1}/k_{+1}$$

K_a is the association constant and is used to quantify affinity. It can be defined as the concentration of drug that produces 50% of the maximum response at equilibrium, in the absence of receptor reserve (p. 10):

$$K_a = 1/K_d$$

Drugs with a high affinity stay bound to their receptor for a relatively long time and are said to have a slow off-rate. This means that at any time the probability that any given receptor will be occupied by the drug is high.

The ability of a drug to combine with one type of receptor is termed specificity. Although no drug is truly specific, most exhibit relatively selective action on one type of receptor.

Agonists

An agonist (A) binds to the receptor (R) and the chemical energy released on binding induces a conformational change that sets off a chain of biochemical events within the cell, leading to a response (AR*). The equation for this is:

$$A + R \xrightarrow{(1)} AR \xrightarrow{(2)} AR^*$$

(1): affinity dependent

(2): efficacy dependent

Partial agonists cannot bring about the same maximum response as full agonists, even if their affinity for the receptor is the same (Figs 1.5 and 1.6).

The ability of agonists, once bound, to activate receptors is termed efficacy. Full agonists have high efficacy, and they are able to produce a maximum response while occupying only a small percentage of the receptors available. Partial agonists have low efficacy, and they are unable to elicit the maximum response even if they are occupying all the available receptors.

Antagonists

Antagonists bind to receptors but they do not activate them; they do not induce a conformational change and so have no efficacy. However, because antagonists occupy the receptor, they prevent agonists from binding and, therefore, block their action.

Two types of antagonist exist, competitive and non-competitive.

Competitive antagonists

These bind to receptors reversibly and effectively produce a dilution of the receptors, such that:

- A parallel shift is produced to the right of the agonist dose–response curve (Fig. 1.7).
- The maximum response is not depressed. This reflects the fact that the antagonist's effect can be overcome by increasing the dose of agonist, i.e. the block is surmountable. Increasing the concentration of agonist increases the probability of the agonist taking the place of an antagonist leaving the receptor.
- The size of the shift in the agonist dose–response curve produced by the antagonist reflects the affinity of the antagonist for the receptor. High-affinity antagonists stay bound to the receptor for a relatively long period of time allowing the agonist little chance to take the antagonist's place.

This concept can be quantified in terms of the dose ratio. The dose ratio is the ratio of the concentration of agonist producing a given response in the presence and

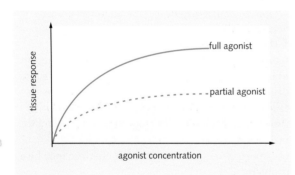

Fig. 1.5 Comparison of the dose–response curve for a partial agonist and a full agonist. (From *Medical Pharmacology at a Glance*, 2nd edn, by MJ Neal. Courtesy of Blackwell Scientific Publications.)

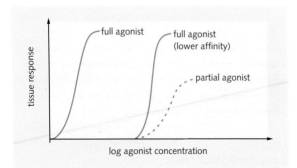

Fig. 1.6 Comparison of the log dose–response curve for a partial agonist and a full agonist. (From *Medical Pharmacology at a Glance*, 2nd edn, by MJ Neal. Courtesy of Blackwell Scientific Publications.)

Fig. 1.7 Comparison of the log dose–response curves for competitive and non-competitive (irreversible) antagonists. (From *Medical Pharmacology at a Glance*, 2nd edn, by MJ Neal. Courtesy of Blackwell Scientific Publications.)

absence of a certain concentration of antagonist, e.g. a dose ratio of 3 tells us that three times as much agonist was required to produce a given response in the presence of the antagonist than it did in its absence.

Non-competitive antagonists:

These are also known as irreversible antagonists. Like competitive antagonists, their presence also produces a parallel shift to the right of the agonist dose–response curve (Fig. 1.7). However, non-competitive antagonists also depress the maximum response, reflecting the fact that the antagonist's effect cannot be overcome by the addition of greater doses of agonist. At low concentrations of antagonist, however, a parallel shift may occur without a reduced maximum response. This tells us that not all of the receptors need be occupied by agonist in order to elicit a maximum response, since irreversible antagonists effectively remove receptors and there must be a number of spare receptors.

Receptor reserve

Although on a log scale the relationship between the concentration of agonist and the response produces a symmetrical sigmoid curve, very rarely does a 50% response correspond to 50% receptor occupancy. This is because there are spare receptors.

This excess of receptors is known as receptor reserve and serves to sharpen the sensitivity of the cell to small changes in agonist concentration.

The low efficacy of partial agonists can be overcome in tissues with a large receptor reserve, and in these circumstances partial agonists may act as full agonists.

The kinetic equations simply demonstrate how drugs act, and how they differ from one another. You are unlikely to be asked about them, though try to work through them as they aid in the building of a good foundation in the subject.

Potency

Potency relates to the concentration of a drug needed to elicit a response.

The EC_{50}, where EC stands for effective concentration, is a number used to quantify potency.

The EC_{50} is the concentration producing 50% of the maximum response. Therefore, the lower the EC_{50}, the more potent the drug.

Where agonists are concerned, potency is related to both the affinity and the efficacy.

Pharmacokinetic variables also affect potency. For example, the acidic pH of the stomach may break down a drug that has been found to be very potent in a test tube. This means that, if given as a tablet, it would have very little potency and would be ineffective.

Pharmacokinetics

Pharmacology can be divided into two disciplines:

- Pharmacokinetics, which considers drug disposition and the way the body affects the drug with time, i.e. the factors that determine its absorption, distribution, metabolism, and excretion.
- Pharmacodynamics, which deals with the effect of the drug on the body.

Compliance

Compliance on the patient's behalf is very important as far as taking drugs is concerned. In order for some drugs to be effective (e.g. antibiotics), they must be taken at regular intervals and for a certain period of time. For certain forms of treatment, patients may even need to come to hospital, in which case transport, work, and having young children may be a problem.

Compliance tends to be more of a problem in paediatric practice since it involves both parents and the child: the parent must remember to give the medication and follow directions accurately; the child must cooperate and not spit out or spill the medicine.

Practical dosage forms are important in achieving compliance. Many tablets are now sugar coated, making them easier to take, and a large number of the drugs manufactured for children are in the form of elixirs or suspensions, which may be available in a variety of different flavours, making their administration less of a problem.

The route of administration of a drug may affect compliance. Taking a drug orally, for example, is more simple than injecting it.

The dosing schedule is also an important aspect of compliance. The easier this is to follow, and the less frequently a drug needs to be taken or administered, the more likely it is that compliance will occur.

Routes of administration

Topical

Topical drugs are placed where they are needed, giving them the advantage that they do not have to cross any barriers or membranes. Examples include skin ointments; ear, nose, or eye drops; and aerosols inhaled in the treatment of asthma.

Enteral

Enteral administration means that the drug reaches its target via the gut. It is the least predictable route of administration, owing to metabolism by the liver, chemical breakdown, and the possible binding to food. Drugs must cross several barriers, which may or may not be a problem according to their physicochemical properties such as charge and size. However, most drugs are administered orally unless the drug is unstable, or is rapidly inactivated in the gastrointestinal tract, or if its efficacy of absorption from the gastrointestinal tract is uncertain owing to metabolism by the liver or the intestines, vomiting, or a disease that may affect drug absorption.

Absorption of drugs via the buccal or sublingual route avoids the portal circulation and it is, therefore, valuable when administering drugs subject to a high degree of first-pass metabolism (which is unavoidable if taken orally). It is also useful for potent drugs with a non-disagreeable taste, such as sublingual nitroglycerin given to relieve acute attacks of angina.

Administration of drugs rectally, such as in the form of suppositories, means that there is less first-pass metabolism by the liver because the venous return from the lower gastrointestinal tract is less than that from the upper gastrointestinal tract. It has the disadvantage, however, of being inconsistent.

Antacids have their effect in the stomach and may be considered as being topical.

Parenteral

Parenteral administration means that the drug is administered in a manner that avoids the gut. The protein drug insulin, for example, is destroyed by the acidity of the stomach and the digestive enzymes within the gut and it must, therefore, be injected, usually subcutaneously.

Intravenous injection of drugs has several advantages:
- It is the most direct route of administration. The drug enters the bloodstream directly and bypasses absorption barriers.
- A drug is distributed in a large volume and acts rapidly.

For drugs that must be given continuously by infusion, or for drugs that damage tissues, this is an important method of administration.

Alternative parenteral routes of administration include subcutaneous, intramuscular, epidural, or intrathecal injections, and transdermal patches such as are used in angina.

The rate of drug absorption from the site of the injection can be decreased by binding the drug to a vehicle or co-administering a vasoconstrictor, such as adrenaline, to reduce blood flow to the site.

Drug absorption

Bioavailability takes into account both absorption and metabolism and describes the proportion of the drug that passes into the systemic circulation. This will, of course, be 100% after an intravenous injection, but following oral administration it will depend on the drug, the individual, and the circumstances under which the drug is given.

Since drugs must cross membranes in order to enter cells or to transfer between body compartments, drug absorption will be affected by both chemical and physiological factors.

Cell membranes

Cell membranes are composed of lipid bilayers and thus absorption is usually proportional to the lipid solubility of the drug. Un-ionized molecules (B) are far more lipid soluble than those that are ionized (BH$^+$) and surrounded by a 'shell' of water.

$$B + H^+ \rightleftharpoons BH^+$$

Size

Small size is another factor that favours absorption. Most drugs are small molecules (molecular weight <1000) that are able to diffuse across membranes in their uncharged state.

pH

Since most drugs are either weak bases, weak acids, or amphoteric, the pH of the environment in which they dissolve, as well as the pK_a value of the drug, will be important in determining the fraction in the un-ionized form that is in solution and able to diffuse across cell membranes. The pK_a of a drug is defined as the pH at which 50% of the molecules in solution are in the ionized form, and is characterized by the Henderson-Hasselbalch equation:

For acidic molecules: $HA \rightleftharpoons H^+ + A^-$

$$pK_a = pH + \log [HA] / [A^-]$$

For basic molecules: $BH^+ \rightleftharpoons B + H^+$

$pK_a = pH + \log [BH^+] / [B]$

Drugs will tend to exist in the ionized form when exposed to an environment with a pH opposite to their own state. Therefore, acids become increasingly ionized with increasing pH (i.e. basic).

It is useful to consider three important body compartments—plasma (pH = 7.4), stomach (pH = 2.0), and urine (pH = 8.0)—in relation to drugs:

- Aspirin is a weak acid (pK_a = 3.5) and its absorption will, therefore, be favoured in the stomach, where it is uncharged, and not in the plasma or the urine, where it is highly charged; aspirin in high doses may even damage the stomach.
- Morphine is a weak base (pK_a = 8.0) that is highly charged in the stomach, quite charged in the plasma, and half charged in the urine. Morphine is able to cross the blood–brain barrier, but it is poorly and erratically absorbed from the stomach and intestines, and metabolized by the liver. It must, therefore, be given by injection or delayed-release capsules. Some drugs, such as quaternary ammonium compounds (e.g. suxamethonium, tubocurarine), are always charged, and must, therefore, be injected.

Drug distribution

Once drugs have reached the circulation, they are distributed around the body. As most drugs are of a very small molecular size, they are able to leave the circulation by capillary filtration to act on the tissues.

The half-life of a drug ($t_{1/2}$) is the time taken for the plasma concentration of that drug to fall to half of its original value.

Bulk transfer in the blood is very quick. Drugs exist either dissolved in blood or bound to plasma proteins such as albumin. Albumin is the most important circulating protein for binding many acidic drugs. Basic drugs tend to be bound to a globulin fraction that increases with age. A drug that is bound is confined to the vascular system and it is unable to exert its actions; this becomes a problem if more than 80% of the drug is bound. Drugs also interact and one drug may displace another. For example, aspirin can displace the benzodiazepine diazepam from albumin.

The apparent volume of distribution (V_d) is the calculated pharmacokinetic space into which a drug is distributed.

$$Vd = \frac{\text{dose administered}}{\text{initial apparent plasma concentration}}$$

V_d values that amount to less than a certain body compartment volume indicate that the drug is contained within that compartment. For example, when the volume of distribution is less than 5 L, it is likely that the drug is restricted to the vasculature. If it is less than 15 L, this implies that the drug is restricted to the extracellular fluid, and greater than 15 L, suggest distribution within the total body water. Some drugs (usually basic) have a volume of distribution that exceeds body weight, in which case tissue binding is occurring. These drugs tend to be contained outside the circulation and may accumulate in certain tissues. Very lipid-soluble substances, such as thiopental, can build up in fat; lead accumulates in bone; and mepacrine, an antimalarial drug, has a concentration in the liver 200 times that in the plasma because it binds to nucleic acids. Some drugs are even actively transported into certain organs.

Highly lipid soluble drugs such as thiopental will accumulate in fat, and as such, its half life will be much longer in obese than in thin patients.

Drug metabolism

Before being excreted from the body, most drugs are metabolized. A small number of drugs exist in their fully ionized form at physiological pH (7.4) and, because of this highly polar nature, they are metabolized to only a minor extent, if at all. The sequential metabolic reactions that occur have been categorized as phases 1 and 2.

Sites of metabolism

The liver is the major site of drug metabolism although most tissues are able to metabolize specific drugs. Other sites of metabolism include the kidney, the lung, and the gastrointestinal tract.

Orally administered drugs, which are usually absorbed in the small intestine, reach the liver via the portal circulation. At this stage, or within the small intestine, the drugs may be extensively metabolized; this is known as first-pass metabolism and means that considerably less drug reaches the systemic circulation than enters the portal vein. This causes problems because it means that higher doses of drug must be given and, owing to individual variation in the degree of first-pass metabolism, the effects of the drug can be unpredictable. Drugs that are subject to a high degree of first-pass metabolism, such as the local anaesthetic lidocaine (lignocaine), cannot be given orally and must be administered by some other route.

Phase 1 metabolic reactions

Phase 1 metabolic reactions include oxidation, reduction, and hydrolysis. These reactions introduce a functional group, such as -OH or NH_2, which increases the polarity of the drug molecule and provides a site for phase 2 reactions.

Oxidations

Oxidations are the most common type of reaction and are catalysed by an enzyme system known as the microsomal mixed function oxidase system, which is located on the smooth endoplasmic reticulum. The enzyme system forms small vesicles known as microsomes when the tissue is homogenized.

Cytochrome P_{450} is the most important enzyme, although other enzymes are involved. This enzyme is a haemoprotein that requires the presence of oxygen, reduced nicotinamide adenine dinucleotide phosphate (NADPH) and NADPH cytochrome P_{450} reductase in order to function. Cytochrome P_{450} exists in several hundred isoforms, some of which are constitutive while others are synthesized in response to specific signals. The substrate specificity of this enzyme depends on the isoform but it tends to be low, meaning that a whole variety of drugs can be oxidized.

Although oxidative reactions usually result in inactivation of the drug, sometimes a metabolite is produced that is pharmacologically active and which may have a duration of action exceeding that of the original drug. In these cases the drug is known as a prodrug, e.g. codeine, which is demethylated to morphine.

Reductions

Reduction reactions also involve microsomal enzymes but are much less common than oxidation reactions. Examples of drugs subject to reduction include prednisone, which is given as a prodrug and reduced to the active glucocorticoid prednisolone, and warfarin, an anticoagulant, which is inactivated by the transformation of a ketone group to a hydroxyl group.

Hydrolysis

Hydrolysis is not restricted to the liver and occurs in a variety of tissues. Aspirin is spontaneously hydrolysed to salicylic acid in moisture.

Phase 2 metabolic reactions

Drug molecules that possess a suitable site that was either present before phase 1 or is the result of a phase 1 reaction, are susceptible to phase 2 reactions. Phase 2 reactions involve conjugation—the attachment of a large chemical group to a functional group on the drug molecule. Conjugation results in the drug being more hydrophilic, and thus more easily excreted from the body. In conjugation it is mainly the liver that is involved, although conjugation can occur in a wide variety of tissues. Chemical groups involved are endogenous activated moieties such as glucuronic acid, sulphate, methyl and acetyl groups, and glutathione. The conjugating enzymes exist in many isoforms, and they show relative substrate and metabolite specificity.

Unlike the products of phase 1 reactions, the conjugate is almost invariably inactive. An important exception is morphine, which is converted to morphine-6-glucuronide, which has an analgesic effect lasting longer than that of its parent molecule.

Factors affecting metabolism

Enzyme induction is the increased synthesis or decreased degradation of enzymes, and it occurs as a result of the presence of an exogenous substance. For example:

- Some drugs are able to increase the activity of certain isoenzyme forms of cytochrome P_{450} and thus increase their own metabolism, as well as that of other drugs.
- Smokers can show increased metabolism of certain drugs because of the induction of cytochrome P_{448} by a constituent in tobacco smoke.
- In contrast, some drugs inhibit microsomal enzyme activity and, therefore, increase their own activity as well as that of other drugs.

Fig. 1.8 gives some examples of enzyme inducing agents, and the drugs whose metabolism is affected.

Competition for a metabolic enzyme may occur between two drugs, in which case there is a decreased metabolism of one or both drugs. This is known as inhibition.

Enzymes that metabolize drugs are affected by many aspects of diet, such as the ratio of protein to carbohydrate, flavonoids contained in vegetables, and

Examples of drugs that induce or inhibit drug-metabolizing enzymes	
Drugs modifying enzyme action	**Drugs whose metabolism is affected**
Enzyme induction Phenobarbitone and other barbiturates Rifampicin Phenytoin Ethanol Carbamazepine	Warfarin Oral contraceptives Corticosteroids Ciclosporin
Enzyme inhibition Allopurinol Chloramphenicol Corticosteroids Cimetidine MAO inhibitors Erythromycin Ciprofloxacin	Azathioprine Phenytoin Various drugs—TCA, cyclophosphamide Many drugs—amiodarone, phenytoin, pethidine Pethidine Ciclosporin Theophylline

Fig. 1.8 Examples of drugs that induce or inhibit drug-metabolizing enzymes. (MAO, monoamine oxidase; TCA, tricyclic antidepressant.) (Adapted from *Pharmacology*, by H Rang, M Dale and J Ritter, 4th edn, 2001. By permission of Churchill Livingstone.)

polycyclic aromatic hydrocarbons found in barbecued foods.

Paracetamol poisoning

Paracetamol is a classic example of a drug that can be lethal at high doses (2–3 times the maximum therapeutic dose), owing to the accumulation of its metabolites.

In phase 2 of the metabolic process, paracetamol is conjugated with glucuronic acid and sulphate. When high doses of paracetamol are taken, these pathways become saturated and the drug is metabolized by the mixed function oxidases. This results in the formation of the toxic metabolite *N*-acetyl-*p*-benzoquinone, which is inactivated by glutathione. However, when glutathione is depleted, this toxic metabolite reacts with nucleophilic constituents in the cell leading to necrosis in the liver and kidneys.

N-Acetylcysteine or methionine can be administered in cases of paracetamol overdose, since they increase liver glutathione formation and the conjugation reactions, respectively.

Drug excretion

Drugs are excreted from the body in a variety of different ways. Excretion can occur by the kidneys into urine, by the gastrointestinal tract into bile and faeces, and by the lungs into exhaled air. Drugs may also leave the body through breast milk and sweat. The most important routes for drug excretion are through the urine and faeces.

The volume of plasma cleared of drug per unit time is known as the clearance rate.

Renal excretion

Glomerular filtration, tubular reabsorption (passive and active), and tubular secretion all determine the extent to which a drug will be excreted by the kidneys.

Glomerular capillaries allow the passage of molecules with a molecular weight <20 000. The glomerular filtrate thus contains most of the substances in plasma except proteins. In the glomerular capillaries:

- The negative charge of the corpuscular membrane also repels negatively charged molecules, including plasma proteins.
- Drugs that bind to plasma proteins such as albumin will not be filtered.

Most of the drug in the blood does not pass into the glomerular filtrate, but passes into the peritubular capillaries of the proximal tubule where it may be transported into the lumen of the tubule by either of two transport mechanisms. One transport mechanism deals with acidic molecules, the other with basic molecules. In the peritubular capillaries:

- Tubular secretion is responsible for most of the drug excretion carried out by the kidneys and, unlike glomerular filtration, allows the clearance of drugs bound to plasma proteins. Competition between drugs that share the same transport mechanism may occur, in which case the excretion of these drugs will be reduced. Probenecid is a drug that was designed to compete with penicillin for excretion and, therefore, increase the duration of action of penicillin.

- Reabsorption of a drug will depend upon the fraction of molecules in the ionized state, which is in turn dependent on the pH of the urine. Intoxification with aspirin (weak acid, $pK_a = 3.5$) can be treated by administering bicarbonate, which makes the urine more alkaline; this ionizes aspirin and renders it less prone to reabsorption.
- Renal disease will affect the excretion of certain drugs. The extent to which excretion is impaired can be deduced by measuring 24-hour creatinine clearance.

Gastrointestinal excretion

Some drug conjugates are excreted into the bile and subsequently released into the intestines where they are hydrolysed back to the parent compound and reabsorbed. This 'enterohepatic circulation' prolongs the effect of the drug.

Mathematical aspects of pharmacokinetics
Kinetic order

Two types of kinetics, related to the plasma concentration of a drug, describe the rate at which a drug leaves the body:

- Zero-order kinetics (Fig. 1.9) describes a decrease in drug levels in the body that is independent of the plasma concentration, and the rate is held constant by a limiting factor, such as availability of an enzyme cofactor. When the plasma concentration is plotted against time, the decrease is a straight line. Alcohol is an example of a drug that displays zero-order kinetics.
- First-order kinetics (Fig. 1.10) is displayed by most drugs. It describes a decrease in drug levels in the body that is dependent on the plasma concentration, as the concentration of the

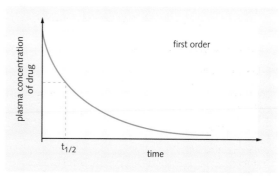

Fig. 1.10 Plasma drug concentration versus time plot for a drug displaying first-order kinetics. ($t_{1/2}$, half-life.)

substrate (drug) is the rate limiting factor. When the plasma concentration is plotted against time, the decrease is exponential.

One-compartment model

The one-compartment model considers the body to be a single compartment. Within this single compartment a drug is absorbed, immediately distributed, and subsequently eliminated by metabolism and excretion.

If the volume of the compartment is V_d and the dose administered D, then the initial drug concentration, C_o, will be:

$$C_o = D/V_d$$

The time taken for the plasma drug concentration to fall to half of its original value is the half-life of that drug. The decline in concentration may be exponential, but this situation expresses itself graphically as a straight line when the log plasma concentration is plotted against the time after intravenous dose (Fig. 1.11).

Half-life is related to the elimination rate constant (K_{el}) by the following equation:

$$t_{1/2} \times K_{el} = \text{natural log 2 (ln 2)}$$

Half-life is related to V_d, but it does not determine the ability of the body to remove the drug from the circulation, since both V_d and half-life change in the same direction. The body's ability to remove a drug from the blood is termed clearance (Cl_p) and is constant for individual drugs:

$$Cl_p = V_d \times K_{el}$$

If the drug is not administered parenterally, plotting the log plasma drug concentration against time will require the consideration of both

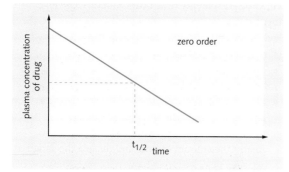

Fig. 1.9 Plasma drug concentration versus time plot for a drug displaying zero-order kinetics. ($t_{1/2}$, half-life.)

Fig. 1.11 Log plasma drug concentration versus time plot compatible with the one-compartment open pharmacokinetic model for drug disposition after a parenteral dose, assuming first-order kinetics. (K_{el}, elimination rate constant; C_0 initial drug concentration; $t_{1/2}$, half-life.)

Fig. 1.13 Log plasma drug concentration versus time plot that requires a two-compartment open model to account for its disposition after a parenteral dose. (K_{el}, elimination rate constant.) (Redrawn from Page et al, 2002.)

• An early, rapid, α-phase, which represents the redistribution of the drug to the peripheral compartment and a modest component of elimination.
• A later, slower, β-phase, which is a combination of elimination and return of the drug from the peripheral compartment to the central compartment, in which the drug then distributes rapidly.

absorption and elimination from the compartment (Fig. 1.12).

The one-compartment model is widely used to determine the dose of drug to be administered.

Two-compartment model

The distribution of drugs between the peripheral compartment (i.e. tissues) and the central compartment (i.e. plasma) occurs at rates varying from rapid to insignificant.

Some drugs distribute slowly or extensively, and in these cases a curvilinear relationship between the log of the plasma concentration and time is seen. Two phases can be observed (Fig. 1.13):

The liver is the main site of drug inactivation, and the kidneys and gastrointestinal tract the main sites for drug excretion—disease of these organs will alter a drug's pharmacokinetics.

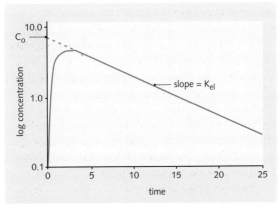

Fig. 1.12 Log plasma drug concentration versus time plot for a drug compatible with the one-compartment open pharmacokinetic model for drug disposition after an oral dose. (K_{el}, elimination rate constant; C_0 initial drug concentration; $t_{1/2}$, half-life.) (Redrawn from Page et al, 2002.)

Model-independent approach

For drugs displaying first-order kinetics, the level of the drug in the body increases until it is equal to the level excreted, at which point steady-state is reached (Fig. 1.14), such that:

• The time to reach steady-state is usually equal to four to five half-lives.
• The amount of drug in the body at steady-state will depend upon the frequency of drug administration—the greater the frequency, the greater the amount of drug and the less the variation between peak and trough plasma concentrations. If the frequency of administration is greater than the half-life, then accumulation of the drug will occur.

Fig. 1.14 Log plasma drug concentration versus time plot for a drug administered by mouth every 6 hours when its terminal disposition half-life is 6 hours.

The loading dose can be calculated according to the desired plasma concentration at steady-state (C_{SS}) and the volume of distribution (V_d) of the drug:

$$\text{Loading dose (mg/kg)} = V_d \, (\text{L/kg}) \times C_{SS} \, (\text{mg/L})$$

Drug interactions and adverse effects

Drug interactions

Drugs interact in a number of ways that may produce unwanted effects. Two types of interactions exist, pharmacodynamic and pharmacokinetic.

Pharmacodynamic interactions

Pharmacodynamic interactions involve a direct conflict between the effects of drugs. This conflict results in the effect of one of the two drugs being enhanced or reduced. For example:

- Propranolol, a β-adrenoceptor antagonist given for angina and hypertension, will reduce the effect of salbutamol, a β_2-adrenoceptor agonist given for the treatment of asthma. The administration of β-blockers to asthmatics should, therefore, be avoided, or undertaken with caution.
- Administration of monoamine oxidase inhibitors, which inhibit the metabolism of catecholamines, enhances the effects of drugs such as ephedrine. This enhancement causes the release of noradrenaline from stores in the nerve terminal and is known as 'potentiation'.

Pharmacokinetic interactions

Absorption, distribution, metabolism, and excretion all affect the pharmacokinetic properties of drugs.

Therefore, any drug that interferes with these processes will be altering the effect of other drugs. For example:

- If administered with diuretics, non-steroidal anti-inflammatory drugs (NSAIDs) will reduce the antihypertensive action of these drugs. NSAIDs bring about this effect by reducing prostaglandin synthesis in the kidney, thus impairing renal blood flow and consequently decreasing the excretion of waste and sodium. This results in an increased blood volume and a rise in blood pressure.
- Enzyme induction, which occurs as a result of the administration of certain drugs, can affect the metabolism of other drugs served by that enzyme (see Fig. 1.8).

Adverse reactions and allergy to a drug are different. Adverse reactions can be minor irritations or upset, though an allergic reaction can be life-threatening.

In some cases, however, drugs are used together so that their interaction can bring about the desired effect. For example, carbidopa prevents the conversion of levodopa (L-dopa) to dopamine and is therefore used with L-dopa in the treatment of Parkinson's disease. L-Dopa is able to cross the blood–brain barrier and enter the brain, where it is converted to dopamine. Carbidopa reduces the peripheral side effects of L-dopa, but it cannot cross the blood–brain barrier.

Adverse effects

As well as interacting with one another and with their target tissue, drugs will also interact with other tissues and organs and alter their function. No drug is without side effects, although the severity and frequency of these will vary from drug to drug and from person to person.

The liver and the kidneys are susceptible to the adverse effects of drugs, as these are the sites of drug metabolism and excretion. Some drugs cause hepatotoxicity or nephrotoxicity.

Those who are more prone to the adverse effects of drugs, include:

- Pregnant women, who must be careful about taking drugs as certain drugs are teratogenic, i.e. cause fetal malformations (e.g. thalidomide taken in the 1960s for morning sickness).

- Breastfeeding women, who must also be careful about which drugs they take, as many drugs can be passed on in the breast milk and consumed by the developing infant.
- Patients with an underlying illness other than the one being treated, such as liver or kidney disease. These illnesses will result in decreased metabolism and excretion of the drug, and they will produce the side effects of an increased dose of the same drug.
- The elderly, who tend to take a large number of drugs, greatly increasing the risk of drug interactions and the associated side effects. In addition, elderly patients have a reduced renal clearance, and a nervous system that is more sensitive to drugs. The dose of drug initially given is usually 50% of the adult dose, and certain drugs are contraindicated.
- Patients with genetic enzyme defects, such as glucose-6-phosphate dehydrogenase deficiency. This deficiency will result in haemolysis if an oxidant drug (e.g. aspirin) is taken.

Certain drugs are carcinogenic, i.e. induce cancer. Genotoxic carcinogens cause mutations, either directly (primary carcinogens) or through their metabolites (secondary carcinogens). Epigenetic carcinogens, such as phorbol esters, do not induce mutations themselves, but they increase the likelihood that a mutagen will do so.

Allergic reactions to certain drugs are common, occurring in 2–25% of cases. Most of these are not serious, e.g. skin reactions; however, rarely, reactions such as anaphylactic shock (type 1 hypersensitivity) occur, which may be lethal unless treated with intravenous adrenaline. The most common allergic reaction is to penicillin, which produces anaphylactic shock in approximately 1 in 50 000 people.

Some drugs, e.g. the vasodilator hydralazine, induce autoimmune reactions similar to systemic lupus erythematosus. Stopping the drug usually puts an end to this reaction, although in some cases glucocorticoid therapy may be needed.

Drug history and drug development

The drug history

A patient's drug history is a crucial component of the clerking process, as drug effects account for a significant proportion of hospital admissions, and foreseeing potential drug interactions and adverse events is crucial.

A complete list of the names and doses of prescribed drugs taken by the patient (noting the proprietary or trade name, and the generic or chemical name, e.g. Viagra® and sildenafil, respectively), and any other medications or supplements they may have bought themselves over the counter at the pharmacy should be documented. Women often forget the contraceptive pill and hormone replacement therapy, and they should be sensitively questioned about these. Non-steroidal anti-inflammatory drugs and paracetamol are often taken by the bucket load in patients with arthritis, and again these should be specifically asked about. Make sure to note how often the drugs were taken, and at what times.

If presented with numerous bottles and packets of tablets, it is important to ensure that they all belong to the patient, and not the partner of the patient, or to someone else; the effects could be devastating. Ask the patient if they were taking all their medicines as prescribed—it is not unusual for people to alter their dosages without consulting a doctor!

Occasionally it is useful to know what drugs have been taken in the recent and distant past; for example, monoamine oxidase inhibitors should be stopped for at least 3 weeks prior to starting a different antidepressant therapy, and the cytotoxic drug bleomycin can cause lung fibrosis years later.

It is essential to ascertain previous adverse reaction to drugs, and to non-drug products such as latex. Explore what happened to the patient, and what was done about it. A simple upset stomach and loose stools just for one day after taking penicillin previously is an acceptable side effect, and it is not grounds for choosing another antibiotic when treating a penicillin-sensitive infection in the future. Widespread cutaneous rash and difficulty breathing, which required adrenaline and hospital admission, is a genuinely worrying adverse effect of a penicillin, and any such drug should be clearly avoided in the future as this was an allergic drug reaction. Allergy to drugs should be clearly marked in the patient's notes and drug charts.

Family history of adverse drug reactions is usually confined to the anaesthetic history, where the concern is largely in relation to the muscle relaxing drugs, particularly suxamethonium.

Asking a patient about recreational or illicit drug use is occasionally important, though on the whole patients find it uncomfortable to talk about, and usually this adds little to the overall drug history.

Knowledge about any hepatic or renal disease, and general health problems, is important when it comes to management and prescribing, as are specific considerations, such as not prescribing aspirin in peptic ulcer disease, or oestrogen to patients with oestrogen-dependent cancers. These aspects are usually brought to light in the rest of the history taking.

> The salient points of the drug history are current and previous drugs and doses, adverse drug reactions and allergies, family history of allergies, recreational drug use, and existing renal, hepatic, or general disease.

Drug development

Hundreds of thousands of substances have been produced by the pharmaceutical industry over the last 50 years, though very few ever get past preclinical screening, and fewer than 10% of these survive clinical assessment.

There are four clinical stages (phases 1–4) a potential drug goes through as part of the assessment of its pharmacokinetics and pharmacodynamics, efficacy, dose–response relationship and safety (Fig. 1.15).

Phase 4 can be regarded as an ongoing phase, where drugs are monitored once licensed for general use. By this stage, the efficacy and dose–response relationship are known, though the side effect profile is often incomplete, and information is gathered on these 'adverse reactions' that are due to, or likely due to, new drugs.

In the United Kingdom, this is known as the yellow card system. *The British National Formulary* (BNF) contains detachable yellow cards, which medical staff complete, documenting adverse drug reactions in their patients, which can then be forwarded to Medicines Control Agency. The Medicines Control Agency collates this data, and uses it for surveillance of unacceptably common or severe adverse effects. This data is publicized in future copies of the BNF, or used in the re-assessment of certain drug licenses.

The five stages of drug development and monitoring		
Phase	**Main aims/means of investigation**	**Subjects**
Preclinical	• Pharmacology • Toxicology	• *In vitro* • In laboratory animals
Phase 1	• Clinical pharmacology and toxicology • Drug metabolism and bioavailability • Evaluate safety	• Healthy individuals and/or patients
Phase 2	• Initial treatment studies • Evaluate efficacy	• Small numbers of patients
Phase 3	• Large randomized controlled trials • Comparing new to old treatments • Evaluate safety and efficacy	• Large numbers of patients
Phase 4	• Post-marketing surveillance • Long-term safety and rare events • Yellow card scheme	• All patients prescribed the drug

Fig. 1.15 The five stages of drug development and monitoring.

- Define what is meant by the term 'drug' and describe how drugs are named.
- Drugs are said to have specific and non-specific actions—explain this.
- What is a cellular receptor? List the types of cellular receptors known.
- By what mechanisms does receptor activation bring about a cellular/physiological response?
- Give an example of a receptor that interacts directly with DNA. How does this receptor bring about its cellular/physiological action?
- What is meant by the terms agonist and antagonist?
- How does the presence of either a competitive or non-competitive antagonist affect the action of an agonist?
- What is receptor reserve? How can it be measured?
- What is potency, and what factors affect the potency of a drug?
- What are the differences between pharmacokinetics and pharmacodynamics?
- What is compliance? How can doctors increase compliance?
- List the common routes by which drugs are administered, and give an example of a drug for each, and its indication.
- What barriers must drugs cross in order to have their effects for each of the routes mentioned above?
- What are the principle steps and location of drug metabolism in the body?
- What is meant by the term enzyme induction? What effects does this have upon a drugs activity?
- Which route out of the body are drugs and their metabolites commonly excreted? What factors accelerate or hinder drug excretion?
- Describe the differences between zero-order and first-order kinetics.
- What is a drug interaction? Give an example.
- What are the main areas of the drug history?
- What is the purpose of the yellow card scheme?

CLINICAL
PHARMACOLOGY

2. Cancer

Concepts of cancer chemotherapy

Cancer

Cancers are malignant neoplasms ('new growths'). Despite their variability, cancers share the characteristics of:
- Uncontrolled proliferation.
- Local invasiveness.
- Tendency to spread (metastasis).
- Changes in some aspects of original cell morphology/retention of other characteristics.

Cancers account for 20–25% of deaths in the Western world; attempts to cure or palliate cancer employ three principal methods: surgery, radiotherapy, and chemotherapy. These methods are not mutually exclusive, often being used in combination, e.g. adjuvant chemotherapy after surgical removal of a tumour.

Chemotherapy

Cancer chemotherapy is the use of drugs to inhibit the rate of growth of, or to kill, cancerous cells, while having minimal effects upon non-neoplastic host cells.

In a fashion similar to antimicrobial chemotherapy, the ideal anticancer drugs target malignant cells in preference to non-malignant cells. This is achieved by exploiting the molecular differences between them.

The most striking difference between cancerous and non-cancerous cells is their accelerated rate of cell division. This remains the main target for therapeutic intervention at present, though newer drugs are being designed which recognize other molecular differences.

The chemotherapeutic techniques currently used include:
- Cytotoxic therapy, which is the main approach.
- Endocrine therapy.
- Immunotherapy.

Cancers differ in their sensitivity to chemotherapy, from the very sensitive (e.g. lymphomas, testicular carcinomas) where complete clinical cures can be achieved, to the resistant (generally solid tumours, e.g. colorectal, squamous cell bronchial carcinoma).

A diagnosis of cancer carries a significant social stigma, and also many myths. Hair loss and sickness are more often the initial concern for patients, rather than other potentially serious side effects of chemotherapy. Nausea and vomiting should be taken seriously in cancer management, as these can have a devastating impact upon patients' quality of life; antiemetic drugs are discussed in Chapter 10.

Cytotoxic chemotherapy
Mechanisms of action

Most cytotoxic drugs affect DNA synthesis. They can be classified according to their site of action on the process of DNA synthesis within the cancer cell (see Fig. 2.1). Cytotoxic drugs are, therefore, most active against actively cycling/proliferating cells, both normal and malignant, and least active against non-dividing cells.

Some drugs are only effective at killing cycling cells during specific parts of the cell cycle. These are known as phase specific (Fig. 2.2). Other drugs are cytotoxic toward cycling cells throughout the cell cycle (e.g. alkylating agents), and these are known as cycle specific.

Selectivity

Cytotoxic drugs are not specifically toxic to cancer cells, and the selectivity they show is marginal at best.

Cytotoxic drugs affect all dividing tissues, both normal and malignant, and, therefore, they are likely to have general toxic side effects (see Fig. 2.4). The side effects of cytotoxic drugs are most often related to the inhibition of division of non-cancerous host cells, namely in the gut, in the bone marrow, and in the reproductive and immune systems.

Relative selectivity can occur with some cancers because:
- In malignant tumours a higher proportion of cells are undergoing proliferation than in normal proliferating tissues.
- Normal cells seem to recover from chemotherapeutic inhibition faster than some cancer cells.
- Synchronized cell cycling may leave discrete periods of vulnerability to cytotoxic drugs.

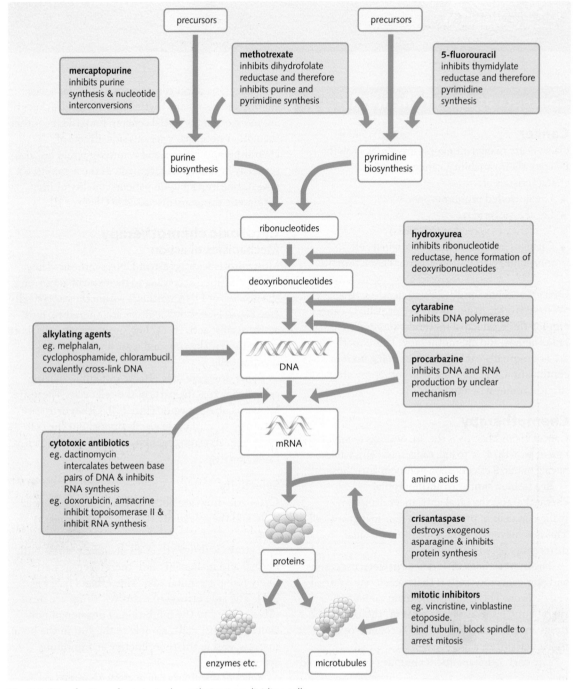

Fig. 2.1 Site of action of cytotoxic drugs that act on dividing cells.

Knowledge of these principles and knowing that cytotoxic drugs kill a constant fraction, not a constant number, of cells, lays down the foundation for chemotherapeutic dosing schedules (Fig. 2.3).

Resistance to cytotoxic drugs

Genetic resistance to cytotoxic drugs can be inherent to the cancer cell line, or acquired during the course of chemotherapy as a result of selection imposed by the chemotherapeutic agent.

Fig. 2.2 Cell cycle and point of action of phase-specific drugs.

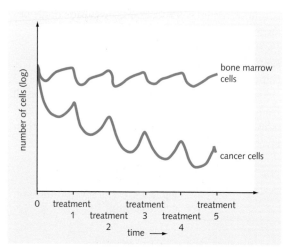

Fig. 2.3 Theoretical anticancer cytotoxic dosing schedule, allowing recovery of normal tissues.

Mechanisms of genetic resistance to cytotoxic drugs

The mechanisms of genetic resistance to cytotoxic drugs include:

- Abnormal transport.
- Decreased cellular retention.
- Increased cellular inactivation (binding/metabolism).
- Altered target protein.
- Enhanced repair of DNA.
- Altered processing.

Some tumours are relatively resistant to chemotherapy because they exist in so-called 'pharmacological sanctuaries'. These occur when a tumour is in a privileged compartment, e.g. protected by the blood–brain barrier, or in large solid tumours when poor blood supply and diffusion limit the penetration of the drug.

In clinical practice, cancers may be treated more successfully with combinations of cytotoxic drugs simultaneously, for example MOPP therapy (melphalan, Oncovin® (vincristine), procarbazine, and prednisolone) for Hodgkin's lymphoma. The theory is that multiple attack with cytotoxic agents acting at different biochemical sites will increase efficacy while reducing the likelihood of resistance.

Cytotoxic agents

Cytotoxic agents, the major group of anticancer drugs, include:

- Alkylating agents.
- Antimetabolites.
- Cytotoxic antibiotics.
- Mitotic inhibitors.
- Miscellaneous agents.

Alkylating agents

Examples of alkylating agents include melphalan, cyclophosphamide, and chlorambucil.

Mechanism of action: Alkylating agents act via a reactive alkyl group that reacts to form covalent bonds with nucleic acids. There follows either cross-linking of the two strands of DNA, preventing replication, or DNA strand breakage (Fig. 2.1).

Route of administration: Melphalan and cyclophosphamide orally and intravenously; chlorambucil orally.

Indications: Melphalan is used in myeloma and in some solid tumours. Cyclophosphamide is used to treat a variety of leukaemias, and lymphomas, and some solid tumours. Chlorambucil is used for leukaemias, lymphomas, and ovarian cancers.

Adverse effects: Generalized cytotoxicity is common with alkylating agents (Fig. 2.4).

A urinary metabolite of cyclophosphamide, acrolein, may cause serious haemorrhagic cystitis.

Damage to gametogenesis and the development of secondary acute non-lymphocytic leukaemias is a particular problem with these alkylating agents.

Therapeutic notes: Extensive clinical experience is available with alkylating agents.

Cytotoxic antibiotics

Dactinomycin (actinomycin D), bleomycin and doxorubicin are examples of cytotoxic antibiotics.

Mechanism of action: Cytotoxic antibiotics act by various means. Dactinomycin prevents transcription by interfering with RNA polymerase. Doxorubicin inhibits transcription and DNA replication by inhibiting topoisomerase II. Bleomycin acts to fragment DNA chains.

Route of administration: Intravenous. Doxorubicin can be given intravesically for bladder cancer.

Indications: Dactinomycin is principally used in paediatric cancers. Doxorubicin is used for acute leukaemias, lymphomas, and a variety of solid tumours. Bleomycin is used for lymphomas and certain solid tumours.

Adverse effects: Generalized cytotoxicity (see Fig. 2.4). Doxorubicin produces dose-dependent cardiotoxicity, as a result of irreversible free radical damage to the myocardium. Bleomycin may cause pulmonary fibrosis.

Mitotic inhibitors

Examples of mitotic inhibitors include the vinca alkaloids, vincristine, vinblastine and vinorelbine, and etoposide.

Mechanism of action: Mitotic inhibitors act by binding tubulin and inhibiting the polymerization of microtubules which is necessary to form the mitotic spindle. This prevents mitosis, and arrests dividing cells at metaphase (Fig. 2.1).

Route of administration: The vinca alkaloids are administered intravenously, and etoposide orally or intravenously.

Indications: Mitotic inhibitors are used for acute leukaemias, lymphomas, and some solid tumours.

Adverse effects: Side effects of mitotic inhibitors result from the fact that tubulin polymerization is relatively indiscriminate, inhibiting other cellular processes that involve microtubules, as well as cell division.

General adverse effects of cytotoxic drugs	
Site	**Effect**
Bone marrow	Myelosuppression can lead to leucopenia, thrombocytopenia and sometimes anaemia, this is often the dose-limiting side effect; there is a high risk of haemorrhage, immunosuppression and infection as a result
Gastrointestinal tract	Inhibition of mucosal cell division may produce anorexia, ulceration or diarrhoea; nausea and vomiting are common, especially with alkylating agents and cisplatin
Skin	Loss of hair (alopecia) may be partial or complete but is usually reversible
Wounds	Impaired wound healing results from cell reproduction inhibition
Reproductive system	Sterility, teratogenesis, and mutagenicity are all possible
Secondary cancers	Many cytotoxic drugs are carcinogenic, additionally the immunosuppression resulting from myelosuppression may reduce immune surveillance of emerging dysplastic cells, leading to an increased risk of development of some cancers after chemotherapy

Fig. 2.4 General adverse effects of cytotoxic drugs.

Generalized cytotoxicity occurs (Fig. 2.4), except that vincristine is unusual in producing little or no bone marrow suppression.

Neurological and neuromuscular effects occur, especially with vincristine, and include peripheral neuropathy leading to paraesthesia, loss of reflexes, and weakness. Recovery from these effects occurs, but it is slow.

Therapeutic notes: The intrathecal administration of vinca alkaloids is contraindicated as it is usually fatal.

As with most drugs, understanding how anticancer agents work allows potential side effects and complications to be predicted.

Antimetabolites

Examples of antimetabolites include the folic acid antagonists (e.g. methotrexate), antipyrimidines (e.g. fluorouracil and cytarabine), and antipurines (e.g. mercaptopurine).

Mechanism of action: Antimetabolites are analogues of normal metabolites and they act by competition, replacing the natural metabolite and then subverting cellular processes (Fig. 2.1).

Methotrexate competitively antagonizes dihydrofolate reductase and prevents the regeneration of intermediates (tetrahydrofolate) essential for the synthesis of purine and thymidylate, thus inhibiting the synthesis of DNA.

Fluorouracil is converted into a fraudulent pyrimidine nucleotide, fluorodeoxyuridine monophosphate, that inhibits thymidylate synthetase, impairing DNA synthesis.

Cytarabine is converted intracellularly to a triphosphate form that inhibits DNA polymerase.

Mercaptopurine is converted into a fraudulent purine nucleotide that impairs DNA synthesis.

Route of administration: Methotrexate is administered orally, intravenously, intramuscularly, and intrathecally. Fluorouracil is usually given intravenously, although it can be given orally and topically. Cytarabine is given subcutaneously, intravenously, and intrathecally. Mercaptopurine is given orally.

Indications: Methotrexate is used for acute lymphoblastic leukaemia, and non-Hodgkin's lymphoma; fluorouracil for solid tumours and some malignant skin conditions; cytarabine for acute myeloblastic leukaemia, and mercaptopurine as maintenance therapy for acute leukaemias.

Adverse effects: Common side effects of antimetabolites are generalized cytotoxicity (Fig. 2.4).

Therapeutic notes: Methotrexate should not be given to people with significant hepatic or renal impairment.

Miscellaneous agents

Several chemotherapeutic cytotoxic agents do not fall into any of the aforementioned groups.

Procarbazine

Mechanism of action: Procarbazine is a methylhydrazine derivative with monoamine oxidase inhibitor actions and cytotoxicity. It inhibits DNA and RNA synthesis by a mechanism that is unclear (Fig. 2.1).

Route of administration: Oral.

Indications: Procarbazine is the first-line drug for lymphomas such as Hodgkin's.

Adverse effects: Generalized cytotoxicity (Fig. 2.4). It causes an adverse reaction in combination with alcohol.

Therapeutic notes: Procarbazine forms part of MOPP therapy for Hodgkin's lymphoma.

Hydroxyurea

Mechanism of action: Hydroxyurea causes the inhibition of ribonucleotide reductase and hence the formation of deoxyribonucleotides (Fig. 2.1).

Route of administration: Oral.

Indications: Hydroxyurea is used for chronic myeloid leukaemia. Polycythemia rubra vera.

Adverse effects: Generalized cytotoxicity (Fig. 2.4).

Crisantaspase

Mechanism of action: Some tumour cells lose the ability to synthesize asparagine, requiring an exogenous source of the substance to grow; normal host cells can synthesize their own. Crisantaspase is a preparation of bacterial asparaginase that breaks down any circulating asparagine, hence inhibiting the growth of some cancers, namely acute lymphoblastic leukaemia (ALL) (Fig. 2.1).

Route of administration: Intramuscular, subcutaneous.

Indications: Crisantaspase is used for ALL.

Adverse effects: The most serious side effects of crisantaspase include severe toxicity to the liver and pancreas. Central nervous system (CNS) depression and anaphylaxis are also risks.

Therapeutic notes: Regular testing of patients given crisantaspase is necessary to monitor organ functions.

Mitotane
Mechanism of action: Mitotane is related to the insecticide dichlorodiphenyltrichloroethane (DDT). It interferes with the formation of adrenocortical steroids and has a selective cytotoxic effect on the cells of the adrenal cortex (Fig. 2.1).
Route of administration: Oral.
Indications: Mitotane is used for tumours of the adrenal cortex.
Adverse effects: Side effects of mitotane include adrenosuppression.

Amsacrine
Mechanism of action: Like doxorubicin, amsacrine works by intercalation between base pairs in the DNA double helix. This stabilizes the DNA structure and stops it being an effective template for RNA synthesis.
Route of administration: Intravenous.
Indications: Amsacrine is used for acute myeloid leukaemia.
Adverse effects: Bone marrow suppression. Cardiotoxicity due to hypokalaemia has been reported.
Therapeutic notes: Electrolytes should be monitored in patients given amsacrine.

Many other anticancer agents are used in the management of malignant tumours, including: altretamine; dacarbazine; pentostatin; platinum compounds; taxanes; thalidomide; topoisomerase I inhibitors; trastuzumab and tretinoin. Detailed information on these can be gained from the BNF or specialist textbooks.

Endocrine therapy
Hormones and antihormones
The growth of some cancers is hormone dependent. Growth of such tumours can be inhibited by surgical removal of the source of the driving hormone, such as the gonads, adrenals, or pituitary. Increasingly, however, administration of hormones or antihormones is preferred.

Endocrine therapy can cause side effects, the nature of which can normally be deduced from the physiological effects of the hormone being given or antagonized. Endocrine therapy generally has the advantage that it carries far fewer serious adverse effects than do cytotoxic agents.

Hormones used in endocrine therapy include:

- Adrenocortical steroids (Ch. 11), e.g. prednisolone, which inhibit the growth of cancers of the lymphoid tissues and blood. In addition they are used to treat some of the complications of the cancer (e.g. oedema).
- Oestrogen antagonists, e.g. tamoxifen, which are competitive inhibitors at oestrogen receptors. Inhibition of the stimulatory effects of oestrogen suppresses the division of breast cancer cells. Tamoxifen is indicated for use in postmenopausal women with metastatic disease, where it has definitely been shown to increase survival times.
- Oestrogens (Ch. 11), e.g. diethylstilbestrol, which have an antiandrogenic effect and can be used to suppress androgen-dependent prostatic cancers.
- Progesterones (Ch. 11), which inhibit endometrial cancer and carcinomas of the prostate and breast.
- Androgen antagonists, e.g. flutamide, which inhibit androgen-dependent prostatic cancers. Gonadotrophin-releasing hormone (GnRH) analogues have a similar effect as they inhibit GnRH release via negative feedback.

Immunotherapy
Immunotherapy of cancer is a recent advance derived from the nineteenth century observation that bacterial infections sometimes provoked the regression of cancer, i.e. indirect immunostimulation.

Approaches of immunotherapy include:
- The use of tumour-specific monoclonal antibodies to target drugs specifically to cancerous cells; the so-called 'magic-bullet' approach.
- The use of vaccines e.g. BCG to provide non-specific immunostimulation.
- The use of specific vaccines prepared using tumour cells from similar cancers, in an attempt to raise an adaptive immune response against the cancer.
- Immunostimulation using drugs, e.g. levamisole.
- The use of cytokines to regulate the immune response so as to favourably target the cancer. Cytokines used include interferon-α, interleukin-2, and tumour necrosis factor.
- The use of recombinant colony stimulating factors to reduce the level and duration of neutropenia after cytotoxic chemotherapy.
- Recombinant human granulocyte colony-stimulating factor (rh-G-CSF; filgrastim) and granulocyte-macrophage colony stimulating factor (GM-CSF; molgramostim) promote the

development of their respective haematopoietic stem cells in the marrow. Their use to raise white blood cell counts after cytotoxic chemotherapy is effective, although this has not been shown to alter overall survival rates.

The future

There are many drugs which are potential candidates as anticancer agents, and numerous in on-going trials across the world. The most promising areas appear to be the use of antisense oligonucleotides, inhibitors of enzymes responsible for cell invasiveness and metastasis, and agents which interfere with tumour angiogenesis (formation of new blood vessels).

Modulation of the host's immune system is believed to become part of cancer therapy in the future, in addition to novel methods of drug delivery, including liposomes and viral vectors.

- What is cancer, and how does it arise? How do malignant cells differ from normal cells?
- What is the definition of chemotherapy? What are the goals of chemotherapy?
- What are the principle targets for cytotoxic chemotherapeutic agents?
- What is resistance to cytotoxic drugs, and how does it arise?
- How do current cytotoxic agents target malignant cells, and have minimal effect upon normal host cells?
- Outline the basis of the cell cycle. Which cells of the normal human actively proliferate regularly?
- What are the common adverse effects of cytotoxic agents?
- What are the main classes of cytotoxic agents?
- What is the role of steroids in the management of malignant disease?
- What future therapies might be used to treat cancer in the future? How are these proposed to work?

3. Infectious Diseases

Concepts of antibacterial chemotherapy

Bacteria belong to the kingdom of prokaryotic organisms. Some bacteria are pathogenic to humans and responsible for a number of medically important diseases.

The principle treatment of infections is chemotherapy, which in its simplest definition is the use of chemicals (drugs) to combat disease (Ch. 2).

The chemotherapy of infections aims to selectively target the invading bacteria while having minimal effect upon the host. This is achieved by exploiting differences that exist between the structure and physiology of the prokaryotic bacterial cells and the host eukaryotic cell (Figs 3.1 and 3.2).

Antibacterial agents can be considered as bacteriostatic (i.e. they inhibit bacterial growth but do not kill the bacteria), or bactericidal (i.e. they kill bacteria).

Note that the distinction is not clear-cut as the ability of an antibacterial agent to inhibit or kill bacteria is partially dependent on its concentration. Also, the distinction is rarely of clinical significance, the exception being immunocompromised patients in whom bactericidal agents are necessary, as the host's immune system is not capable of final elimination of the bacteria.

Antibiotics: definition

The term antibiotic strictly refers to antimicrobial agents that are synthesized and released by microorganisms, e.g. penicillins from fungi. In practice, the term antibiotic has become synonymous with all antibacterial agents, whether natural or synthetic, and it is used as such in this chapter.

Spectrum of activity: definition

Antibiotics have a narrow or broad spectrum of activity. Broad-spectrum antibiotics are active against many bacterial species, whereas narrow-spectrum antibiotics are active against only one or a few species.

Classification of antibiotics

There are three main ways of classifying antibiotics:

Fig. 3.1 Site of action of cytotoxic drugs that act on dividing cells.

Differences between prokaryotic and eukaryotic cells		
Site	Exploitable difference	Antibacterial drugs
Peptidoglycan cell wall	Peptidoglycan cell walls are a uniquely prokaryotic feature not shared by eukaryotic (mammalian) cells. Drugs that act here are therefore very selective	Penicillins Cephalosporins Glycopeptides
Cytoplasmic membrane	Bacteria possess a plasma membrane within the cell wall which is a phospholipid bilayer, as in eukaryotes. However in bacteria the plasma membrane does not contain any sterols and this results in differential chemical behaviour that can be exploited	Polymyxins
Protein synthesis	The bacterial ribosome (50S+30S subunits) is sufficiently different from the mammalian ribosome (60S+40S subunits) that sites on the bacterial ribosome are good targets for drug action	Aminoglycosides Tetracyclines Chloramphenicol Macrolides Fusidic acid
Nucleic acids	The bacterial genome is in the form of a single circular strand of DNA plus ancillary plasmids unenclosed by a nuclear envelope, in contrast to the eukaryotic chromosomal arrangement within the nucleus. Drugs may interfere directly or indirectly with microbial DNA and RNA metabolism, replication and transcription	Antifolates Quinolones Rifampicin

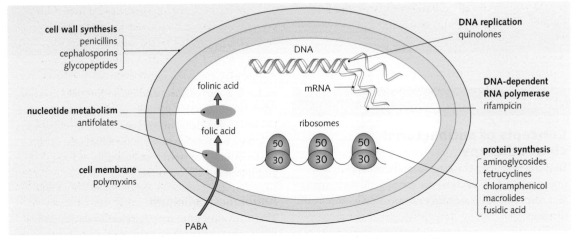

Fig. 3.2 Sites of action of different types of antibiotic agent. (PABA, *para*-aminobenzoic acid.)

- Whether they are bactericidal or bacteriostatic.
- By their site of action.
- By their chemical structure.

Antibiotics will be described according to their site of action in this chapter.

Antibiotic resistance

When an antibiotic is ineffective against a bacterium, that bacterium is said to be resistant. Resistance to antibiotics can be acquired or innate.

Innate resistance

Innate resistance is a long-standing characteristic of a particular species of bacteria. For instance, *Pseudomonas aeruginosa* has always been resistant to treatment with several antibiotics, including benzylpenicillin, vancomycin, and fusidic acid.

Acquired resistance

Acquired resistance is when bacteria that were sensitive to an antibiotic become resistant.

Biochemical mechanisms responsible for resistance to an antibiotic include:

- Production of enzymes that inactivate the drug, e.g. β-lactamases produced by many bacteria, which inactivate penicillin.
- Alteration of drug binding site, e.g. aminoglycosides and erythromycin bind to the bacterial ribosome and inhibit protein synthesis. Resistant organisms have modified the sites of drug binding so that they no longer have affinity for the drugs.
- Reduction in drug uptake and accumulation, e.g. some bacteria are resistant to tetracycline because they have altered their cell membrane to make it impermeable to the drug. Other bacteria may use active transport mechanisms to pump a drug out of the cell before it accumulates to an effective level.
- Development of altered metabolic pathways, e.g. bacteria can become resistant to trimethoprim because of acquired changes in their dihydrofolate reductase enzyme that gives it very little affinity for the drug.

The major stimulus for the development of acquired resistance is the use of antibiotics themselves. Antibiotic use exerts selective pressure on bacteria to 'acquire' resistance in order to survive.

Acquired resistance to antibiotics can develop in bacterial populations in many ways, although all involve genes that code for the resistance mechanism located either on the bacterial chromosome or on plasmids.

The 'acquisition' of resistance by a bacterium can either be achieved *de novo* by spontaneous mutation, or by being transferred from another bacterium.

The development of clinical antibiotic drug resistance is a major problem imposing serious constraints upon the medical treatment of many bacterial infections. Methicillin-resistant *Staphylococcus aureus* (MRSA) and some strains of *Mycobacteria tuberculosis* are real examples of multiple drug-resistant bacteria that are not uncommon in hospitals across the world.

Prescribing antibiotics

Like most drugs, many antibiotics have side effects, some more serious than others (Ch. 1). When prescribing antibiotics there are many considerations to take into account that determine which antibiotic to use, by which route, for how many days, etc. These include:

- Organism responsible for, or likely to be responsible for the symptoms e.g. *Staphylococcus* infection of a pierced belly-button.
- Severity of illness e.g. oral or parenteral antibiotics.
- Previous antibiotic therapy e.g. symptoms have not responded to a 7-day course of a penicillin.
- Previous adverse/allergic response to antibiotics e.g. penicillin rash.
- Other medications being taken e.g. warfarin, phenytoin, oral contraceptive pill.
- On-going medical considerations e.g. pregnancy, breastfeeding, renal failure.

Always try to get a sample for microbial culture prior to starting antibiotics unless there is a threat to life by withholding antibiotics.

Antibacterial drugs that inhibit cell wall synthesis

Examples of antibacterial drugs that inhibit bacterial cell wall synthesis include the penicillins and the cephalosporins (the β-lactam antibiotics), and the glycopeptides (Fig. 3.2).

Penicillins

Examples of penicillins include benzylpenicillin, phenoxymethylpenicillin, flucloxacillin, amoxicillin, and ampicillin.

Mechanism of action: Penicillins are bactericidal. Structurally they possess a thiazolidine ring connected to a β-lactam ring. The side chain from the β-lactam ring determines the unique pharmacological properties of the different penicillins.

Penicillins bind to penicillin-binding proteins on susceptible microorganisms. This interaction results in inhibition of peptide cross-linking within the microbial cell wall, and indirect activation of autolytic enzymes. The combined result is lysis (Fig. 3.2).

Spectrum of activity: Penicillins exhibit considerable diversity in their spectrum of activity (Fig. 3.3).

Benzylpenicillin is active against aerobic Gram-positive and Gram-negative cocci and many anaerobic organisms. Many staphylococci are now resistant to benzylpenicillin. Flucloxacillin is used against penicillin resistant staphylococci as it is not inactivated by their β-lactamase. Phenoxymethylpenicillin is similar to benzylpenicillin but less active. Amoxicillin and ampicillin are broad-spectrum penicillins.

Route of administration: Benzylpenicillin must be administered parenterally as it is inactivated when given orally. Phenoxymethylpenicillin, flucloxacillin, amoxicillin, and ampicillin are active when given orally. Consult BNF for parenteral routes.

Contraindications: Known hypersensitivity to penicillins or cephalosporins.

Adverse effects: Generally very specific and safe antibiotics. Hypersensitivity reactions are the main adverse effect, including rashes (common) and anaphylaxis (rare). Neurotoxicity occurs at excessively high cerebrospinal fluid (CSF) concentrations. Diarrhoea is common, owing to disturbance of normal colonic flora.

Therapeutic notes: Resistance to penicillins is often due to production of β-lactamase by some microorganisms, which hydrolyses the β-lactam ring. This resistance gene is located in a plasmid and is transferable. Flucloxacillin is resistant to β-lactamase.

Cephalosporins

The cephalosporins comprise a large group of drugs. The three main subgroups include:

- First-generation drugs, e.g. cefadroxil (oral) and cefradine (parenteral).
- Second-generation drugs, e.g. cefuroxime (oral) and cefamandole (parenteral).
- Third-generation drugs, e.g. cefixime (oral) and cefotaxime (parenteral).

Mechanism of action: Cephalosporins are bactericidal. They are β-lactam-containing antibiotics and inhibit bacterial cell-wall synthesis in a manner similar to the penicillins. Structurally, cephalosporins possess a dihydrothiazine ring connected to the β-lactam ring that makes them more resistant to hydrolysis by β-lactamases than are the penicillins.

Spectrum of activity: The cephalosporins are broad-spectrum antibiotics that are second-choice agents for many infections (Fig. 3.3).

Route of administration: Oral, intravenous or intramuscular. Consult BNF.

Drugs of choice and alternatives for selected common bacterial pathogens			
Bacterium	Drug(s) of choice	Alternatives	Comments
Streptococcus species	Penicillin	First-generation cephalosporins Erythromycin Clindamycin Vancomycin	A few strains are penicillin resistant, especially some *S. pneumoniae* Erythromycin is only for mild infections Vancomycin is only for serious infections
Enterococcus species	Penicillin or ampicillin plus gentamicin	Vancomycin plus gentamicin	There are some strains for which streptomycin is synergistic but gentamicin is not Some strains are resistant to synergy with any aminoglycoside
Staphylococcus species	Antistaphylococcal penicillin e.g. flucloxacillin	First-generation cephalosporins Vancomycin	Vancomycin is required for methicillin-resistant strains Rifampicin is occasionally used to eradicate the nasal carriage state
Neisseria meningitidis	Penicillin	Chloramphenicol Third-generation cephalosporins	Rare strains are penicillin resistant
Neisseria gonorrhoeae	Cefixime	Ciprofloxacin Third-generation cephalosporins	Some strains are fluoroquinolone resistant (especially in Asia)
Bordetella pertussis	Erythromycin	Trimethoprim with sulfamethoxazole	
Haemophilus influenzae	Aminopenicillin (ampicillin, amoxicillin)	Cefuroxime Third generation cephalosporins Chloramphenicol	Approximately 30% are aminopenicillin-resistant; aminopenicillins should not be used empirically in serious infections until susceptibility results are available Rifampicin is used to eradicate the nasal carriage state
Enterobacteria in urine	Trimethoprim with sulfamethoxazole	Ciprofloxacin Gentamicin Nitrofurantoin	β-lactams are less effective than trimethoprim with sulfamethoxazole or fluoroquinolones for the treatment of urinary tract infection
Enterobacteria in cerebrospinal fluid	Third-generation cephalosporin	Trimethoprim with sulfamethoxazole	In neonates only, aminoglycosides are equivalent to third generation cephalosporins Experience with trimethoprim with sulfamethoxazole in meningitis is limited

Fig. 3.3a Drugs of choice and alternatives for selected common bacterial pathogens.

Contraindications: Known hypersensitivity to cephalosporins or penicillins.

Adverse effects: Side effects of the cephalosporins include hypersensitivity reactions, which occur in a similar and cross-reacting fashion to the penicillins. Diarrhoea is common, owing to disturbance of normal colonic flora. Nausea and vomiting may also occur.

Therapeutic notes: The cephalosporins can be inactivated by the β-lactamase enzyme, though the later generation drugs are more resistant to hydrolysis.

Glycopeptides

Vancomycin and teicoplanin are the classical glycopeptides.

Mechanism of action: Glycopeptides are bactericidal. They inhibit peptidoglycan synthesis, with possible effects on RNA synthesis (Fig. 3.2).

Spectrum of activity: Vancomycin is active only against aerobic and anaerobic Gram-positive bacteria. Glycopeptides are reserved for resistant staphylococcal infections and *Clostridium difficile* in antibiotic-associated pseudomembranous colitis (see Fig. 3.3).

Route of administration: Glycopeptides are usually administered intravenously as are not well absorbed orally. Oral administration is reserved for when a local gastrointestinal tract effect is required, e.g. in colitis.

Adverse effects: Side effects of glycopeptides include ototoxicity and nephrotoxicity at high plasma levels, and fever, rashes, and local phlebitis at the site of infection.

Therapeutic notes: Acquired resistance to vancomycin is rare, but reports of vancomycin-resistant enterococci are becoming more common.

Bacterium	Drug(s) of choice	Alternatives	Comments
Enterobacteria elsewhere (blood, lung, etc.)	Gentamicin Third-generation cephalosporins Ciprofloxacin	Trimethoprim with sulfamethoxazole	Two-drug therapy is sometimes used in serious infection Monotherapy with a third-generation cephalosporin should be avoided if the pathogen is *Enterobacter cloacae*, *E. aerogenes*, *Serratia marcescens* or *Citrobacter freundii*
Pseudomonas aeruginosa	Antipseudomonal penicillin plus aminoglycoside	Ceftazidime Ciprofloxacin	Two-drug therapy recommended except for urinary tract infection
Bacteroides fragilis	Metronidazole or clindamycin	Imipenem Penicillin β-lactamase inhibitors	*B. fragilis* is usually involved in polymicrobial infections; therefore another antibiotic active against Enterobacteriaceae is often required
Mycoplasma pneumoniae	Macrolides e.g. erythromycin	Tetracycline	Although tetracyclines are as effective as macrolides, the latter are recommended because of better activity against *Pneumococcus*, which can mimic this infection
Chlamydia trachomatis	Tetracycline	Azithromycin Erythromycin	Azithromycin is the only therapy effective in a single dose Erythromycin is used in pregnancy
Rickettsial species	Tetracycline	Chloramphenicol	
Listeria monocytogenes	Ampicillin plus gentamicin	Vancomycin plus gentamicin	
Legionella species	Erythromycin	Tetracycline	Rifampicin is occasionally used as a second agent in severe cases
Clostridium difficile	Metronidazole	Vancomycin (oral)	
Mycobacterium tuberculosis	Isoniazid plus rifampicin plus pyrazinamide plus ethambutol	Streptomycin Fluoroquinolones Cycloserine Clarithromycin Capreomycin	Directly observed therapy is recommended Isoniazid is used alone for preventive therapy
Mycobacterium leprae	Dapsone plus rifampicin ± clofazimine	Clarithromycin	Thalidomide is useful for erythema nodosum leprosum

Drugs of choice and alternatives for selected common bacterial pathogens (continued)

Fig. 3.3b Drugs of choice and alternatives for selected common bacterial pathogens.

Monobactam and carbapenems

Aztreonam is a monobactam antibiotic, and imipenem is an carbapenem antibiotic. Both groups contain β-lactam rings, though are resistant to many β-lactamases. For indications, spectrum of activity and adverse effects consult BNF.

Antibacterial drugs that inhibit bacterial nucleic acids

Antibacterial drugs that inhibit bacterial nucleic acids include (Fig. 3.2):

- The antifolates, which affect DNA metabolism.
- The quinolones, which affect DNA replication and packaging.
- Rifampicin, which affects transcription (p. 39).

Antifolates

Examples of antifolates include the sulphonamides (e.g. sulfadiazine), and trimethoprim.

Mechanism of action: Folate is an essential cofactor in the synthesis of purines and hence of DNA. Bacteria, unlike mammals, must synthesize their own folate from para-aminobenzoic acid (Fig. 3.2). This pathway can be inhibited at two points: the sulphonamides inhibit dihydrofolate synthetase, while trimethoprim inhibits dihydrofolate reductase. These drugs are bacteriostatic.

Spectrum of activity: The sulphonamides are used for 'simple' urinary tract infections (UTIs). Trimethoprim and co-trimoxazole (trimethoprim

and sulfamethoxazole) are used for UTIs and respiratory tract infections (see Fig. 3.3).
Route of administration: Oral, intravenous.
Contraindications: Pregnant women, as theoretical teratogenic risk with antifolates. Neonates, as bilirubin displacement can damage the neonatal brain (kernicterus).
Adverse effects: Nausea, vomiting and hypersensitivity reactions, e.g. rashes, fever, Stevens–Johnson syndrome. The sulphonamides are relatively insoluble and can cause crystalluria, while trimethoprim can cause myelosuppression/ agranulocytosis.
Therapeutic notes: Antifolates are often used in combined preparations as they have synergistic effects. Resistance is common, and it is due to the production of enzymes that have reduced affinity for the drugs. Resistance can be acquired on plasmids in Gram-negative bacteria.

Quinolones
Ciprofloxacin and nalidixic acid are quinolones.
Mechanism of action: Quinolones are bactericidal. They act by inhibiting prokaryotic DNA gyrase. This enzyme packages DNA into supercoils and is essential for DNA replication and repair (Fig. 3.2).
Spectrum of activity: Ciprofloxacin has a broad spectrum of activity, while nalidixic acid is more narrowly active against Gram-negative organisms (see Fig. 3.3).
Route of administration: Oral, intravenous. Ciprofloxacin is so well absorbed orally that intravenous administration is rarely required unless the patient is unable to tolerate oral medication.
Contraindications: Quinolones should not be given with theophylline as theophylline-toxicity may be precipitated.
Adverse effects: Gastrointestinal upset. Rarely, hypersensitivity and CNS disturbances occur.

Antibacterial drugs that inhibit protein synthesis
Antibacterial drugs that inhibit protein synthesis are summarized in Fig. 3.4, and include:
- Aminoglycosides.
- Tetracyclines.
- Chloramphenicol.
- Macrolides.
- Lincosamides.
- Fusidic acid.

Aminoglycosides
Examples of aminoglycosides include gentamycin, streptomycin, netilmicin, and amikacin.
Mechanism of action: Aminoglycosides are bactericidal. They bind irreversibly to the bacterial ribosome. This inhibits the translation of mRNA to protein and causes more frequent misreading of the prokaryotic genetic code (Fig. 3.4).
Spectrum of activity: Aminoglycosides have a broad spectrum of activity but with low activity against anaerobes, streptococci, and pneumococci (see Fig. 3.3). Streptomycin is used against *Mycobacterium tuberculosis* (p. 39).
Route of administration: Parenteral only.
Contraindications: Acute neuromuscular blockade can occur if an aminoglycoside is used in combination with anaesthesia or other neuromuscular blockers.
Adverse effects: Dose-related ototoxicity and nephrotoxicity at high plasma levels.
Therapeutic notes: Resistance to aminoglycosides is increasing and is primarily due to plasmid-borne genes encoding degradative enzymes.

Tetracyclines
Examples of tetracyclines include tetracycline, minocycline, and doxycycline.
Mechanism of action: Tetracyclines are bacteriostatic. They work as a result of selective uptake into bacterial cells by active bacterial transport systems not possessed by mammalian cells. The tetracycline then binds reversibly to the bacterial ribosome, interfering with the attachment of tRNA to the mRNA ribosome complex (Fig. 3.4).
Spectrum of activity: Tetracyclines have broad-spectrum activity against Gram-positive and Gram-negative bacteria, as well as intracellular pathogens (see Fig. 3.3).
Route of administration: Oral, intravenous. Oral absorption is incomplete and can be impaired by calcium (e.g. milk), and magnesium or aluminium salts (e.g. antacids).
Contraindications: Tetracyclines should not be given to children or pregnant women.
Adverse effects: Gastrointestinal disturbances are common after oral administration. In children, tetracyclines depress bone growth, and produce permanent discoloration of teeth.
Therapeutic notes: Resistance to tetracyclines is slow to develop, but it is now widespread. In the majority

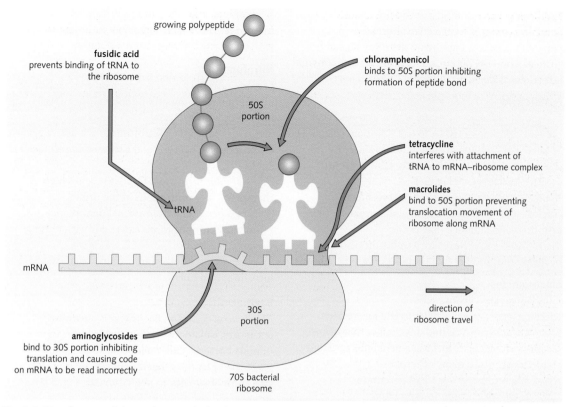

Fig. 3.4 Site of action of the antibiotics which inhibit bacterial protein synthesis.

of cases, resistance is due to decreased uptake of the drug, and is plasmid borne.

Chloramphenicol

Mechanism of action: Chloramphenicol is both bactericidal and bacteriostatic, depending on the bacterial species. It reversibly binds to the bacterial ribosome, inhibiting the formation of peptide bonds (Fig. 3.4).

Spectrum of activity: Chloramphenicol has a broad spectrum of activity against many Gram-positive cocci and Gram-negative organisms (see Fig. 3.3). Because of its toxicity, it is reserved for life-threatening infections, especially typhoid fever and meningitis.

Route of administration: Oral, intravenous.

Contraindications: Chloramphenicol should not be given to pregnant women or neonates.

Adverse effects: Myelosuppression and reversible anaemia. Neutropenia and thrombocytopenia may occur during chronic administration. Fatal aplastic anaemia is rare.

Neonates cannot metabolize chloramphenicol and 'grey baby syndrome' may develop, which comprises pallor, abdominal distension, vomiting, and collapse.

Therapeutic notes: Resistance to chloramphenicol is due to a plasmid-borne gene encoding an enzyme that inactivates the drug by acetylation. Blood monitoring is necessary.

Macrolides

Erythromycin, clarithromycin and azithromycin are examples of macrolides.

Mechanism of action: Macrolides are bacteriostatic/bactericidal. They reversibly bind to the bacterial ribosome, preventing the translocation movement of the ribosome along mRNA (Fig. 3.3).

Spectrum of activity: Erythromycin is effective against most Gram-positive bacteria and spirochaetes. Clarithromycin is active against *Haemophilus influenzae*, *Mycobacterium avium cellulare* and *Helicobacter pylori*.

Route of administration: Oral, intravenous.

Adverse effects: Side effects of erythromycin include gastrointestinal disturbance, which is common after oral administration. Liver damage and jaundice can occur after chronic administration.

Therapeutic notes: Resistance to erythromycin results from a mutation of the binding site on the ribosome.

Erythromycin has a similar spectrum of activity to penicillin, and it is an effective alternative in penicillin-sensitive patients. Azithromycin can be given as a one-off dose for uncomplicated chlamydial infections of the genital tract.

Fusidic acid
Mechanism of action: Fusidic acid is a steroid that prevents binding of tRNA to the ribosome (Fig. 3.4).
Spectrum of activity: Fusidic acid has a narrow spectrum of activity, particularly against Gram-positive bacteria (see Fig. 3.3).
Route of administration: Oral, intravenous.
Adverse effects: Gastrointestinal disturbance. Skin eruptions and jaundice may occur.
Therapeutic notes: Resistance to fusidic acid can occur via mutation or by plasmid-borne mechanisms.

Lincosamides
Clindamycin is a lincosamide.
Mechanism of action: Similar to the macrolides.
Spectrum of activity: Clindamycin is active against Gram-positive cocci, including penicillin-resistant staphylococci, and many anaerobes.
Route of administration: Oral, parenteral.
Adverse effects: Antibiotic-associated (pseudomembranous) colitis; greater risk than for other antibiotics.
Therapeutic notes: Clindamycin is used for staphylococcal joint and bone infections.

Miscellaneous antibacterials
Miscellaneous antibacterials include:
- Metronidazole.
- Nitrofurantoin.
- Bacitracin.
- Polymyxins.

Metronidazole and tinidazole
Mechanism of action: Metronidazole is bactericidal. It is metabolized to an intermediate that inhibits bacterial DNA synthesis and degrades existing DNA. Its selectivity is due to the fact that the intermediate toxic metabolite is not produced in mammalian cells.
Spectrum of activity: Metronidazole is antiprotozoal (p. 47), and it has antibacterial activity against anaerobic bacteria (see Fig. 3.3).
Route of administration: Oral, rectal, intravenous, and topical.
Contraindications: Metronidazole should not be given to pregnant women.
Adverse effects: Mild headache and gastrointestinal disturbance. Adverse drug reactions occur with alcohol.

Therapeutic notes: Acquired resistance to metronidazole is rare. Tinidazole is similar to metronidazole but has a longer duration of action.

Nitrofurantoin
Mechanism of action: The mechanism of action of nitrofurantoin is uncertain though it possibly interferes with bacterial DNA metabolism.
Spectrum of activity: Nitrofurantoin is active against Gram-positive bacteria and *Escherichia coli* (see Fig. 3.3).
Route of administration: Oral; it reaches high therapeutic concentrations in the urine.
Adverse effects: Gastrointestinal disturbance. Pulmonary complications can occur with chronic therapy.
Therapeutic notes: Rarely, chromosomal resistance to nitrofurantoin can occur.

Bacitracin
Mechanism of action: Bacitracin is a natural antibiotic, isolated from *Bacillus subtilis*, that inhibits bacterial cell-wall formation.
Spectrum of activity: Bacitracin is similar in its spectrum of activity to penicillin (see Fig. 3.3).
Route of administration: Topical.
Adverse effects: Well tolerated when used topically. Serious nephrotoxicity can occur if it is used systemically.
Therapeutic notes: Bacitracin is much less likely to cause hypersensitivity reactions than penicillin. Acquired resistance is rare.

Polymyxins
Colistin is an example of a polymyxin, though this class is seldom prescribed due to its toxicity.
Mechanism of action: Polymyxins are bactericidal. They are peptides that interact with phospholipids on the outer plasma cell membranes of Gram-negative bacteria, disrupting their structure. This disruption destroys the bacteria's osmotic barrier, leading to lysis (Fig. 3.2).
Spectrum of activity: Polymyxins are active only against Gram-negative bacteria including *Pseudomonas aeruginosa* (see Fig. 3.3).
Route of administration: Intravenous, intramuscular, inhalation. Oral polymyxins are given to sterilise the bowel in neutropenic patients.
Adverse effects: Perioral and peripheral, paraesthesia, vertigo, nephrotoxicity, and neurotoxicity.
Therapeutic notes: Resistance to polymyxins is rare.

Antimycobacterial drugs

The mycobacteria are slow-growing intracellular bacilli that cause tuberculosis (*Mycobacterium tuberculosis*) and leprosy (*Mycobacterium leprae*) in humans.

Mycobacteria differ in their structure and lifestyle from Gram-positive and Gram-negative bacteria, and they are treated with different drugs.

Antituberculosis therapy

The first-line drugs used in the treatment of tuberculosis are:

- Isoniazid, which inhibits the production of mycolic acid, a component of the cell wall unique to mycobacteria, and is bactericidal against growing organisms. Taken orally it penetrates tuberculous lesions well. Adverse effects occur in about 5% of patients and include peripheral neuropathy, hepatotoxicity, and autoimmune phenomena. Resistance is rare in developed countries, but not in less-developed areas.
- Rifampicin, which inhibits DNA-dependent RNA polymerase, causing a bactericidal effect. It is a potent drug, active orally. Adverse effects are infrequent, but they can be serious, e.g. hepatotoxicity and 'toxic syndromes'. Orange-discolouration of the urine is a common side effect. There are many drug interactions, and resistance can develop rapidly.
- Ethambutol, which is bacteriostatic. The mechanism of action is uncertain, involving impaired synthesis of the mycobacterial cell wall. Ethambutol is administered orally. Adverse effects are uncommon, but reversible optic neuritis may occur. Resistance often develops.
- Pyrazinamide, the mechanism of action of which is uncertain but it may involve metabolism of drug within *Mycobacterium tuberculosis* to produce a toxic product, pyrazinoic acid, which works as a bacteriostatic agent in the low pH environment of the phagolysosome. It is active orally. Adverse effects are hepatotoxicity and raised plasma urate levels that can lead to gout. Resistance can develop rapidly.
- Streptomycin, which is now rarely used in the UK for tuberculosis (p. 36).

The second-line drugs used for tuberculosis infections when first-line drugs have been discontinued owing to resistance or adverse effects are:

- Capreomycin, which is a peptide drug given intramuscularly. It can cause ototoxicity and kidney damage.
- Cycloserine, which is a broad-spectrum drug that inhibits peptidoglycan synthesis. This drug is administered orally, and can cause CNS toxicity.
- New macrolides, e.g. azithromycin and clarithromycin.
- Quinolones, e.g. ciprofloxacin.

To reduce the emergence of resistant organisms, a compound drug therapy is used to treat tuberculosis, involving:

- An initial phase of about 2 months consisting of three drugs: isoniazid, rifampicin, and pyrazinamide.
- Continuation phase of 4 months consisting of two drugs: isoniazid and rifampicin. Longer treatment regimens may be needed for patients with meningitis or bone/joint involvement.

Antileprosy therapy

Tuberculoid leprosy is treated with dapsone and rifampicin for 6 months.

Lepromatous leprosy is treated with dapsone, rifampicin, and clofazimine for up to 2 years.

Dapsone resembles sulphonamides chemically, and it may inhibit folate synthesis in a similar way. It is active orally. Adverse effects are numerous, and some fatal. Consult BNF.

Clofazimine is a chemically complex dye that accumulates in macrophages, possibly acting on mycobacterial DNA. As a dye, clofazimine can discolour the skin and urine red. Other adverse effects are numerous. It is active orally.

Grouping of antibacterial drugs by their mechanism of action rather than chemical structure is easier, more important, and more relevant to your understanding.

Antiviral drugs

Concepts of viral infection

Viruses are obligate intracellular parasites that lack independent metabolism and can only replicate within the host cells they enter and infect. A virus particle, or virion, consists essentially of DNA or RNA enclosed in a protein coat (capsid). In addition, certain viruses may possess a lipoprotein envelope and replicative enzymes (see Fig. 3.5).

Viruses are classified largely according to the architecture of the virion and the nature of their genetic material. Viral nucleic acid may be single stranded (ss) or double stranded (ds) (Fig. 3.6).

Antiviral agents

Because viruses have an intracellular replication cycle and they share many of the metabolic processes of the host cell, it has proved extremely difficult to find drugs that are selectively toxic to them. Additionally, by the time a viral infection becomes detectable clinically, the viral replication process tends to be very far advanced, making chemotherapeutic intervention difficult. All current antiviral agents are virustatic rather than virucidal and, therefore, they rely upon host immunocompetence for a complete clinical cure.

Nevertheless, antiviral chemotherapy is clinically effective against some viral diseases (identified with an asterisk in Fig. 3.6). The viruses include:

- Herpesviruses (herpes simplex virus, HSV; varicella zoster virus, VZV; cytomegalovirus, CMV).
- Influenza viruses A and more recently B.
- Respiratory syncytial virus, arenaviruses.
- Human immunodeficiency virus 1 (HIV-1).

The selective inhibition of these viruses by drugs depends on either:

- Inhibition of unique steps in the viral replication pathways, such as adsorption of the virion to the cell receptor, penetration, uncoating, assembly, and release.
- Preferential inhibition of steps shared with the host cell, which include transcription and translation.

In addition to chemotherapy, immune based therapies, such as the use of immunoglobulins and cytokines in viral infection, are also mentioned below.

Inhibition of attachment to or penetration of host cells

Amantadine

Mechanism of action: Amantadine blocks a primitive ion channel in the viral membrane (named M_2) preventing fusion of a virion to host cell membranes, and inhibits the release of newly synthesized viruses from the host cell (Fig. 3.7).
Route of administration: Oral.

Indications: Amantadine is used for the prophylaxis and treatment of acute influenza A in groups at risk. It is not effective against influenza B.
Adverse effects: Some patients (5–10%) report non-serious dizziness, slurred speech, and insomnia. Neurological side effects and renal failure can occur at high concentrations.
Therapeutic notes: Emergence of resistance to amantadine associated with clinical failure has been reported in 25–50% of patients. Amantadine is not used widely because of problems with resistance, its narrow spectrum of activity, and because influenza vaccines are often preferred.

Neuraminidase inhibitors

Zanamivir belongs to the neuraminidase inhibitor class of drugs.
Mechanism of action: Zanamivir inhibits the release of newly synthesized viruses from the host cell by inhibiting the enzyme—neuraminidase—that is responsible for cleaving the peptide links between virus and host.
Route of administration: Zanamivir is delivered by inhalation, though its sister drug oseltamivir may be given orally.
Indications: Treatment of influenza A or B virus within 48 hours after onset of symptoms when influenza is endemic in the community.
Contraindications: Breastfeeding.
Adverse effects: Gastrointestinal disturbances.

Immunoglobulins

Examples of immunoglobulins include human normal immunoglobulin (HNIG/γ-globulin) and specific immunoglobulins, e.g. hepatitis B (HBIG), rabies (RIG), varicella zoster (VZIG), and cytomegalovirus (CMVIG) immunoglobulins.
Mechanism of action: Immunoglobulins bind specifically to antigenic determinants on the outside of virions. By specifically binding to a virus, the immunoglobulins may neutralize it by coating the virus and preventing its attachment and entry into host cells.

HNIG is prepared from pooled plasma of ~1000 donors and contains antibodies to measles, mumps, varicella, and hepatitis A.

Specific immunoglobulins are prepared by pooling the plasma of selected donors with high levels of the antibody required.
Route of administration: Intramuscular, though intravenous immunoglobulins can be given.
Indications: HNIG is administered for the protection of susceptible contacts against hepatitis A, measles, mumps, and rubella. Specific

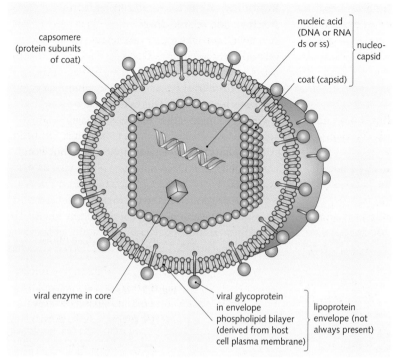

Fig. 3.5 Diagrammatic representation of the components of a virion.

capsomere
(protein subunits
of coat)

nucleic acid
(DNA or RNA
ds or ss) } nucleo-
capsid

coat (capsid)

viral enzyme in core

viral glycoprotein
in envelope
phospholipid bilayer
(derived from host
cell plasma membrane) } lipoprotein
envelope (not
always present)

Fig. 3.6 Classification of selected medically important viruses and the diseases they cause. (*, viruses for which effective chemotherapy exists; ds, double stranded; ss, single stranded.)

Classification of medically important viruses and the diseases they cause

Family	ss/ds	Viruses	Diseases
DNA viruses			
Herpes viruses	ds	Herpes simplex (HSV)*	Cold sores, genital herpes
		Varicella-zoster (VZV)*	Chickenpox, shingles
		Cytomegalovirus (CMV)*	Cytomegalic disease
		Epstein–Barr virus (EBV)*	Infectious mononucleosis
Poxviruses	ds	Variola	Smallpox
Adenoviruses	ds	Adenoviruses	Acute respiratory disease
Hepadnaviruses	ds	Hepatitis B	Hepatitis
Papovaviruses	ds	Papilloma	Warts
Parvoviruses	ss	B19	Erythema infectiosum
RNA viruses			
Orthomyxoviruses	ss	Influenza A* and B*	Influenza
Paramyxoviruses	ss	Measles virus	Measles
		Mumps virus	Mumps
		Parainfluenza	Respiratory infection
		Respiratory syncytial*	Respiratory infection
Coronaviruses	ss	Coronavirus	Respiratory infection
Rhabdoviruses	ss	Rabies virus	Rabies
Picornaviruses	ss	Enteroviruses	Meningitis
		Rhinoviruses	Colds
		Hepatitis A	Hepatitis
Calciviruses	ss	Norwalk virus	Gastroenteritis
Togaviruses	ss	Alphaviruses	Encephalitis, haemorrhagic fevers
		Rubivirus	Rubella
Reoviruses	ds	Rotavirus	Gastroenteritis
Arenavirus	ss	Lymphocytic choriomeningitis	Meningitis
		Lassavirus*	Lassa fever
Retroviruses	ss	HIV I, II*	AIDS

immunoglobulins may attenuate or prevent hepatitis and rabies following known exposure, and before the onset of signs and symptoms, e.g. following exposure to a rabid animal. VZIG and CMVIG are indicated for prophylactic use to prevent chickenpox, and cytomegalic disease in immunosuppressed patients at risk.

Contraindications: Immunoglobulins should not be given to people with known antibody against IgA.

Adverse effects: Malaise, chills, fever, and (rarely) anaphylaxis.

Therapeutic notes: Protection with immunoglobulins is immediate and lasts several weeks. HNIG may interfere with vaccinations for 3 months.

Inhibition of nucleic acid replication
Aciclovir and related drugs

Aciclovir, famciclovir and valaciclovir are all closely related anti-viral drugs.

Mechanism of action: Aciclovir and related drugs are characterized by their selective phosphorylation in herpes-infected cells. This takes place by a viral thymidine kinase rather than host kinase, as a first step.

Phosphorylation yields a triphosphate nucleotide that inhibits viral DNA polymerase and viral DNA synthesis.

These drugs are selectively toxic to infected cells because, in the absence of viral thymidine kinase, the host kinase activates only a small amount of the drug. In addition, the DNA polymerase of herpes virus has

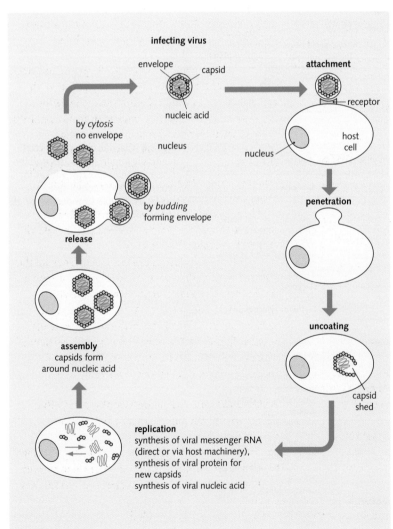

Fig. 3.7 Stages in the infection of a host's cell and replication of a virus. Several thousand virus particles may be formed from each cell. (Redrawn from *Medical Microbiology*, 2nd edn, by Mims et al, 1998. By permission of Mosby.)

a much higher affinity for the activated drug than has cellular DNA polymerase (Fig. 3.7).

Route of administration: Topical, oral, parenteral.

Indications: Aciclovir and related drugs are used for the prophylaxis and treatment of herpes simplex virus (HSV) and varicella zoster virus (VZV) infections, superficial and systemic, particularly in the immunocompromised.

Adverse effects: Side effects are minimal. Rarely, renal impairment and encephalopathy occur.

Therapeutic notes: The herpes genome in latent (non-replicating) cells is not affected by aciclovir therapy, and so recurrence of infection after cessation of treatment is to be expected.

Cytomegalovirus (CMV) is resistant to aciclovir because its genome does not encode thymidine kinase.

Ganciclovir

Mechanism of action: Ganciclovir is a synthetic nucleoside analogue, structurally related to aciclovir. It also requires conversion to the triphosphate nucleotide form, though by a different kinase. Ganciclovir acts as a substrate for viral DNA polymerase and as a chain terminator, aborting virus replication.

Route of administration: Oral, intravenous.

Indications: While as active as aciclovir against HSV and VZV, ganciclovir is reserved for the treatment of severe CMV infections in immunocompromised people, owing to its side effects.

Adverse effects: Reversible neutropenia in 40% of patients. There is occasional rash, nausea, and encephalopathy.

Therapeutic notes: Maintenance therapy with ganciclovir at a reduced dose may be necessary to prevent recurrence of CMV.

Ribavirin (tribavirin)

Mechanism of action: Ribavirin is a nucleoside analogue that selectively interferes with viral nucleic acid synthesis in a manner similar to aciclovir.

Route of administration: For respiratory syncytial virus (RSV) by inhalation; for Lassa virus intravenously.

Indications: Severe respiratory syncytial virus bronchiolitis in infants. Lassa fever.

Adverse effects: Reticulocytosis; respiratory depression.

Therapeutic notes: The necessity of aerosol administration for RSV limits the usefulness of this effective drug.

Nucleoside analogue reverse transcriptase inhibitors

Examples of nucleoside reverse transcriptase inhibitors include zidovudine (AZT), and the newer drugs, abacavir, didanosine (ddI), lamivudine (3TC), stavudine (d4T) and zalcitabine (ddC).

Mechanism of action: These nucleotide analogues all require intracellular conversion to the corresponding triphosphate nucleotide for activation. The active triphosphates competitively inhibit reverse transcriptase, and they cause termination of DNA chain elongation once incorporated. Affinity for viral reverse transcriptase is 100 times that for host DNA polymerase (Fig. 3.8, site 3).

Route of administration: Oral.

Indications: Nucleoside reverse transcriptase inhibitors are used for the management of asymptomatic and symptomatic HIV infections, and the prevention of maternal–fetal HIV transmission.

Adverse effects: Side effects of AZT are uncommon at the recommended low dosage in patients with asymptomatic or mild HIV infections, but more common in AIDS patients on higher dosage regimes.

Toxicity to human myeloid and erythroid progenitor cells commonly causes anaemia and neutropenia, i.e. bone-marrow suppression. Other common side effects include nausea, insomnia, headaches, and myalgia.

The major dose-limiting effects of ddI are pancreatitis and peripheral neuropathy, and of ddC and d4T, peripheral neuropathy.

Therapeutic notes: Drug resistance evolves to all the current nucleoside reverse transcriptase inhibitors by the development of mutations in reverse transcriptase, although the kinetics of resistance development varies for the different drugs (e.g. 6–18 months for AZT). Combined therapies may have a place in increasing efficacy synergistically and reducing emergence of resistant strains.

Non-nucleoside reverse transcriptase inhibitors

Efavirenz and nevirapine are examples of drugs within this class.

Mechanism of action: Efavirenz and nevirapine both bind to reverse transcriptase near the catalytic site, leading to a conformational change that inactivates this enzyme.

Route of administration: Oral.

Contraindications: Breastfeeding.

Adverse effects: Generally well tolerated. Rash, dizziness, and headache may occur.

Therapeutic notes: Resistance can develop quickly when sub-therapeutic doses are employed.

Inhibition of post-translational events
Protease inhibitors

Examples of protease inhibitors include saquinavir, and the newer drugs, ritonavir, indinavir, nelfinavir and amprenavir.

Mechanism of action: Protease inhibitors prevents the virus-specific protease of HIV cleaving the inert polyprotein product of translation into various structural and functional proteins (Fig. 3.8, site 5).

Route of administration: Oral.

Indications: Protease inhibitors are used for the management of asymptomatic and symptomatic HIV infections, in combination with nucleoside reverse transcriptase inhibitors.

Adverse effects: Protease inhibitors are well tolerated. Nausea, vomiting, and diarrhoea are common. In addition, indinavir and ritonavir may cause taste disturbances, and saquinavir may cause buccal and mucosal ulceration.

Therapeutic notes: Combination treatment between protease inhibitors and nucleoside reverse transcriptase inhibitors produces additive antiviral effects and reduces the incidence of resistance. Such combination therapy is termed highly active antiretroviral therapy (HAART).

Immunomodulators
Interferons

Mechanism of action: Interferons (IFNs) are endogenous cytokines with antiviral activity, which are normally produced by leucocytes and other cells in response to viral infection. Three major classes have been identified (α, β, and γ) and they have been shown to have immunoregulatory and antiproliferative effects.

The mechanism of the antiviral effect of IFN varies for different viruses and cells. IFNs have been shown to bind to cell-surface receptors and signal a cascade of events that interfere with viral penetration, uncoating, synthesis, or methylation of mRNA, translation of viral protein, viral assembly, and viral release (Fig. 3.7).

Probably the most important effect of IFNs is the induction of enzymes in the host cell that inhibit the translation of viral mRNA.

The relatively recent production of IFNs in large quantities by cell culture and recombinant DNA technology has allowed their evaluation and prescription as antiviral agents.

Route of administration: Intravenous, intramuscular.

Indications: The exact role of interferons (IFNs) in the treatment of viral infections remains unclear. They have a wide spectrum of activity and have been shown to be effective in the treatment of chronic hepatitis (B and C), amongst others.

Adverse effects: Influenza-like syndrome with fatigue, fever, myalgia, nausea, and diarrhoea is the commonest side effect. Chronic administration can cause bone-marrow depression and neurological effects.

Therapeutic notes: The role of IFNs remains to be clearly established. Their usefulness has been limited by the need for repeated injections and dose-limiting adverse effects.

Drugs used in HIV infection

Infection with the human immunodeficiency virus (HIV) ultimately results in progression to the acquired immunodeficiency syndrome (AIDS). There are currently no drugs which can prevent this progression, though there are numerous agents on the market and in clinical trials which delay the rate of progression.

There are a variety of potential sites for antiviral drug action in the HIV-1 replicative cycle (Fig. 3.8).

The three main classes of drug used in the treatment of HIV have already been discussed. These are:

- Nucleoside reverse transcriptase inhibitors (Fig. 3.8, site 3).
- Non-nucleoside reverse transcriptase inhibitors (Fig. 3.8, site 3).
- Protease inhibitors (Fig. 3.8, site 5).

Future anti-HIV drug therapy

A number of strategies are being pursued in research laboratories across the world in the quest for effective drugs to treat HIV infection. These strategies include:

- Drugs which interrupt HIV binding to host cells, notably the gp120 envelope protein.
- Drugs designed specifically to 'smother' and prevent its entry into cells.
- Antisense oligonucleotides to complement specific portions of the viral genome and inhibit transcription and replication.

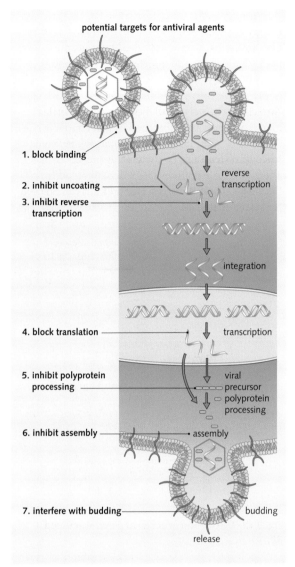

potential targets for antiviral agents

1. block binding

2. inhibit uncoating

3. inhibit reverse transcription

reverse transcription

integration

4. block translation — transcription

5. inhibit polyprotein processing — viral precursor polyprotein processing

6. inhibit assembly — assembly

7. interfere with budding — budding

release

Fig. 3.8 The HIV replicative cycle and potential sites of antiviral drug action.

The development of antiviral drugs is a rapidly-moving field and, with HIV especially, one that is currently topical. Keep up to date, as knowledge of recent developments in this area should impress examiners.

Antifungal drugs

Concepts of fungal infection

Fungi are members of a kingdom of eukaryotic organisms that live as saprophytes or parasites. A few species of fungi are pathogenic to humans.

Fungal infections are termed mycoses, and they may be superficial, affecting the skin, nails, hair, mucous membranes, or systemic, affecting deep tissues and organs.

Three main groups of fungi cause disease in humans (Fig. 3.9).

Fungal pathogenicity results from mycotoxin production, allergenicity/inflammatory reactions, and tissue invasion. Opportunistic fungal infections are important causes of disease in the immunosuppressed.

Antifungal drugs

There are four main classes of antifungal drugs. These are the:

- Polyene macrolides.
- Imidazole antifungals.
- Triazole antifungals.
- Other antifungals.

The sites of action of the antifungal drugs are summarized in Fig. 3.10.

Fig. 3.9 Main groups of fungi causing disease in humans.

Fungi causing disease in humans			
Fungal class	**Form**	**Example**	**Disease caused**
Moulds	Filamentous branching mycelia	Dermatophytes e.g. *Tinea spp.* *Aspergillus fumigatus*	Athlete's foot, ringworm and other superficial mycoses Pulmonary or disseminated aspergillosis
True yeasts	Unicellular (round or oval)	*Cryptococcus neoformans*	Cryptococcal meningitis and lung infections in the immunocompromised
Yeast-like fungi	Similar to yeasts but can also form long (non-branching) filaments	*Candida albicans*	Oral and vaginal thrush, endocarditis and septicaemias

Polyene macrolides

Examples of polyene macrolides include amphotericin B and nystatin.

Mechanism of action: Polyene macrolides bind to ergosterol in the fungal cell membrane, forming pores through which cell constituents are lost. This results in fatal damage (Fig. 3.11). These drugs are selectively toxic because in human cells the major sterol is cholesterol, not ergosterol.

Route of administration: Amphotericin B is administered topically and intravenously. Nystatin is too toxic for intravenous use. It is not absorbed orally at all, and so it is applied topically as a cream, vaginal pessaries, or tablets sucked so as to deliver the drug via the oral membranes.

Indications: Amphotericin is a broad-spectrum antifungal used in potentially fatal systemic infections. Nystatin is used to suppress candidiasis (thrush) on the skin and mucous membranes (oral and vaginal).

Adverse effects: Fever, chills, and nausea. Long-term therapy invariably causes renal damage. Nystatin may cause oral sensitization.

Therapeutic notes: Creatinine clearance must be monitored during amphotericin therapy to exclude renal damage. Resistance can develop *in vivo* to amphotericin, but not to nystatin.

Imidazoles

Examples of imidazoles include clotrimazole, miconazole, and ketoconazole.

Mechanism of action: Imidazoles have a broad spectrum of activity. They inhibit fungal lipid (especially ergosterol) synthesis in cell membranes.

Interference with fungal oxidative enzymes results in the accumulation of 14α-methyl sterols, which may disrupt the packing of acyl chains of phospholipids, inhibiting growth and interfering with membrane-bound enzyme systems.

Route of administration: Intravenous, topical. Ketoconazole is given orally as, unlike the other imidazoles, it is well absorbed by this route.

Indications: Candidiasis and dermatophyte mycoses. Miconazole can also be used intravenously as an alternative to amphotericin in disseminated mycoses. Because ketoconazole is active orally, it can be used for systemic mycoses.

Fig. 3.11 Mechanism of action of polyene antifungal agents.

Fig. 3.10 Sites of action of antifungal drugs.

Adverse effects: Topical use of imidazoles tends to be unproblematic. Intravenous miconazole is often limited by side effects of nausea, faintness, and haematological disorders. Oral ketoconazole can cause serious hepatotoxicity and adreno-suppression.

Therapeutic notes: Resistance rarely develops to imidazoles.

Triazoles

Examples of triazoles include fluconazole and itraconazole.

Mechanism of action: Triazoles are similar to imidazoles (see above), although they have greater selectivity against fungi, and they cause less endocrinological problems.

Route of administration: Oral.

Indications: Fluconazole can be used for a wide range of systemic and superficial infections, including cryptococcal meningitis, as it reaches the CSF in high concentrations. Itraconazole is similarly indicated, although unlike fluconazole, it can be used against Aspergillus.

Adverse effects: Nausea, diarrhoea, and rashes. Itraconazole is well tolerated though nausea, headaches, and abdominal pain can occur, but it should not be given to patients with liver damage.

Therapeutic notes: Resistance rarely develops to the triazoles.

Other antifungals
Allylamines

Terbinafine is an example of an allylamine.

Mechanism of action: Terbinafine prevents ergosterol synthesis by inhibiting the enzyme squalene oxidase, resulting in squalene accumulation, which leads to membrane disruption and cell death. It is lipophilic and penetrates superficial tissues well, including the nails.

Route of administration: Oral, topical.

Indications: Terbinafine has been recently introduced against dermatophyte infections including ringworm, where oral therapy is appropriate because of the site and severity of extent of infection.

Adverse effects: Mild nausea, abdominal pain, and skin reactions. Loss of taste has been reported.

Therapeutic notes: Resistance rarely develops. Initial trials with terbinafine show impressive clinical and mycological cure rates.

Flucytosine

Mechanism of action: Flucytosine is imported into fungal, but not human, cells, where it is converted into 5-fluorouracil, a potent inhibitor of DNA synthesis.

Route of administration: Intravenous.

Indications: Flucytosine is most active against yeasts, and it is indicated for use in systemic candidiasis and as an adjunct to amphotericin in cryptococcal meningitis.

Adverse effects: Nausea and vomiting are common. Rare side effects include hepatotoxicity, hair loss, and bone-marrow suppression.

Therapeutic notes: Weekly blood counts of patients on flucytosine are necessary to monitor bone marrow suppression.

Griseofulvin

Mechanism of action: The action of griseofulvin is not fully established, but it probably interferes with microtubule formation or nucleic acid synthesis and polymerization. It is selectively concentrated in keratin and, therefore, it is suitable for treating dermatophyte mycoses.

Route of administration: Oral.

Indications: Griseofulvin is the drug of choice for widespread or intractable dermatophyte infections, where topical therapy has failed.

Adverse effects: Hypersensitivity reactions, headaches, rashes, and photosensitivity.

Therapeutic notes: Because griseofulvin is fungistatic rather than fungicidal, treatment regimes are long amounting to several weeks or months. Griseofulvin is more effective for skin than nail infections.

Superficial mycoses (e.g. 'athletes foot', 'thrush') are common and usually easily treated with topical drugs that have few adverse effects. Deep mycoses are rare (except in the immunocompromised), serious, and may be fatal despite therapy with systemic drugs, which often have adverse effects.

Antiprotozoal drugs

Concepts of protozoal infection

Protozoa are members of a phylum of unicellular organisms, some of which are parasitic pathogens in humans causing several diseases of medical and global importance. Parasitic protozoa replicate within the host's body; they are usually divided into four subphyla according to their type of locomotion (Fig. 3.12).

Malaria

Malaria is the most important protozoan disease in tropical medicine. It is responsible for two million deaths per year and much morbidity in the 200 million people worldwide who are infected.

Malaria is caused by four species of plasmodial parasites (see below) that are transmitted by female anopheline mosquitoes.

Antimalarial drugs target different phases of the malarial life cycle (Fig. 3.13). This life cycle proceeds as follows:

- When an infected mosquito feeds on a human it injects sporozoites into the bloodstream from its salivary glands.
- The sporozoites rapidly penetrate the liver where they transform and grow into tissue schizonts containing large numbers of merozoites. In the case of *Plasmodium vivax* and *P. ovale*, some schizonts remain dormant in the liver for years (hypnozoites), before rupturing to cause a relapse.
- The large tissue schizonts rupture after 5–20 days, releasing thousands of merozoites that invade circulating red blood cells (RBCs), and multiply inside the cell.
- The host's RBCs rupture, leading to the release of more merozoites. These then invade and destroy more RBCs. This cycle of invasion and destruction causes the episodic chills and fever that characterize malaria.

- Some merozoites develop into gametocytes. If these are taken up by a feeding mosquito, the insect becomes infected, thus completing the cycle.

The clinical features and severity of malaria depend upon the species of parasite and the immunological status of the person infected. Clinically significant malaria is less common in adults who have always lived in endemic areas, as partial immunity develops.

The four types of plasmodium causing malaria are:

- *P. falciparum*, which is widespread and causes malignant tertian (fever every third day) malaria. There is no exo-erythrocytic stage, so that, if the erythrocytic forms are eradicated, relapses do not occur.
- *P. vivax*, which is widespread and causes benign, tertian relapsing malaria. Exo-erythrocytic forms may persist in the liver for years and cause relapses.
- *P. malariae*, which is rare and causes benign quartan (fever every fourth day) malaria. There is no exo-erythrocytic stage, so that, if the erythrocytic forms are eradicated, relapses do not occur.
- *P. ovale*, which is mainly African and causes a rare form of benign relapsing malaria. Exo-erythrocytic forms may persist in the liver for years and cause relapses.

Approaches to antimalarial chemotherapy

Antimalarial drugs are usually classified in terms of their action against different stages of the parasite (Fig. 3.13). They are used to protect against or cure malaria or to prevent transmission.

Classification of medically important protozoan species causing disease in humans			
Sub-phyla	Defining characteristics	Medically important species	Disease
Amoebae (sarcodina)	Amoeboid movement with pseudopods	*Entamoeba histolytica*	Amoebiasis (amoebic dysentery)
Flagellates (mastigophora)	Flagella that produces a whip-like movement	*Giardia lamblia* *Trichomonas vaginalis* *Leishmania spp.* *Trypanosoma spp.*	Giardiasis Trichomonal vaginitis Leishmaniasis Trypanosomiasis (sleeping sickness and Chagas' disease)
Ciliates (ciliophora)	Cilia beat to produce movement	—	—
Sporozoans (sporozoa)	No locomotor organs in adult stage	*Plasmodium spp.*	Malaria

Fig. 3.12 Classification of medically important protozoan species causing disease in humans.

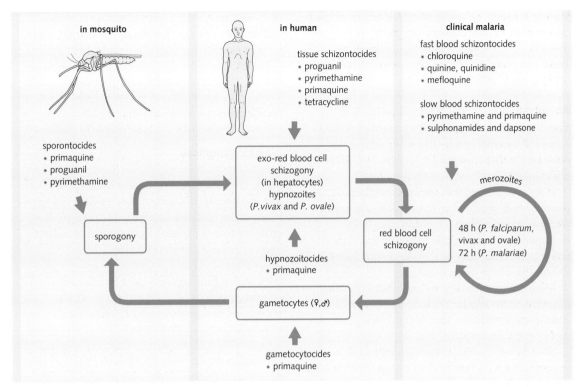

in mosquito

in human

clinical malaria

fast blood schizontocides
* chloroquine
* quinine, quinidine
* mefloquine

slow blood schizontocides
* pyrimethamine and primaquine
* sulphonamides and dapsone

tissue schizontocides
* proguanil
* pyrimethamine
* primaquine
* tetracycline

sporontocides
* primaquine
* proguanil
* pyrimethamine

exo-red blood cell
schizogony
(in hepatocytes)
hypnozoites
(*P.vivax* and *P. ovale*)

merozoites

sporogony

red blood cell
schizogony

48 h (*P. falciparum*,
vivax and ovale)
72 h (*P. malariae*)

hypnozoitocides
* primaquine

gametocytes (♀,♂)

gametocytocides
* primaquine

Fig. 3.13 Malarial life cycle and point of action of chemotherapeutic agents.

Prophylactic use

The aim of prophylactic use is to prevent the occurrence of infection in a previously healthy individual who is at potential exposure risk.

Suppressive prophylaxis involves the use of blood schizonticides to prevent acute attacks; causal prophylaxis involves the use of tissue schizonticides or drugs against the sporozoite to prevent the parasite becoming established in the liver.

Curative (therapeutic use)

Antimalarial drugs can be used curatively (therapeutically) against an established infection.

Suppressive treatment aims to control acute attacks, usually with blood schizonticides; radical treatment aims to kill dormant liver forms, usually with a hypnozonticide, to prevent relapsing malaria.

Antimalarial drugs
4-aminoquinolines

Chloroquine is an example of a 4-aminoquinoline.
Mechanism of action: Chloroquine is a rapidly acting blood schizonticide (Fig. 3.13). It is concentrated 100-fold in erythrocytes that contain plasmodial parasites; this occurs because ferriprotoporphyrin IX, a degradation product of haemoglobin digestion by the parasites, acts as a chloroquine receptor. It is unclear how the high chloroquine concentrations kill the parasites; possibly, the digestion of haemoglobin is inhibited.
Route of administration: Oral. In severe falciparum malaria infections, injections or infusions can be used.
Indications: Suppressive chemoprophylaxis and treatment of susceptible strains of plasmodium.
Adverse effects: Nausea, vomiting, headache, rashes, and, rarely, neurological effects.
Therapeutic notes: Chloroquine is considered safe for use in pregnant women. It rapidly controls fever (24–48 hours) but it cannot produce a lasting radical cure in *P. vivax* and *P. ovale* infections as it does not affect hypnozoites.

In most areas, *P. falciparum* is resistant to chloroquine, necessitating combination chemoprophylaxis with antifolates (see later).

Quinoline–methanols

Examples of quinoline–methanols include quinine and mefloquine.
Mechanism of action: Quinoline–methanols are rapidly acting blood schizonticides (Fig. 3.13). It is not precisely known how the quinoline–methanols

work but, like chloroquine, they are known to bind to a product of haemoglobin digestion.

Route of administration: Quinine is administered orally or by rate-controlled infusion in severe cases. Mefloquine is only given orally.

Indications: Quinine is the drug of choice for treating the acute clinical attack of falciparum malaria resistant to chloroquine. Mefloquine is effective against all malarial species including multidrug-resistant *P. falciparum*, and it can also be used for chemoprophylaxis.

Adverse effects: Quinine: tinnitus, headache, nausea, blurring of vision, hypoglycaemia, and, rarely, blood disorders. Overdose results in profound hypotension due to peripheral vasodilatation and myocardial depression (see Ch. 7). Quinine is safe in pregnancy.

Mefloquine: nausea, vomiting, gastrointestinal disturbance, and postural hypotension. Rarely, acute neuropathic conditions may occur. Mefloquine may cause fetal abnormalities.

Therapeutic notes: The quinoline–methanols are used in combination therapy with other agents such as the sulphonamides or tetracyclines.

Antifolates

Examples of antifolates include type 1 drugs, e.g. sulphonamides and dapsone, and type 2 drugs, e.g. pyrimethamine and proguanil.

Mechanism of action: Antifolates are slow-acting (in comparison with chloroquine, quinine, and mefloquine) blood schizonticides, tissue schizonticides, and sporonticides. These drugs inhibit the formation of folate compounds and thus inhibit DNA synthesis and cell division. All growing stages of the malarial parasite are affected.

The sulphonamides and dapsone are known as type 1 antifolate drugs. They compete with *p*-aminobenzoic acid (PABA) for the enzyme dihydropteroate synthetase, which is found only in the parasites.

Proguanil and pyrimethamine are known as type 2 antifolate drugs. They selectively inhibit malarial dihydrofolate reductase.

These two groups of drug act on the same pathway but at different points; they are used in combination as their synergistic blockade is more powerful than any one drug acting alone.

Route of administration: Oral.

Indications: Antifolates are used in combination for the causal chemoprophylaxis of malaria, or in combination with quinine for the treatment of acute chloroquine-resistant malaria.

Adverse effects: Antifolates have almost no side effects if used in therapeutic doses. In toxic doses, type 2 antifolates can inhibit mammalian dihydrofolate reductase and cause a megaloblastic anaemia. Skin rashes occasionally occur.

Therapeutic notes: Common chemoprophylactic combinations include chloroquine plus pyrimethamine with a sulphonamide or dapsone.

8-aminoquinolines

Primaquine is an example of an 8-aminoquinoline.

Mechanism of action: Primaquine is an hypnozonicide and gametocide. It is unclear how the drug works, but it may cause oxidative damage to the parasite. It is effective against the non-growing stages of malaria, i.e. hypnozoites and gametocytes (Fig. 3.13).

Route of administration: Oral.

Indications: Primaquine is used for the radical cure of relapsing malarias (*P. ovale* and *P. vivax*) and prevention of transmission of *P. falciparum*.

Contraindications: Pregnancy.

Adverse effects: Nausea, vomiting, and bone-marrow depression. Intravenous haemolysis can occur in people with glucose-6-phosphate deficiency.

Therapeutic notes: Primaquine is usually used in combination with chloroquine. Resistance is rare.

Treatment of other protozoal infections

Amoebiasis

Amoebic dysentery is caused by infection with *Entamoeba histolytica*, which is ingested in a cystic form. Dysentery results from invasion of the intestinal wall by the parasite. Occasionally, the organism encysts in the liver, forming abscesses.

Metronidazole (p. 38) is the drug of choice for acute invasive amoebic dysentery, it kills the trophozoites though has no activity against the cyst forms. Diloxanide and tinidazole are also used to treat amoebiasis.

Giardiasis

Giardiasis is a bowel infection caused by the flagellate *Giardia lamblia*. Infection follows ingestion of contaminated water or food and involves flatulence and diarrhoea.

Metronidazole (p. 38) is the drug of choice for giardiasis.

Trichomonas vaginitis

Trichomonas vaginitis is caused by the flagellate *Trichomonas vaginalis*. It is a sexually transmitted inflammatory condition of the female vagina and, occasionally, male urethra.

Metronidazole (p. 38) is the drug of choice for trichomonas vaginitis.

Trypanosomiasis and leishmaniasis
Trypanosomiasis
African sleeping sickness and South American Chagas' disease are caused by species of flagellate trypanosome.

Insect vectors introduce the parasites into the human host, where they reproduce, causing bouts of parasitaemia and fever. Toxins released cause damage to organs—the CNS in the case of sleeping sickness, and the heart, liver, spleen, bone, and intestine in Chagas' disease.

Leishmaniasis
Leishmania species are flagellated parasites that are transmitted by a sandfly vector, assuming a non-flagellated intracellular form that resides within macrophages on infecting humans.

Clinical infections range from simple, resolving cutaneous infections to systemic 'visceral' forms with hepatomegaly, splenomegaly, anaemia, and fever.

The prophylaxis and treatment of trypanosomiasis and leishmaniasis are difficult and of variable efficacy. The drugs used are generally toxic and dangerous, making specialised knowledge essential.

Pneumocystis pneumonia
Pneumocystis pneumonia is most often associated with HIV infection, and is now considered an AIDS-defining illness. The infective agent *Pneumocystis carinii* is not truly a protozoa, though it has similarities with both protozoa and fungi, and it remains difficult to classify.

Signs and symptoms of *Pneumocystis carinii* pneumonia (PCP) are similar to other pneumonias, but culture is not possible, and the microorganism must be visualized by direct microscopy.

High dose oral or parenteral co-trimoxazole (trimethoprim and sulfamethoxazole) is the drug of choice, with parenteral pentamidine as an alternative.

A decent knowledge of the plasmodial life cycle is a prerequisite to understanding the mechanism and site of action of antimalarial drugs.

Anthelminthic drugs

Concepts of helminthic infection
Helminth is derived from the Greek *helmins*, meaning worm. Anthelminthic drugs are, therefore, medicines acting against parasitic worms.

The three groups of helminths that parasitize humans are:
- Cestoda (tapeworms).
- Nematoda (roundworms).
- Trematoda (flukes).

Fig. 3.14 lists medically important helminth infections and the main drugs used in their treatment.

Anthelminthic drugs
To be effective, an anthelminthic drug must be able to penetrate the cuticle of the worm, or gain access to its alimentary tract, so that it may exert its pharmacological effect upon the physiology of the worm.

Anthelminthic drugs act on parasitic worms by a number of mechanisms. These include:
- Damaging or killing the worm directly.
- Paralysing the worm.
- Damaging the cuticle of the worm so that host defences, such as digestion and immune rejection, can affect the worm.
- Interfering with worm metabolism.

Because there is great diversity across the different helminth classes, drugs highly effective against one species of worm are often ineffectual against another species.

Niclosamide
Mechanism of action: Niclosamide, a salicylamide derivative, is the most used drug for tapeworm infestations. It blocks glucose uptake at high concentrations, irreversibly damaging the scolex (attachment end) of the tapeworm, leading to the release and expulsion of the tapeworm. It is a safe, selective drug since very little is absorbed from the gastrointestinal tract.
Route of administration: Oral.
Indications: Tapeworm infestation (Fig. 3.14).
Adverse effects: Mild gastrointestinal disturbance.
Therapeutic notes: Patients are fasted before treatment with niclosamide. Purgatives to expel the dead worm segments (proglottides) can be used, but

Classification of medically important helminth infection and the main drugs in their treatment		
	Helminth species	**Drugs used in treatment**
• **Cestodes**		
Beef tapeworm	*Taenia saginata*	Niclosamide, praziquantel
Pork tapeworm	*Taenia solium*	Niclosamide, praziquantel
Fish tapeworm	*Diphyllobothrium latum*	Niclosamide, praziquantel
Hydatid tapeworm	*Echinococcus granulosus*	Albendazole
• **Nematodes**		
Intestinal species	*Ascaris lumbricoides*	Mebendazole, piperazine
Common round worms	*Enterobius vermicularis*	Mebendazole, piperazine
Threadworm/pin worm	*Strongyloides stercoralis*	Thiabendazole, albendazole
Threadworm (USA)	*Trichuris trichiura*	Mebendazole
Whipworm	*Necator americanus*	Mebendazole
Hookworms	*Ankylostoma duodenale*	Mebendazole
Tissue species		
Trichinella	*Trichinella spiralis*	Thiabendazole
Guinea worm	*Dracunculus medinesis*	Metronidazole*
Filariaroidea	*Wucheria bancrofti*	Diethylcarbamazine
	Loa loa	Diethylcarbamazine
	Brugia malayi	Diethylcarbamazine
	Onchocerca volvulus	Ivermectin
• **Trematodes**		
Blood flukes/	*Schistosoma japonicum*	Praziquantel
Schistosomes	*Schistosoma mansoni*	Praziquantel
	Schistosoma haematobium	Praziquantel

Fig. 3.14 Classification of medically important helminth infections and the main drugs used in their treatment. (*see p. 38.)

these are probably unnecessary, since the worm may be digested after the effects of the drug.

Praziquantel

Mechanism of action: Praziquantel increases the permeability of the helminth plasma membrane to calcium. At low concentrations this causes contraction and spastic paralysis and, at higher concentrations, vesiculation and vacuolization damage is caused to the tegument of the worm.

Route of administration: Oral.

Indications: Praziquantel is the drug of choice for all schistosome infections (Fig. 3.14), and for cysticercosis (a rare cestode condition caused by encystation of larvae of the tapeworm *Taenia solium*, in human organs).

Adverse effects: Mild gastrointestinal disturbance, and headache and dizziness may occur shortly after administration.

Therapeutic notes: Praziquantel should be taken after meals three times a day for 2 days only.

Piperazine

Mechanism of action: Piperazine is a reversible neuromuscular blocker that causes a flaccid paralysis in worms, leading to their expulsion by gastrointestinal peristalsis. It has very little effect on the host.

Route of administration: Oral.

Indications: Piperazine is used for roundworm and threadworm gastrointestinal infestation.

Adverse effects: Gastrointestinal disturbance, and neurotoxic effects (dizziness) may occur.

Therapeutic notes: A single dose of piperazine is usually effective for treating roundworm infection; threadworm infestation may require a longer course (7 days).

Benzimidazoles

Examples of benzimidazoles include mebendazole, thiabendazole, and albendazole.

Mechanism of action: Benzimidazoles bind with high affinity to a site on tubulin dimers, thus preventing the polymerization of microtubules. Subsequent depolymerization leads to complete breakdown of the microtubule.

The selectivity of benzimidazoles arises because they are 250–400 times more potent in helminth than in mammalian tissue. The process takes time to have effect, and the worm may not be expelled for days.

Route of administration: Oral.

Indications: Benzimidazoles are used in the treatment of hydatid disease, and many nematode infestations (Fig. 3.14).

Contraindications: Benzimidazoles should not be given to pregnant women as they are teratogenic and embryotoxic.

Adverse effects: Occasional gastrointestinal disturbance. Thiabendazole causes more frequent gastrointestinal disturbance, headache, and dizziness. Serious hepatotoxicity rarely occurs.

Therapeutic notes: Dosage regimes of benzimidazoles range from a single dose for pinworm infestation to multiple doses for up to 5 days for trichinosis.

Diethylcarbamazine

Mechanism of action: It is not clear exactly how diethylcarbamazine exerts its filaricidal effect. It has been suggested that it damages or modifies the parasites in such a way as to make them more susceptible to host immune defences.

Diethylcarbamazine kills both microfilariae in the peripheral circulation and adult worms in the lymphatics.

Route of administration: Oral.

Indications: Diethylcarbamazine is the drug of choice for lymphatic filariasis caused by *Wucheria bancrofti*, *Loa loa*, and *Brugia malayi* (Fig. 3.14).

Adverse effects: Gastrointestinal disturbance, headache, and lassitude.

Material from the damaged and dead worms causes allergic side effects, including skin reactions,

lymph gland enlargement, dizziness, and tachycardia, lasting from 3 to 7 days.

Therapeutic notes: To minimize the dangerous sudden release of dead worm material, the initial dose of diethylcarbamazine is started low and then increased and maintained for 21 days.

Ivermectin

Mechanism of action: Ivermectin immobilizes the tapeworm *Onchocerca volvulus* by causing tonic paralysis of the peripheral muscle system. It does this by potentiating the effect of γ-amino butyric acid (GABA) at the worm's neuromuscular junction.

Route of administration: Oral.

Indications: Ivermectin is the drug of choice for *Onchocerca volvulus*, which causes river blindness (Fig. 3.14).

Adverse effects: Ocular irritation, transient electrocardiographic changes, and somnolence. An immediate immune reaction to dead microfilariae (Mazzotti reaction) can be severe.

All the anthelminthic drugs described in this chapter are administered orally.

- What are the differences between bacterial (prokaryotic) and mammalian (eukaryotic) cells, and how are these differences exploited by selective antibacterial agents?
- Describe the differences between innate and acquired antibiotic resistance, the biochemical mechanisms of resistance, and the genetic mechanisms by which it is acquired.
- Outline the classification of mycobacterial diseases and the drugs used in their treatment.
- List some of the more common side effects of antibiotic drugs, and the likely mechanisms responsible for these.
- List the main routes of administration for antibiotic drugs, and give an example of an antibiotic drug that would be administered by this route, the microbial organism responsible for the disease, and the clinical features of the disease.
- What are the peculiar features of viruses as infective pathogens, and how does their life cycle make selective chemotherapy difficult?
- What is the broad classification of viruses, and what are the major human diseases caused by viruses?
- Describe the mechanism of action of the different classes of antiviral drugs, and the point in the viral replication cycle they act upon.

- Name the drugs currently used in the treatment of HIV infection.
- By what routes can antiviral drugs be administered, and what would be the indications for each route given?
- Describe the classification of fungi and the types of infections that fungi can cause in humans.
- What are the main classes of antifungal drugs? Describe their mechanism and site of action.
- What is an opportunistic infection, and who is susceptible to this type of disease? Name some of the more common opportunistic infections.
- Name three protozoan subphyla and the medically important diseases they cause.
- Draw a simple diagram illustrating the life cycle of the malaria parasite.
- Add the site of action of the antimalarial drugs to this life cycle.
- Describe the classification of the helminths that parasitize humans.
- Name the medically important helminths in each group, the disease they cause, and the drugs used in their treatment.
- Discuss the mechanisms of action of the drugs used in the treatment of helminth infections.
- List the more common infections that present to the health profession, the likely infective agents, and the most suitable drugs to treat these infections, considering all microbiological and viral species.

4. Inflammation, Pain, and Immunosuppression

Inflammation and pain

Inflammation and pain go hand-in-hand, and probably result in the majority of doctor–patient consultations.

In practice, the holistic approach allows the doctor to assess which therapeutics should be employed when a patient presents with pain or inflammation, though for the purpose of this chapter the two are described individually for simplicity. Arthritis provides an excellent example of where pain and inflammation are intimately married, and so the anti-rheumatic drugs are also described in this chapter.

Inflammation

Inflammation describes the changes seen in response to tissue injury or insult, as originally defined by the Latin words dolor, rubor, calor, and tumor, meaning pain, redness, heat, and swelling. Some add a fifth phrase, *functio laesa* (loss of function).

These changes result from alterations in local blood vessels. This leads to dilatation of the blood vessels, their increased permeability, and increased receptiveness for leucocytes, resulting in the accumulation of inflammatory cells at the site of injury. The main cells seen in an acute inflammatory response are polymorphonuclear neutrophil leucocytes and macrophages. Lymphocytes, as well as basophils and eosinophils, also accumulate, especially in certain types of inflammation.

Inflammatory responses are produced and controlled by the interaction of a wide range of inflammatory mediators, some derived from leucocytes, some from the damaged tissues. Examples include histamine, kinins (bradykinin), neuropeptides (substance-P, calcitonin gene-related peptide), cytokines (e.g. interleukins), and the arachidonic acid metabolites (eicosanoids).

Arachidonic acid metabolites: the eicosanoids

Of the inflammatory mediators mentioned above, the eicosanoids are of special importance because:

- They are involved in the majority of inflammatory reactions.

- Most anti-inflammatory therapy is based on the manipulation of their biosynthesis—i.e. non-steroidal anti-inflammatory drugs (NSAIDs) and steroidal anti-inflammatory drugs (glucocorticoids).

The eicosanoids are a family of polyunsaturated fatty acids formed from arachidonic acid. The biosynthetic pathway is shown in Fig. 4.1.

Arachidonic acid is derived mainly from phospholipids of cell membranes, from which it is mobilized by the action of the enzyme phospholipase A_2.

Arachidonic acid is then further metabolized:

- By cyclooxygenase to produce the 'classical prostaglandins', thromboxane and prostacyclin, collectively known as the prostanoids.
- By lipoxygenase to produce the leukotrienes.

The actions of eicosanoids in inflammatory reactions are listed in Fig. 4.2.

Anti-inflammatory drugs

The main drugs used for their broad-spectrum anti-inflammatory effects are:

- Non-steroidal anti-inflammatory drugs.
- Steroidal anti-inflammatory drugs (glucocorticoids) (Ch. 11 and p. 59).

Both these classes of anti-inflammatory drug exert their effect by inhibiting the formation of eicosanoids (see Fig. 4.1).

In addition, a number of other drug classes, used clinically under certain circumstances, have more restricted anti-inflammatory actions. These are:

- Disease-modifying antirheumatic drugs (DMARDs) (p.59).
- Drugs used to treat gout (p. 60).
- Antihistamines (p. 157).

Non-steroidal anti-inflammatory drugs

NSAIDs are a chemically diverse group of drugs that all possess the ability to inhibit both forms of the enzyme cyclooxygenase (see Fig. 4.1), an action that is responsible for their pharmacological effects (see Fig. 4.4).

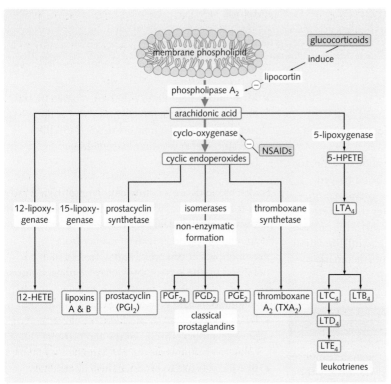

Fig. 4.1 Biosynthetic pathway of the eicosanoids. (LT, leukotrienes; HETE, hydroxyeicosatetraenoic acid; PG, prostaglandin; HPETE, hydroperoxyeicosatetraenoic acid; NSAID, non-steroidal anti-inflammatory drug.)

Actions of the eicosanoids in the inflammatory reaction	
Eicosanoid	**Actions in inflammation**
• **Prostanoids**	
'Classical prostaglandins' e.g. PGD_2, PGE_2, PGF_2	Produce increased vasodilatation, vascular permeability and oedema in an inflammatory reaction; prostaglandins also sensitize nociceptive fibres to stimulation by other inflammatory mediators
Thromboxane A_2 (TXA_2)	Platelet aggregation and vasoconstriction
Prostacyclin (PGI_2)	Inhibition of platelet aggregation and vasodilatation
• **Leukotrienes**	
e.g. LTB_4, LTC_4	Increase vascular permeability, promote leucocyte chemotaxis (and cause contraction of bronchial smooth muscle)

Fig. 4.2 Actions of the eicosanoids in the inflammatory reaction.

The first drugs of this type were the salicylates (e.g. aspirin) extracted from the bark of the willow tree. Subsequently, many synthetic and semi-synthetic NSAIDs have been created by pharmacologists. Chemically and structurally heterogeneous, they are related through their common mechanism of action (Fig. 4.3).

Mechanism of action: The main action of all the NSAIDs is inhibition of the enzyme cyclooxygenase. This enzyme is involved in the metabolism of arachidonic acid to form the prostanoids, i.e. the 'classical prostaglandins', prostacyclin and thromboxane A_2.

Inhibition of cyclooxygenase can occur by several mechanisms:
- Irreversible inhibition—e.g. aspirin causes acetylation of the active site.
- Competitive inhibition—e.g. ibuprofen acts as a competitive substrate.
- Reversible, non-competitive inhibition—e.g. paracetamol has a free-radical trapping action that interferes with the production of hydroperoxidases, which are believed to have an essential role in cyclooxygenase activity.

Cyclooxygenase exists in two enzyme isoforms:
- COX-1, which is expressed in most tissues, especially platelets, gastric mucosa, and renal vasculature; it is involved in physiological cell signalling. Most adverse effects of NSAIDs are caused by inhibition of COX-1.

- COX-2, which is induced at sites of inflammation and produces the prostanoids involved in inflammatory responses. Analgesic and anti-inflammatory effects of NSAIDs are largely a result of inhibition of COX-2.

COX-2-specific inhibitors are now licensed for use in several countries for symptomatic relief in osteoarthritis and rheumatoid arthritis; evaluation of their therapeutic effects and reduced side effect profile remains under scrutiny.

> Always remember the reasons behind the conflict over NSAIDs. The cardiologist will want every patient on aspirin—for its anti-platelet action. The gastroenterologist and the nephrologist will want to stop aspirin—as it causes GI upset and ulceration, and potentially worsens renal blood flow.

Clinical effects: NSAIDs work by the inhibition of cyclooxygenase and resulting inhibition of prostaglandin synthesis, producing three major clinical actions of potential therapeutic benefit: analgesia, an anti-inflammatory action, and an antipyretic (fever reducing) action (Fig. 4.4).

Not all NSAIDs possess these three actions to exactly the same extent, an example being the lack of anti-inflammatory activity possessed by paracetamol (see Fig. 4.3).

In addition to these three main categories of effect, aspirin has a pronounced effect on inhibiting platelet aggregation, due to reduced thromboxane synthesis. This has led to its successful use in primary and secondary prevention of cardiovascular and cerebrovascular events (Ch. 7).

Indications: NSAIDs are widely used for a variety of complaints. They are available on prescription and 'over the counter'. Their use includes musculoskeletal and joint diseases (strains, sprains, rheumatic problems, arthritis, gout, etc.), analgesia for mild to moderate pain relief including headaches and dysmenorrhoea, and symptomatic relief in fever.

Contraindications: NSAIDs should not be given to people with gastrointestinal ulceration or bleeding, or a previous hypersensitivity to any NSAID. Caution should be used in asthma and when renal function is impaired.

Adverse effects: Generalized adverse effects of NSAIDs are common, especially in the elderly and in chronic users, and these mostly arise from the non-selective inhibition of COX-1 and COX-2 (Fig. 4.5).

Less commonly, liver disorders and bone marrow depression are seen.

Other unwanted effects that are relatively specific to individual compounds are also seen (see below).

Therapeutic notes on individual NSAIDs

Salicylic acids, e.g. aspirin, which is cheap, and is still the drug of choice for many sorts of mild pain despite a relatively high incidence of gastrointestinal side effects. It is also used for its antiplatelet action. However, it produces tinnitus in toxic doses.

Propionic acids, e.g. ibuprofen, which is effective and well tolerated. It is the drug of choice for inflammatory joint disease, owing to its low incidence of side effects.

Acetic acids, e.g. indometacin (indomethacin), which is a highly potent inhibitor of COX that is effective but associated with a high incidence of side effects. It commonly causes neurological effects such as dizziness and confusion, as well as gastrointestinal upsets.

Non-steroidal anti-inflammatory drugs				
Chemical class	Examples	Analgesic	Antipyretic	Anti-inflammatory
Salicylic acids	Aspirin	+	+	+
Propionic acids	Ibuprofen Fenuprofen	+	+	+
Acetic acids	Indometacin	+	+	++
Oxicams	Piroxicam	+	+	++
Pyrazolones	Phenylbutazone	+/−	+	++
Fenemates	Mefenamic acid	+	+	+/−
para-Aminophenols	Paracetamol	+	+	−

Fig. 4.3 Classes of non-steroidal anti-inflammatory drugs and comparison of their main actions.

Major clinical effects of NSAIDs	
Clinical action	Mechanism of action
Analgesic action	• The analgesic effect is largely a peripheral effect that is due to the inhibition of prostaglandin synthesis at the site of pain and inflammation • Prostaglandins do not produce pain directly, but sensitize nociceptive fibre nerve endings to other inflammatory mediators (bradykinin, histamine, 5-HT), amplifying the basic pain message; prostaglandins of the E and F series are implicated in this sensitizing action • Thus NSAIDs are most effective against pain where there is an inflammatory component • A small component of the analgesic action of NSAIDs is a consequence of a central effect in reducing prostaglandin synthesis in the CNS; paracetamol especially works in this manner
Anti-inflammatory action	• Prostaglandins produce increased vasodilatation, vascular permeability and oedema in an inflammatory reaction • Inhibition of prostaglandin synthesis therefore reduces this part of the inflammatory reaction • NSAIDs do not inhibit the numerous other mediators involved in an inflammatory reaction; thus inflammatory cell accumulation, for example, is not inhibited
Antipyretic action	• During a fever, leucocytes release inflammatory pyrogens (e.g. interleukin-1) as part of the immune response; these act on the thermoregulatory centre in the hypothalamus to cause an increase in body temperature • This effect is believed to be mediated by an increase in hypothalamic prostaglandins (PGEs), the generation of which is inhibited by NSAIDs • NSAIDs do not affect temperature under normal circumstances or in heat stroke

Fig. 4.4 Three major clinical actions of non-steroidal anti-inflammatory drugs (NSAIDs).

General adverse effects of NSAIDs		
System	Adverse effect	Cause
GI	Dyspepsia, nausea, vomiting	Inhibition of the normal protective actions of prostaglandins on the gastric mucosa
	Ulcer formation and potential haemorrhage risk in chronic users	PGE_2 and PGI_2 normally inhibit gastric acid secretion, increase mucosal blood flow, and have a cytoprotective action
Renal	Renal damage/nephrotoxicity Renal failure can occur after years of chronic abuse	Inhibition of PGE_2- and PGI_2-mediated vasodilatation in the renal medulla and glomeruli
Other	Bronchospasm, skin rashes, other allergic-type reactions	Hypersensitivity reaction/allergy to drug

Fig. 4.5 General adverse effects of non-steroidal anti-inflammatory drugs (NSAIDs). (GI, gastrointestinal; PG, prostaglandin.)

Oxicams, e.g. piroxicam, which is a potent drug widely used for chronic inflammatory conditions. It is given only once daily, but causes a relatively high incidence of gastrointestinal problems.

Pyrazolones, e.g. phenylbutazone, which is an extremely potent agent but can produce a fatal bone marrow aplasia. For this reason it is reserved for the treatment of intractable pain in ankylosing spondylitis.

Fenemates, e.g. mefenamic acid, which is a moderately potent drug, but it commonly causes gastrointestinal upsets and occasionally skin rashes.

para-Aminophenols, e.g. paracetamol, which is used as an analgesic only and not as an anti-inflammatory drug. It is effective for pain, especially headaches, and fever. This is probably due to its mechanism of action in trapping free radicals and interfering with the production of hydroperoxidases, which are believed to have an essential role in cyclooxygenase activity. In areas of inflammation, phagocytic cells produce high levels of peroxide that swamp this effect.

Paracetamol causes a serious, potentially fatal, hepatotoxicity in toxic doses (2–3 times therapeutic) that saturate the normal liver conjugation systems, leading to the formation of a toxic metabolite, N-acetyl-p-benzoquinone (Ch. 1).

COX-2 specific inhibitors, e.g. rofecoxib and celecoxib, which preferentially inhibit the inducible COX-2 enzyme, limiting COX-1-mediated side effects observed with other, non-specific NSAIDs.

The COX-2 inhibitors are licensed in the United Kingdom for symptomatic relief in osteoarthritis and rheumatoid arthritis, but they are contraindicated in inflammatory bowel disease.

Steroidal anti-inflammatory drugs (glucocorticoids)

Glucocorticoids possess powerful anti-inflammatory actions that make them useful in several diseases, e.g. rheumatoid arthritis, inflammatory bowel conditions, bronchial asthma, and inflammatory conditions of the skin.

Their profound generalized inhibitory effects on inflammatory responses result from the effects of corticosteroids in altering the activity of certain corticosteroid-responsive genes. The anti-inflammatory action results from:

- Reduced production of acute inflammatory mediators, especially the eicosanoids (see Fig. 4.1). Corticosteroids prevent the formation of arachidonic acid from membrane phospholipids by inducing the synthesis of a polypeptide called lipocortin. Lipocortin inhibits phospholipase A_2, the enzyme normally responsible for mobilizing arachidonic acid from cell membrane phospholipids, and thus inhibits the subsequent formation of both prostaglandins and leukotrienes.
- Reduced numbers and activity of circulating immunocompetent cells, neutrophils, and macrophages.
- Decreased activity of macrophages and fibroblasts involved in the chronic stages of inflammation, leading to decreased inflammation and decreased healing.

Glucocorticoids are discussed in detail in Chapter 11.

Disease-modifying antirheumatic drugs

DMARDs are a diverse group of agents that are mainly used in the treatment of rheumatoid arthritis, which is a chronic, progressive, and destructive inflammatory disease of the joints (Fig. 4.6).

The mechanism of action of the DMARDs is often unclear—they appear to have a long-term depressive effect upon the inflammatory response as well as possibly modulating other aspects of the immune system.

All DMARDs have a slow onset of action, with clinical improvement not becoming apparent until 4–6 months after the initiation of treatment. DMARDs have been shown to improve symptoms and reduce disease activity. Whether they alter the long-term outcome of the disease is controversial.

DMARDs are generally indicated for use in severe, active, progressive rheumatoid arthritis when NSAIDs alone have proved inadequate. DMARDs are frequently used in combination with an NSAID and/or low dose glucocorticoids.

Gold salts

Examples of gold salts include sodium aurothiomalate and auranofin.

Mechanism of action: The mechanism of action of gold salts is unknown—they may be taken up by, and inhibit, mononuclear macrophages, or they may affect the production of free radicals.

Route of administration: Sodium aurothiomalate is given by intramuscular injection, and auranofin orally.

Adverse effects: Rashes, proteinuria, ulceration, diarrhoea, and bone marrow suppression.

Therapeutic notes: When administering gold salts, careful patient monitoring, including blood counts and urine analysis, is necessary. If any serious adverse effects develop, treatment must be stopped.

Disease-modifying anti-rheumatic drugs (DMARDs)	
Class	**Example**
Gold salts	Sodium aurothiomalate, auranofin
Penicillamine	Penicillamine
Antimalarials	Chloroquine, hydroxyquinine
Sulfasalazine	Sulfasalazine
Immunosuppressants	Cytotoxic drugs: methotrexate, azathioprine, ciclosporin

Fig. 4.6 Disease-modifying antirheumatic drugs.

Penicillamine

Mechanism of action: The mechanism of action of penicillamine is unknown. It chelates metals, and it has immunomodulatory effects, including suppression of immunoglobulin production and effects on immune complexes. Penicillamine may also decrease interleukin 1 (IL-1) synthesis.

Route of administration: Oral.

Adverse effects: Rashes, proteinuria, ulceration, gastrointestinal upsets, fever, transient loss of taste, and bone marrow suppression.

Therapeutic notes: When administering penicillamine, careful patient monitoring, including blood counts and urine analysis, is necessary. If any serious adverse effects develop, treatment must be stopped.

Antimalarials

Examples of antimalarials include chloroquine and hydroxychloroquine (Ch. 3).

Mechanism of action: The mechanism of antimalarials is unclear. They interfere with a wide variety of leucocyte functions, including IL-1 production by macrophages, lymphoproliferative responses, and T cell cytotoxic responses.

Route of administration: Oral.

Adverse effects: At the low doses currently recommended for antimalarials, toxicity is rare. The major adverse effect is retinal toxicity.

Therapeutic notes: People on antimalarials should have their vision monitored.

Sulfasalazine

Mechanism of action: Sulfasalazine is broken down in the gut into its two component molecules, 5-aminosalicylate (5-ASA) and sulfapyridine. The 5-ASA moiety is believed to be a free radical scavenger and responsible for most of this drugs antirheumatic effects.

Route of administration: Oral.

Adverse effects: Side effects of sulfasalazine are mainly due to sulfapyridine; they are common, but rarely serious. These include nausea, vomiting, headache, and rashes. Rarely, blood disorders and oligospermia are reported.

Therapeutic notes: People on sulfasalazine should have their blood counts monitored.

Immunosuppressants

Certain drugs with immunosuppressive actions have been shown to be effective in rheumatoid arthritis. These include azathioprine, ciclosporin (cyclosporin A), and corticosteroids, which may work by suppressing the autoimmune component of rheumatoid arthritis (p. 67).

 The DMARDs are usually prescribed by a specialist. Their mechanisms of action are largely unknown, but remember most patients taking these agents require regular blood tests to assess their renal and liver function, and to monitor their red and white blood cell counts.

Drugs used in gout

Gout is a condition in which uric acid (monosodium urate) crystals are deposited in tissues, especially in the joints, provoking an inflammatory response that manifests as an extremely painful acute arthritis. Uric acid crystallizes in the tissues when plasma urate levels are high, as a result of either excessive production or reduced renal excretion.

There are two treatment strategies for gout—treatment of an acute attack and prophylaxis against further attacks (Fig. 4.7).

Treatment of an acute attack
Non-steroidal anti-inflammatory drugs

At the onset of an acute attack of gout, NSAIDs are used for their general anti-inflammatory and analgesic effects (p. 55).

Aspirin and other salicylates are not used in gout as they inhibit uric acid excretion in the urine, exacerbating serum concentrations.

Drugs used in the treatment of gout	
• **Treatment of an acute attack**	**Example**
NSAIDs	Indometacin
Immunosuppressive	Colchicine
• **Prophylaxis against recurrent attacks** (reduction of plasma uric acid concentration)	
Agents that reduce uric acid synthesis	Allopurinol
Agents that increase uric acid excretion (uricosurics)	Sulfinpyrazone, probenecid

Fig. 4.7 Drugs used in the treatment of gout.

Colchicine

Mechanism of action: Colchicine helps in gouty arthritis by inhibiting the migration of leucocytes such as neutrophils into the inflamed joint. This effect is achieved as a result of the action of colchicine binding to tubulin, the protein monomer of microtubules, resulting in their depolymerization. The end result is that cytoskeletal movements and cell motility are severely inhibited.

The inhibition of microtubular function inhibits mitotic spindle formation, giving colchicine a cytotoxic effect on dividing cells. This cytotoxic effect is responsible for side effects of colchicine.

Route of administration: Oral, rarely intravenously.

Adverse effects: Side effects of colchicine include gastrointestinal toxicity, with nausea, vomiting, and diarrhoea, occurring in 80% of people. Rarely, bone marrow suppression and renal failure occur.

Therapeutic notes: Colchicine is rapidly effective. It is given for the first 24 hours of an attack and then no further for 7 days. Nausea and vomiting are extremely common side effects.

Prophylaxis against recurrent attacks

Preventative management of gout includes diet and lifestyle changes, as well as the use of drugs that reduce plasma uric acid concentration. These drugs should not be used during an acute attack, as they will initially worsen symptoms. NSAIDs or colchicine should be co-administered for the first 3 months of treatment, as initiation of prophylactic treatment may precipitate an acute attack.

Agents that reduce uric acid synthesis

Allopurinol is an example of a drug that reduces uric acid synthesis.

Mechanism of action: Allopurinol inhibits the enzyme xanthine oxidase, which converts purines (from DNA breakdown) into uric acid, thus reducing uric acid production.

Route of administration: Oral.

Adverse effects: Headaches, dyspepsia, diarrhoea, rash, drug interactions, and acute exacerbation of gout initially. Rarely, life-threatening hypersensitivity occurs.

Agents that increase uric acid excretion

Uricosurics are drugs that increase uric acid excretion. Examples of uricosurics include sulfinpyrazone and probenecid.

Mechanism of action: Uricosurics compete with uric acid for reabsorption in the proximal tubules, preventing uric acid reabsorption and resulting in uricosuria.

Route of administration: Oral.

Adverse effects: Gastrointestinal upset, deposition of uric acid crystals in the kidney, interference with excretion of certain drugs, and acute exacerbation of gout initially.

Therapeutic notes: Uricosurics should not be used during an acute attack of gout. NSAIDs or colchicine should be co-administered for the first 3 months of treatment, as initiation of treatment may precipitate an acute attack.

Pain

Pain is a common everyday experience that performs an essential defensive function. However, uncontrolled pain can severely diminish quality of life, and it may then be amenable to pharmacotherapy.

Pain, which may be acute or chronic, is defined as an unpleasant sensory and emotional experience associated with actual or potential tissue damage. Pain is a subjective experience, as there are currently no means of accurately and objectively assessing the degree of pain a patient is experiencing.

An analgesic drug is one that effectively removes (or at least lessens) the sensation of pain.

Pain perception

Pain perception is best viewed as a three-stage process—activation of nociceptors, followed by the transmission, and onward passage, of pain information.

Activation of nociceptors in the peripheral tissues

Noxious thermal, chemical, or mechanical stimuli can trigger the firing of primary afferent fibres (type C / Aδ), through the activation of nociceptors (pain-specific receptors) in the peripheral tissues (Fig. 4.8).

Transmission of pain information

Transmission of pain information from the periphery to the dorsal horn of the spinal cord is inhibited or amplified by a combination of local (spinal) neuronal circuits and descending tracts from higher brain centres. This constitutes the 'gate-control mechanism'.

In the gate-control mechanism:
- The primary afferent fibres synapse in lamina I and II of the dorsal horn of the spinal cord.

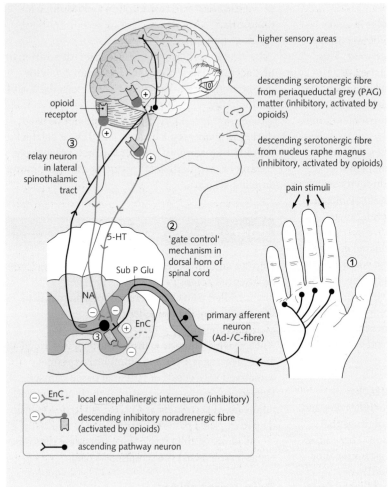

Fig. 4.8 Diagram showing nociceptive pathways and sites of opioid action. 1. Activation of nociceptors in the peripheral tissues; 2. Transmission of pain information; 3. Onward passage of pain information to higher centres. (Glu, glutamate; 5-HT, 5-hydroxytryptamine (serotonin); NA, noradrenaline; Sub P, substance P.).

- Transmitter peptides (substance P, calcitonin gene-related peptide, bradykinin, glutamate) and nitric oxide (NO) are involved in the ascending pain pathways, though the interactions are complex and have not yet been fully defined.
- The activity of the dorsal horn relay neurons is modulated by several inhibitory inputs. These include: local inhibitory interneurons, which release opioid peptides; descending inhibitory noradrenergic fibres from the locus ceruleus area of the brainstem, which are activated by opioid peptides; and descending inhibitory serotonergic fibres from the nucleus raphe magnus and periaqueductal grey areas of the brainstem, which are also activated by opioid peptides (Fig. 4.8).

Onward passage of pain information

The onward passage of pain information is via the spinothalamic tract, to the higher centres of the brain. The higher centres of the brain coordinate the cognitive and emotional aspects of pain and control appropriate reactions. Opioid peptide release in both the spinal cord and the brainstem can reduce the activity of the dorsal horn relay neurons and cause analgesia, known as 'shutting the gate' (Fig. 4.8).

Opioid receptors

All opioids, whether endogenous peptides, naturally occurring drugs, or chemically synthesized drugs, interact with specific opioid receptors to produce their pharmacological effects.

Drugs interact with opioid receptors as either full agonists, partial agonists, mixed agonists (full agonists on one opioid receptor, but partial agonists on another), or as antagonists. Opioid analgesics are agonists.

There are three major opioid receptor subtypes—μ, δ, and κ. The existence of a fourth receptor (σ) remains controversial.

The distinctions between the actions associated with μ- and δ-receptors are relatively unclear, because selective agonists and antagonists have only recently been discovered. However:

- μ-receptors are thought to be responsible for most of the analgesic effects of opioids and for some major adverse effects, e.g. respiratory depression. Most of the analgesic opioids in use are μ-receptor agonists.
- δ-receptors are probably more important in the periphery, but they may also contribute to analgesia.
- κ-receptors contribute to analgesia at the spinal level, and may elicit sedation and dysphoria, but they produce relatively few adverse effects, and do not contribute to physical dependence.
- σ-receptors are not selective opioid receptors, but they are the site of action of psychomimetic drugs, such as PCP. They may account for the dysphoria produced by some opioids.

Opioid receptor activation has an inhibitory effect on synapses in the CNS and in the gut (Fig. 4.9).

Secondary-messenger systems associated with opioid receptor activity include:

- μ / δ-receptors, the activation of which causes hyperpolarization of a neuron by opening potassium channels and inhibiting calcium channels.
- k-receptors, the activation of which inhibits calcium channels.

Activation of all opioid receptors causes a decrease in cAMP production, the functional significance of which is not clear.

Endogenous opioids

Physiologically, the CNS has its own 'endogenous opioids' that are the natural ligands for opioid receptors.

There are three main families of endogenous opioid peptides occurring naturally in the CNS:

- Endorphins.
- Dynorphins.
- Enkephalins.

They are derived from three separate gene products (precursor molecules), but all possess homology at their amino end.

The expression and anatomical distribution of the products of these three precursor molecules within the CNS is varied, and each has a distinct range of affinities for the different types of opioid receptor (Fig. 4.10).

Though it is known that the endogenous opioids possess analgesic activity, their precise function in the CNS and elsewhere is poorly defined. They are not used therapeutically.

Opioid analgesic drugs

Opioid analgesics are drugs, either naturally occurring (e.g. morphine) or chemically synthesized,

When treating pain, remember the analgesic ladder. Start with non-opioid drugs such as paracetamol or other NSAIDs; if these are ineffective move up a step to weak opioid drugs such as codeine with paracetamol. If these agents are not controlling the pain, then move up the final step to the strong opioid drugs such as morphine and diamorphine.

Fig. 4.9 Actions mediated by opioid receptor subtypes. (GIT, gastrointestinal tract.)

Receptor subtypes			
Action	μ/δ	κ	σ
Analgesia	Supraspinal and spinal	Spinal	—
Respiratory depression	Marked	Slight	—
Pupil	Constricts	—	Dilates
GIT mobility	Reduced (constipating)	—	—
Mood/effect	Euphoria inducing but also sedating	Dysphoria inducing mildly sedating	Marked dysphoric and psychomimetic actions
Physical dependence	+++	+	—

Endogenous opioid peptides		
Precursor molecules	Products	Relative opioid receptor affinity
Pro-opiomelanocortin (POMC)	Endorphins e.g. β-endorphin and other non-opioid peptides e.g. ACTH	μ
Proenkephalin	Enkephalins e.g. Leu^5 enkephalin, Met^5 enkephalin, extended Met^5 enkephalins	δ μ μ
Prodynorphin	Dynorphins e.g. dynorphin A	κ

Fig. 4.10 Endogenous opioid peptides.

that interact with specific opioid receptors to produce the pharmacological effect of analgesia.

The first opioid drug was opium, the crude exudate of the seed head of the opium poppy *Papaver somniferum*; simple extraction yields morphine. Subsequently, many synthetic and semi-synthetic opioids have been created by pharmacologists.

Examples of opioid analgesics are given in Fig. 4.11.
Mechanism of action: Opioid analgesic drugs work by agonist action at opioid receptors (see above).

Note that the sense of euphoria produced by strong opioids undoubtedly contributes to their analgesic activity by helping to reduce the anxiety and stress associated with pain. This effect also accounts for the illicit use of these drugs.
Route of administration: Oral, rectal, intravenous, or intramuscular.

Oral absorption is irregular and incomplete, necessitating larger doses; 70% is removed by first-pass hepatic metabolism.
Indications: Strong opioids are used in moderate to severe pain, particularly visceral, postoperative, or cancer-related; in myocardial infarction and acute pulmonary oedema; and in perioperative analgesia (p. 111).

Weak opioids are used in the relief of 'mild to moderate' pain, as antitussives (Ch. 8), and as antidiarrhoeal agents (Ch. 10), taking advantage of these 'side effects' of opioid analgesics.
Contraindications: Opioid analgesics should not be given to people in acute respiratory depression, with acute alcoholism, at risk of paralytic ileus, and with

head injuries prior to neurological assessment (interferes with assessment of the level of consciousness).
Adverse effects: Opioid analgesics share many side effects, though qualitative and quantitative differences exist. These can be subdivided into central adverse actions and peripheral adverse actions.

Central adverse actions include the following:
- Drowsiness and sedation, in which initial excitement is followed by sedation and finally coma (on overdose).
- Reduction in sensitivity of the respiratory centre to CO_2, leading to shallow and slow respiration.
- Tolerance and dependence (Ch. 6).
- Suppression of cough, an effect exploited clinically in antitussives (Ch. 8).
- Vomiting due to stimulation of the chemoreceptor trigger zone (CTZ).
- Pupillary constriction due to stimulation of the parasympathetic third cranial nerve nucleus.
- Hypotension and reduced cardiac output, which are partly due to reduced hypothalamic sympathetic outflow.

Peripheral adverse actions include the following:
- Constipation, which is partly due to stimulation of cholinergic activity in gut wall ganglia that results in smooth wall spasm.
- Contraction of smooth muscle in the sphincter of Oddi and in the ureters, which results in an increase in blood amylase and lipase due to pancreatic stasis.
- Histamine release, which produces bronchospasm, flushing, and arteriolar dilatation.
- Lowered sympathetic discharge and direct arteriolar dilatation, which results in lowered cardiac output and hypotension.

Adverse effects of opioids tend to limit the dose that can be given, and the level of analgesia that can be

Opioid analgesics	
Weak opioid analgesics	Strong opioid analgesics
Pentazocine Codeine Dihydrocodeine Dextropropoxyphene	Morphine Diamorphine Phenazocine Pethidine Buprenorphine Nalbuphine

Fig. 4.11 Opioid analgesics.

maintained. The most serious of all these effects is respiratory depression, which is the most common cause of death from opioid overdose.

Constipation and nausea are also common problems and clinically it is common to co-administer laxatives and an antiemetic (Ch. 10). Tolerance and dependence: Tolerance to opioid analgesics can be detected within 24–48 hours from the onset of administration, and it results in larger and larger doses of the drug being needed to achieve the same clinical effect.

Dependence involves μ-receptors and is both physical and psychological in nature and is discussed in Chapter 6.

If physical dependence develops, it is characterized by a definite withdrawal syndrome following cessation of drug treatment. This syndrome comprises a complex mixture of irritable, and sometimes aggressive, behaviour combined with extremely unpleasant autonomic symptoms such as fever, sweating, yawning, and pupillary dilatation. The withdrawal syndrome is relieved by the administration of μ-receptor agonists, and worsened by the administration of μ-receptor antagonists.

Psychological dependence of opioid analgesics is based on the positive reinforcement provided by euphoria.

In the clinical context, especially in terminal care, where tolerance and dependence can be monitored, they are not inevitably problematic. However, the fear of tolerance and dependence often leads to over-caution in the use of opioid analgesics, and inadequate pain control in some patients. It is not uncommon for palliative care patients to take over 1000 mg of morphine sulphate twice daily and remain alert and active.

Therapeutic notes: Strong opioid analgesics include morphine, diamorphine (heroin), phenazocine, pethidine, buprenorphine, and nalbuphine:

- Morphine remains the most valuable drug for severe pain relief, though it frequently causes nausea and vomiting. It is the drug of choice for severe pain in terminal care. Morphine is the standard against which other opioid analgesics are compared.
- Diamorphine (heroin) is twice as potent as morphine, owing to its greater penetration of the blood–brain barrier. It is metabolized to 6-acetylmorphine and thence morphine in the body. Diamorphine causes less nausea and hypotension than morphine, but more euphoria.
- Phenazocine has a more prolonged action than morphine, and it can be administered sublingually.

It can be useful in biliary colic as it has less of a tendency to increase biliary spasm than other opioids.
- Pethidine is more lipid soluble than morphine, and it has a rapid onset and short duration of action, making it useful in labour. Pethidine is equianalgesic compared with morphine, but it produces less constipation. Interaction with MAOIs is serious, causing fever, delirium, and convulsions or respiratory depression.
- Buprenorphine has both agonist and antagonist actions at opioid receptors, and it may precipitate withdrawal symptoms in patients dependent on other opioids. It has a longer duration of action than morphine and its lipid solubility allows sublingual administration. Vomiting may be a problem. Unlike most opioid analgesics, the effects of buprenorphine are only partially antagonized by naloxone owing to its high-affinity attraction to opioid receptors.
- Nalbuphine is an agonist at κ-receptors and an antagonist at μ-receptors. It is equianalgesic compared with morphine, but it produces less nausea and vomiting. High doses cause dysphoria.

Weak opioid analgesics include pentazocine, codeine, dihydrocodeine, and dextropropoxyphene:
- Pentazocine has both κ / σ-receptor agonist and μ-antagonist actions, and it may precipitate withdrawal symptoms in patients dependent on other opioids. Pentazocine is weak orally, but, by injection, it has a potency between that of morphine and codeine. It is not recommended because of the side effects of thought disturbances and hallucinations, which probably are due to its action on σ-receptors.
- Codeine has about one twelfth of the analgesic potency of morphine. The incidence of nausea and constipation limit the dose and duration that can be used. Codeine is also used for its antitussive and antidiarrhoeal effects.
- Dihydrocodeine has an analgesic efficacy similar to that of codeine. It may cause dizziness and constipation.
- Dextropropoxyphene has an analgesic efficacy about half that of codeine (i.e. very mild), and so it is often combined with aspirin or paracetamol. Such mixtures can be dangerous in overdose, with dextropropoxyphene causing respiratory depression and acute heart failure, while the paracetamol is hepatotoxic.

Opioid antagonists

Examples of opioid antagonists include naloxone and naltrexone.

Mechanism of action: These drugs act by specific antagonism at opioid receptors: μ-, δ-, and κ-receptors are blocked more or less equally. They block the actions of endogenous opioids as well as of morphine-like drugs.

Naloxone is short acting (half-life: 2–4 hours) while naltrexone is long acting (half-life: 10 hours).

Route of administration: Intravenous.

Indications: Opioid antagonists are given to reverse opioid-induced analgesia and respiratory depression rapidly, mainly after overdose, or to improve breathing in newborn babies that have been affected by the opioids given to their mother.

Adverse effects: Precipitation of withdrawal in those with physical dependence on opioids. Reversal of analgesic effects of opiate agonist.

Headache and neuralgic pain
Headache

Headache is a very common presenting symptom, yet one which can be difficult to manage. The most common causes of headache include:

- Tension-type headache.
- Migraine.
- Headache associated with eye or sinus disease.

More sinister causes of headache (including meningitis and neoplasia) are less common, and these can often be confidently excluded by the history and by examination.

The pathophysiology underlying headache is unclear, though symptomatic relief is often obtained from NSAIDs and paracetamol (see above). Some headaches are related to stress and anxiety, and these patents may benefit from antidepressant drugs (Ch. 6).

The management of migraine can address the acute attacks, or attempt to prevent migrainous episodes (prophylaxis) in those who experience frequent attacks.

Drugs used for acute migrainous attacks:
- NSAIDs and paracetamol (see above).
- Antiemetics (Ch. 10).
- Serotonin (5-HT$_1$) agonists.

Drugs used in migraine prophylaxis:
- Antihistamine/serotonin (5-HT) antagonists.
- Beta-antagonists (Ch. 7).
- Tricyclic antidepressants (Ch. 6).

Serotonin (5-HT$_1$) agonists

Sumatriptan and rizatriptan are serotonin agonists.

Mechanism of action: Serotonin agonists are believed to reverse the dilatation of cerebral blood vessels in the acute attack, which may be responsible for some of the symptoms of migraine.

Route of administration: Oral, intranasal, subcutaneous.

Indications: Acute migrainous attacks.

Contraindications: Caution in coronary artery disease (may cause vasoconstriction or coronary vessels), hepatic impairment, pregnancy, and breastfeeding.

Adverse effects: Sensations of tingling, heat, chest tightness.

Antihistamine/serotonin antagonists

Pizotifen is the main drug in this class.

Mechanism of action: Unlike the serotonin agonists, pizotifen appears to limit the initial pro-inflammatory and vascular changes which precede migrainous episodes.

Route of administration: Oral.

Indications: Prevention of vascular headache.

Contraindications: Cautions in urinary retention, angle-closure glaucoma, renal impairment, pregnancy, and breastfeeding.

Adverse effects: Antimuscarinic effects, drowsiness, increased appetite.

 Headache is a common complaint and, more often than not, it does not represent a sinister pathology. Analgesics will simply help to control the symptoms so, if a patient frequently returns with pain, be sure to look for a treatable underlying cause.

Neuralgic pain

Neuralgic pain is classically nerve pain, in the distribution of a particular nerve or nerve root. The more common pathologies, which come into this category, include sciatica and trigeminal neuralgia.

Neuralgia commonly occurs because of compression or entrapment of the nerve or nerve root, and definitive management relies on surgical release of the nerve.

Pharmacological options can be employed when surgery is ill advised, or ineffective, or as an adjunct. NSAIDs are not particularly effective for neuralgic pain, and they have usually been self-prescribed prior to the patient consulting a professional opinion.

Antidepressants, in particular amitriptyline, often have an 'analgesic' effect in neuralgic pain, and often at a dose lower than their antidepressant effect (Ch. 6).

The other main class of drug used orally in neuralgic pain are the antiepileptics, notably carbamazepine, phenytoin, and more recently lamotrigine (Ch. 6). These potentially stabilize the neurons involved, and limit their activation.

Injection of the nerve in question with local anaesthetic can provide relief for some patients (Ch. 5), though nerve ablation with drugs or by surgical means can be performed to alleviate symptoms.

Immunosuppression

Introduction
Deliberate pharmacological suppression of the immune system is used in the following three main clinical areas:

- To suppress inappropriate autoimmune responses (e.g. systemic lupus erythematosus or rheumatoid arthritis), where the host immune system is 'attacking' host tissue.
- To suppress host immune rejection to donor organ grafts or transplants.
- To suppress donor immune responses against host antigens (prevention of graft-versus-host disease (GVHD) after bone marrow transplant).

The main pharmacological agents used for immunosuppression are:

- Ciclosporin (cyclosporin A).
- Azathioprine.
- Glucocorticoids (Ch. 11).

Immunosuppressant drugs
Ciclosporin (cyclosporin A)
Mechanism of action: Ciclosporin is a cyclic peptide, derived from fungi, that has powerful immunosuppressive activity. It has a selective inhibitory effect on T cells by inhibiting the T cell receptor (TCR)-mediated signal-transduction pathway. It is believed to exert its actions after entering the T cell and preventing the transcription of specific genes (Fig. 4.12).

After entry into the T cell, ciclosporin specifically binds to its cytoplasmic binding protein, cyclophilin. This ciclosporin–cyclophilin complex then binds to a serine/threonine phosphatase called calcineurin, inhibiting its phosphatase activity. Calcineurin is normally activated when intracellular calcium ion levels rise following T cell receptor binding to the appropriate major histocompatibility complex:antigen complex. When calcineurin is active it dephosphorylates the cytoplasmic component of the nuclear factor of activated T cells (NF-ATc) into a form that migrates to the nucleus and induces transcription of genes, such as that for IL-2, that are involved in T cell activation.

Inhibition of calcineurin by the ciclosporin–cyclophilin complex, therefore, prevents the nuclear translocation of NF-ATc and the transcription of certain genes essential for the activation of T cells. Hence the production of IL-2 by T helper cells, the maturation of cytotoxic T cells, and the production of some other lymphokines, such as interferon-γ, are all inhibited.

The overall action of ciclosporin is to suppress reversibly both cell-mediated and antibody-specific adaptive immune responses.

Indications: Ciclosporin is used for the prevention of graft and transplant rejection, and prevention of GVHD.

Route of administration: Oral, intravenous.

Adverse effects: Unlike most immunosuppressive agents, ciclosporin does not cause myelosuppression. It is markedly nephrotoxic to the proximal tubule of the kidney, and renal damage almost always occurs. This may be reversible or permanent. Hypertension occurs in 50% of people.

Less serious side effects include mild hepatotoxicity, anorexia, lethargy, gastrointestinal upsets, hirsutism, and gum hypertrophy.

Therapeutic notes: Ciclosporin is often used as part of a post-transplantation 'triple therapy' regime with oral corticosteroids and azathioprine.

Azathioprine
Mechanism of action: Azathioprine is a prodrug that is converted into the active component 6-mercaptopurine in the liver. Mercaptopurine is a fraudulent purine nucleotide that impairs DNA synthesis, and it has a cytotoxic action on dividing cells.

Indications: Azathioprine is used for the prevention of graft and transplant rejection, and autoimmune conditions when corticosteroid therapy alone is inadequate.

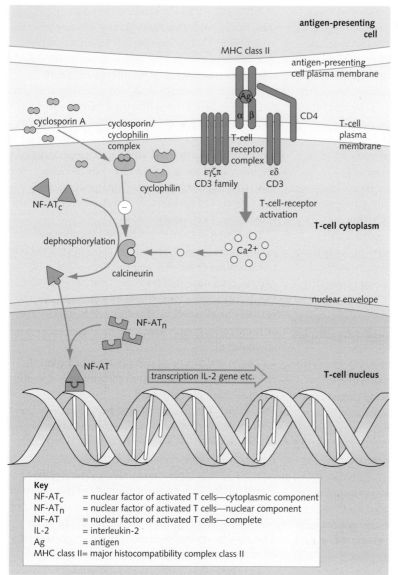

Fig. 4.12 Ciclosporin and T cell suppression.

Route of administration: Oral, intravenously.

Adverse effects: Side effects of azathioprine include bone marrow suppression, which can lead to leucopenia, thrombocytopenia, and sometimes anaemia. This is often the dose-limiting side effect.

Increased susceptibility to infections (often opportunistic pathogens), and to certain cancers (lymphomas) can occur. Common side effects include gastrointestinal disturbances, nausea, vomiting, and diarrhoea. Loss of hair (alopecia) may be partial or complete, but this is usually reversible.

Drug interaction with allopurinol necessitates lowering the dose of azathioprine.

Therapeutic notes: Azathioprine is used as part of a post-transplantation 'triple therapy' regime with oral corticosteroids.

Immunosuppressant drugs are toxic agents, with adverse effects common, serious, and frequently dose limiting. Knowledge of these adverse effects and why they occur is, therefore, important.

Glucocorticoids

The use of glucocorticoids as immunosuppressant agents involves both their anti-inflammatory actions and their effects on the immune system (Ch. 11).

- What are the cardinal clinical features of inflammation?
- How do these arise physiologically?
- What are the principle chemical mediators of the acute inflammatory response?
- Outline the conversion of arachidonic acid to its pro-inflammatory metabolites.
- How do non-steroidal anti-inflammatory drugs act? Name some examples of these drugs.
- Why are cyclooxygenase 2 inhibitors believed to be superior to non-specific inhibitors of cyclooxygenase?
- What are the common adverse effects and contraindications to non-steroidal anti-inflammatory drugs?
- How do steroids act as anti-inflammatory agents?
- Classify the drugs used in the treatment of rheumatoid arthritis. List their adverse effects.
- Why might the immunosuppressant drugs have a role to play in the management of rheumatoid arthritis?
- What is the underlying cause of gout? Which joints does it classically involve?
- List the drugs used in the treatment of acute and chronic gout.
- What is pain, and what is the definition of an analgesic?
- How do opioid analgesic drugs act? What are their principal adverse effects?
- How can these adverse effects be minimized?
- Name an opiate antagonist, and list indications for its use.
- What are the main treatment options for headache?
- What important clinical diagnoses should be excluded in the patient with headache, and what are the likely differential diagnoses?
- What drugs are used to treat neuralgic pain? How might these act?
- What are the indications for immunosuppressant drugs, and how do they act? Gives examples of such agents.

5. Peripheral Nervous System

Nerve conduction

Conduction of impulses through nerves occurs as an all-or-none event called the action potential. The action potential is caused by voltage-dependent opening of sodium and potassium channels in the cell membrane.

The sodium equilibrium potential (Eq Na$^+$) is +60 mV and the potassium equilibrium potential (Eq K$^+$) is –90 mV. Since a resting nerve has 50–75 more potassium channels open than sodium channels, the resting membrane potential is –70 mV.

Fig. 5.1 shows the concentrations of sodium and potassium inside and outside a resting nerve. The Na$^+$/K$^+$ pump (Na$^+$/K$^+$ ATPase) is an energy-dependent pump that functions to maintain the concentration gradient of these two ionic species across the membrane. Three sodium ions are pumped out of the cell for every two potassium ions pumped in, and thus the excitability of the cell is retained.

Figs 5.2 and 5.3 summarize the events that occur during a nerve action potential. During a nerve action potential:

Fig. 5.1 Intracellular and extracellular sodium and potassium concentrations. The Na$^+$/K$^+$ ATPase pump maintains these concentration gradients across the cell membrane.

Fig. 5.2 Nerve action potential. For explanation of points 1–6, see Fig. 5.3.

Fig. 5.3 State of sodium and potassium channels and membrane potential at different stages of the neuronal action potential.

	Sodium channels	Potassium channels	Membrane potential
	State of sodium and potassium channels and membrane potential at different stages of the nerve action potential		
1	Closed resting	Closed resting	Resting (–70 mV)
2	Open	Closed resting	Depolarization (action potential upstroke)
3	More channels open	Closed resting	More depolarization
4	Channels close (inactive)	Special set of channels start opening	Peak of action potential reached
5	All inactivated	More channels open	Re-polarization
6	Closed resting	Channels close	Resting membrane potential re-established

- The rate of sodium entry into the nerve axon becomes greater than the rate of potassium out of the axon, at which point the membrane becomes depolarized (the loss of a electrical gradient across the membrane).
- Depolarization sets off a sodium-positive feedback whereby more voltage-gated sodium channels open and the membrane becomes more depolarized.
- A threshold, which is usually 15 mV greater than the resting membrane potential, must be reached if an action potential is to be generated.
- The membrane repolarizes when the sodium channels become inactivated; a special set of potassium channels open and potassium leaves the axon.
- The sodium channels eventually regain their resting excitable state and the Na^+/K^+ ATPase restores the membrane potential back to -70 mV.

Fig. 5.4 shows the voltage-operated sodium channels in their inactivated, activated, and resting states. Two types of gate exist within the channel, the m-gates and the h-gates. These gates are open or closed according to the state of the channel.

Sodium channel

The voltage-operated sodium channel is present in all excitable tissues. It is a transmembrane protein made up of four domains, each with six transmembrane regions. It is sensitive to membrane potential and selectively passes sodium ions.

Local anaesthetics block the sodium channel, and thus nerve conduction, by binding to the sixth transmembrane region of the fourth domain.

Size of the nerve fibre

Small nerve fibres are preferentially blocked because of their high surface-area to volume ratio. This results in a differential block whereby the small nociceptive (pain) and autonomic fibres are blocked but not the larger fibres responsible for the mediation of movement and touch.

Local anaesthetics
History

Local anaesthetics are drugs used to inhibit pain sensation. These drugs work by reversibly blocking nerve conduction.

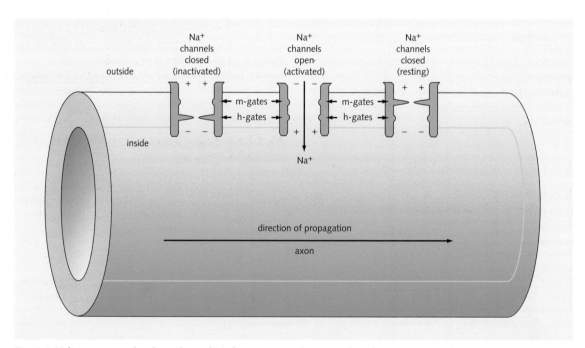

Fig. 5.4 Voltage-operated sodium channels in their inactivated, activated, and resting states. The m-gates and h-gates open or close according to the state of the channel. In the resting sodium channel, the m-gates are held closed by the strongly negative (-70 mV) electrical gradient across the membrane. Once an action potential begins to propagate, the loss of the membrane potential causes the m-gates to open, allowing sodium into the cell, further propagating the action potential. After a very short time, a further conformational change causes the h-gates to close, inactivating the sodium channel. The membrane then re-polarizes, and once at -70 mV, the m-gates again close, and the h-gates open so the sodium channel is back in its resting state.

South American Indians have been chewing the leaves of the coca plant, *Erythroxylon coca*, for thousands of years. When they chewed the plant, they found that their mouth and tongue went numb, and that euphoria and excitement were induced. Cocaine was found to be the active ingredient, and it was first isolated from the coca plant in 1860.

Freud was the first to use cocaine clinically to treat patients, but this was unsuccessful. In 1884, however, Koller obtained some cocaine from Freud and was able to demonstrate its local anaesthetic effects upon the cornea.

Procaine was first synthesized in 1905 as a synthetic substitute for cocaine.

Chemistry

All local anaesthetics have the same basic structure:
- An aromatic group (lipophilic end) linked to a basic side chain (hydrophilic end) by an ester or amide bond (Fig. 5.5).
- The basic side chain (usually a secondary or tertiary amine) is important since only the uncharged molecule can enter the nerve axoplasm.

Potency and duration of action are correlated with high lipid solubility.

Pharmacokinetics

Elimination of local anaesthetics is dependent upon the nature of the chemical bond:
- Local anaesthetics with ester bonds are inactivated by plasma cholinesterases.
- Local anaesthetics with amide bonds are degraded by N-dealkylation in the liver.

Metabolites can often be pharmacologically active.

Mechanism of block

Importance of pH and ionization

Local anaesthetics are weak bases ($pK_a = 8$–9). Only the uncharged form can penetrate lipid membranes;

thus, quaternary ammonium compounds, which are fully protonated, must be injected directly into the nerve axon if they are to work.

The proportion of uncharged local anaesthetic is governed by the pH, the pK_a, and the Henderson–Hasselbalch equation (Ch. 1):

$$B + H^+ = BH^+$$

$$pK_a = pH + \log [BH^+]/[B]$$

A local anaesthetic with a pK_a of 8.0 will be 10% uncharged at pH 7.0, 50% uncharged at pH 8.0, and 5% uncharged at pH 6.0.

Routes of block

The majority of local anaesthetics block by two routes (Fig. 5.6):
- By the hydrophobic route, the uncharged form enters the membrane and blocks the channel from a site in the protein membrane interface.
- By the hydrophilic route, the uncharged form crosses the membrane to the inside where the charged form blocks the channel. This pathway depends on the channel being open and, therefore, this type of block is use dependent. Use dependency is especially important in the antiarrhythmic action of local anaesthetics.

Nerve block occurs when the number of non-inactivated channels (those unaffected by the drug) is insufficient to bring about depolarization to threshold.

Routes of administration

Surface anaesthesia

In surface anaesthesia, the local anaesthetic is applied directly to the mucous membranes, e.g. cornea, bronchial tree, oesophagus, and genitourinary tract. The local anaesthetic, e.g. lidocaine (lignocaine),

Fig. 5.5 General structure of ester- and amide-linked local anaesthetics.

Fig. 5.6 Hydrophobic and hydrophilic routes of block for local anaesthetics.

must be able to penetrate the tissues easily. For skin tetracaine (amethocaine) is used to anaesthetize the skin prior to venepuncture, especially in children and anxious adults.

Problems occur when large areas, e.g. the bronchial tree, are anaesthetized.

Infiltration anaesthesia

Infiltration anaesthesia involves direct injection of a local anaesthetic into tissue. Often, a vasoconstrictor such as adrenaline is used with the local anaesthetic to prevent the spread of the local anaesthetic into the systemic circulation. Vasoconstrictors must never be used at extremities as ischaemia could result.

Intravenous regional anaesthesia (IVRA) involves the injection of the local anaesthetic distal to a cuff inflated above arterial pressure. It is important that the cuff is not released prematurely as this could cause the release of a potentially toxic bolus into the circulation. This type of local anaesthetic block is now seldom used.

Nerve block anaesthesia

In nerve block anaesthesia, local anaesthetic is injected close to the appropriate nerve trunk, e.g. the brachial plexus. The injection must be accurate in location.

Spinal and epidural anaesthesia

Spinal anaesthesia involves the injection of a local anaesthetic into the cerebrospinal fluid (CSF) in the subarachnoid space. A certain amount of spread can be controlled by increasing the specific gravity of the solution and tilting the patient.

In epidural anaesthesia, the local anaesthetic is injected into the space between the dura mater and the spinal cord.

In both spinal and epidural anaesthesia, the local anaesthetic acts by blocking mainly spinal roots, as opposed to the spinal cord itself. Problems arise from the block of preganglionic sympathetic fibres supplying the vasculature (causing vasodilatation) and the heart (causing bradycardia), both leading to hypotension. Rostral spread can lead to the blocking of intercostal and phrenic nerves and result in respiratory depression.

Unwanted effects

Unwanted effects of local anaesthetics are mainly associated with the spread of the drug into the systemic circulation. These include:

- Effects on the central nervous system (CNS) such as restlessness, tremor, confusion, and agitation.

At high doses, CNS depression can occur. Procaine is worse than lidocaine (lignocaine) or prilocaine for causing CNS depression, and is seldom used. The exception is cocaine, which, owing to its monoamine-uptake blocking activity, produces euphoria.

- Respiratory depression.
- Possible effects on the cardiovascular system, including myocardial depression and vasodilatation.
- Visual disturbances and twitching. Severe toxicity causes convulsions and coma.

Properties and uses

Fig. 5.7 shows the properties and uses of the main local anaesthetics, and Fig. 5.8 lists other compounds that block sodium channels.

Somatic nervous system

Neuromuscular junction
Physiology of transduction

Skeletal (voluntary) muscle is innervated by motor neurons, the axons of which are able to propagate action potentials at high velocities.

The area of muscle that lies below the axon terminal is known as the motor end-plate, and the chemical synapse between the two is known as the neuromuscular junction (NMJ).

The axon terminal incorporates membrane-bound vesicles containing the neurotransmitter acetylcholine (ACh). Depolarization of the presynaptic terminal of the nerve by an action potential (generated by sodium influx) causes voltage-sensitive calcium channels to open, allowing calcium ions into the terminal. Normally, the level of calcium ions inside the nerves is very low—10 000 times lower than the external concentration. This calcium influx causes the release of ACh by exocytosis from vesicles. ACh diffuses across to the muscle membrane where it binds to the nicotinic acetylcholine receptor (nicAChR) and/or is inactivated by acetylcholinesterase (Fig. 5.9). Several events then occur:

- During association, ACh binds to the nicAChR, which is an ion channel that allows cations into the muscle (mainly sodium but also potassium to a lesser extent).
- During the conformational change, the pore of the ion channel is open for 1 ms, during which approximately 20 000 sodium ions enter the cell.

Properties and uses of the main local anaesthetics

	Rate of onset	Duration	Tissue penetration	Chemistry	Common use
Cocaine	Rapid	Moderate	Rapid	Ester bond	ENT
Procaine	Moderate	Short	Slow	Ester bond	Little used, CNS effects
Tetracaine (amethocaine)	Slow	Long	Moderate	Ester bond	Topical, pre-venepuncture
Oxybuprocaine (benoxinate)	Rapid	Short	Rapid	Ester bond	Surface, ophthalmology
Benzocaine	Very slow	Very long	Rapid	Ester bond, no basic side chain	Surface ENT
Lidocaine (lignocaine)	Rapid	Moderate	Rapid	Amide bond	Widely used in all applications, EMLA
Prilocaine	Moderate	Moderate	Moderate	Amide bond	Many uses, IVRA, EMLA. Low toxicity
Bupivacaine	Slow	Long	Moderate	Amide bond	Epidural and spinal anaesthesia

Fig. 5.7 Properties and uses of the main local anaesthetics. (ENT, ear, nose and throat; IVRA, intravenous regional anaesthetic.)

Fig. 5.8 Naturally occurring and synthetic sodium channel blockers.

Sodium channel blockers

Compound	Source	Type of block
Tetrodotoxin	Puffer fish	Outside only
Saxitoxin	Plankton	Outside only
μ-conotoxins	Piscivorous marine snail	Affects inactivation
μ-agatoxins	Funnel web spider	Affects inactivation
α-, β-, and γ-toxins	Scorpions	Complex
QX314 and QX222	Synthetic, permanently charged local anaesthetics	Inside only (hydrophilic pathway)
Benzocaine	Synthetic, uncharged local anaesthetic	From within the membrane (hydrophobic pathway)
Local anaesthetics	Plant (cocaine), others synthetic	Inside and from within the membrane

The resulting depolarization, called an end-plate potential (EPP), depolarizes the adjacent muscle fibre.

- If the cellular response is large enough, an action potential is generated in the rest of the muscle fibre (sodium influx), resulting in the opening of voltage-operated calcium channels, but this time the calcium influx mediates contraction.

- ACh is rapidly inactivated by an enzyme called acetylcholinesterase (AChE) which hydrolyses ACh into the inactive metabolites choline and acetic acid.
- In the synthesis of ACh, the choline generated is taken up by the nerve terminal where another enzyme, choline acetyl transferase (ChAT), converts it back to ACh to be re-used.

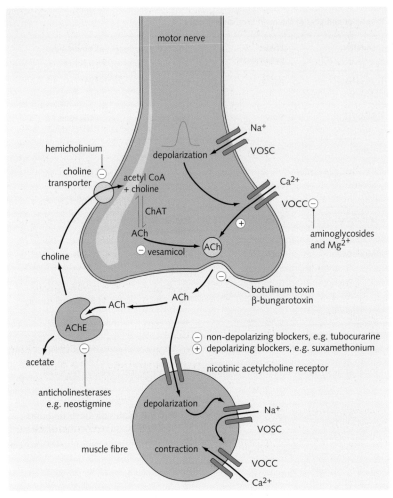

Fig. 5.9 Physiology of impulse transduction at the neuromuscular junction (NMJ) showing the site of action of drugs used in conjunction with the NMJ. (VOSC, voltage-operated sodium channel; VOCC, voltage-operated calcium channel; AChE, acetylcholinesterase; ChAT, choline acetyl transferase; vesamicol, an experimental drug.)

Nicotinic acetylcholine receptor

The nicAChR is made up of five subunits (two α, one β, one γ, and one δ) that traverse the membrane and surround a central pore. The four different subunits show high sequence identity.

ACh must bind to both of the α-subunits in order to open a channel.

Each subunit has four membrane-spanning regions (helices), i.e. each receptor has a total of 20. One of the transmembrane helices (M_2) from each subunit forms the lining of the channel pore.

Pharmacological targets

There are three major targets within the NMJ for clinically useful drugs (Fig. 5.10):

- The presynaptic release.
- The nicotinic acetylcholine receptor.
- Acetylcholinesterase.

Targets for clinically useful drugs at the neuromuscular junction		
Site	**Action**	**Use**
nicAChR	Block transmission	Neuromuscular blockers for surgery
AChE	Enhance transmission	Peripheral neuropathy, e.g. myasthenia gravis
Release	Block transmission	Spasms, e.g. squints, tics, tremors, etc.

Fig. 5.10 Targets for clinically useful drugs at the neuromuscular junction. Myasthenia gravis is an autoimmune disease in which there are decreased numbers of available receptors at the end-plate due to antibody binding. To allow normal neuromuscular function, drugs that increase the amount of acetylcholine in the cleft are given. (AChE, acetylcholine esterase; nicAChR, nicotinic acetylcholine receptor.)

The neuromuscular junction is a very important site for therapeutic manipulation. The electrical impulse from the neuron is converted into a chemical signal that mediates the effect—largely muscular contraction.

Drugs affecting the neuromuscular junction
Presynaptic agents
Drugs inhibiting ACh synthesis: The rate-limiting step in the synthesis of ACh is the uptake of choline into the nerve terminal.

Hemicholinium is an analogue of choline that blocks the choline transporter and causes a depletion of ACh stores. Because of the time taken for the stores to run down, the onset of this drug is slow. This, and the frequency-dependent nature of the block (depletion of stores is related to release of ACh), means that it is not useful clinically. The block is reversed by the addition of choline.

Drugs inhibiting vesicular packaging of ACh: Vesamicol inhibits the active transport of ACh into storage vesicles and results in neuromuscular block.

Drugs inhibiting ACh release: Calcium entry into the nerve terminal is necessary for the release of ACh; thus, agents such as aminoglycoside antibiotics (e.g. streptomycin) that prevent this step will cause neuromuscular blockade. Muscle paralysis is occasionally a side effect of aminoglycoside antibiotics, but it can be reversed by the administration of calcium salts.

Botulinum toxin is a neurotoxin produced by the anaerobic bacillus *Clostridium botulinum*. The toxin is very potent and it is believed to inhibit ACh release by inactivating actin, which is necessary for exocytosis. In botulism, a serious type of food poisoning caused by this toxin, victims experience progressive parasympathetic and motor paralysis. Botulinum toxin type A is sometimes used clinically in the treatment of excessive muscle contraction disorders (dystonias) such as strabismus (squint), spasticity, and tremors.

Beta-bungarotoxin contained in snake venom acts in a similar manner to botulinum toxin.

Postsynaptic agents
Non-depolarizing blockers: These act as competitive antagonists by binding to the nicAChR but not activating it, and producing motor paralysis. Details of the most commonly used non-depolarizing blockers are given in Fig. 5.11.

Approximately 80–90% of receptors must be blocked to prevent transmission, since the amount of

Non-depolarizing blockers of postsynaptic receptors at the neuromuscular junction				
Drug	Approximate duration (mins)	Side effects		Elimination
		Ganglion block	Histamine release	Other	
Tubocurarine	60–120	Partial	Sometimes	Hypersensitivity (rare)	Mainly hepatic
Pancuronium	40–60	X	Minimal	Block of muscarinic receptors in the heart → tachycardia	Mainly renal
Gallamine	15	X	X	Block of muscarinic receptors in the heart → tachycardia	Mainly renal: avoid in patients with renal disease
Alcuronium	20	X	X	Dose dependency	Mainly hepatic
Vecuronium	20–30	X	X		Mainly hepatic
Atracurium	15–30	X	Sometimes		Degradation in plasma at body pH (Hofmann elimination)

Fig. 5.11 Non-depolarizing blockers of postsynaptic receptors at the neuromuscular junction.

ACh released by nerve terminal depolarization usually greatly exceeds that required to generate an action potential in the muscle. The drugs are all quaternary ammonium compounds and, therefore, do not cross the blood–brain barrier or the placenta. They are poorly absorbed orally and they must be administered by intravenous injection. 'Tetanic fade' (i.e. non-maintained muscle tension during brief nerve stimulation) is seen with some of these drugs. This can be explained by the blocking of presynaptic autoreceptors which usually maintain the release of ACh during repeated stimulation.

The block can be reversed by anticholinesterases and depolarizing drugs. It is also enhanced in patients with myasthenia gravis. The main side effect from these drugs is hypotension caused by the blocking of ganglionic transmission. Histamine release from mast cells, resulting in bronchospasm, may be a problem in certain individuals (Fig. 5.11).

Depolarizing (non-competitive) blockers: Depolarizing blockers initially activate receptors, causing depolarization, but in doing so block further activation.

Depolarizing blockers act on the motor end-plate in the same manner as ACh, i.e. they are agonists and increase the cation permeability of the end-plate. However, unlike ACh, which is released in brief spurts and rapidly hydrolysed, depolarizing blockers remain associated with the receptors long enough to cause a sustained depolarization and a resulting loss of electrical excitability (phase I).

Repeated or continuous administration of depolarizing blockers leads to the block becoming more characteristic of non-depolarizing drugs. This is known as phase II and is probably due to receptor desensitization, whereby the end-plate becomes less sensitive to ACh. The block starts to show tetanic fade and it is partly reversed by anticholinesterase drugs.

Suxamethonium is the only depolarizing blocker used clinically because of its rapid onset time and short duration of action (approximately 4 minutes). Suxamethonium is a quaternary ammonium compound, and it must be given by intravenous injection. It is rapidly hydrolysed by plasma cholinesterase, although certain people with a genetic variant of this enzyme may experience a neuromuscular block that may last for hours.

Depolarizing blockers have no effect in patients with myasthenia gravis, since these patients have a decreased number of receptors at the end-plate. In this instance, the blocking potency of depolarizing blockers is reduced.

The side effects of depolarizing blockers include:
- Initial spasms, which occur prior to paralysis, often resulting in postoperative muscle pain.
- Muscarinic receptor activation resulting in bradycardia. Bradycardia can be prevented by the administration of atropine.
- Potassium release from muscle resulting in elevated plasma potassium levels. This is usually a problem only in the case of trauma.

Anticholinesterases

Anticholinesterases inhibit AChE and thus increase the amount of ACh in the synaptic cleft and enhance cholinergic transmission.

Most of the anticholinesterases used are quaternary ammonium compounds and, therefore, they do not penetrate the blood–brain barrier.

Short-acting anticholinesterases include edrophonium. This is selective for the NMJ and clinically relevant in the diagnosis of myasthenia gravis. Edrophonium's duration of action is only 2–10 minutes because it binds by electrostatic forces (no covalent bonds) to the active site of the enzyme. Edrophonium is, therefore, not used therapeutically.

Intermediate-acting anticholinesterases include neostigmine, pyridostigmine, and physostigmine.

Neostigmine is used intravenously to reverse the effects of non-depolarizing blockers. Its duration of action is 2–4 hours, and it is used orally in the treatment of myasthenia gravis. Although neostigmine shows some selectivity for the NMJ, atropine is sometimes co-administered to block the muscarinic effects of the drug.

Pyridostigmine has a duration of action of 3–6 hours, and it is also used orally in the treatment of myasthenia gravis. It has few parasympathetic actions.

Physostigmine shows selectivity for the postganglionic parasympathetic junction. It is a tertiary amine and its use is, therefore, associated with central effects such as initial excitation followed by depression, and possibly respiratory depression and unconsciousness. The central effects can be antagonized by atropine. Physostigmine is used in the form of eye drops to constrict the pupil and contract the ciliary muscle in the treatment of glaucoma.

Most of the long-lasting or irreversible anticholinesterases are organophosphorous compounds. For example, sarin and tabun were developed as nerve gases, and parathion was developed as an insecticide, as well as for clinical use. These drugs have many adverse effects, such as bradycardia, hypotension, breathing problems, depolarizing neuromuscular block, central effects, and possible death from peripheral nerve demyelination. Ecothiopate shows selectivity for the postganglionic parasympathetic junction, and it is used in the treatment of glaucoma.

While myasthenia gravis is a rare disease, its pathophysiology and clinical features are very interesting, and as such it is commonly asked about in exams and vivas.

Autonomic nervous system

Basic concepts

The autonomic nervous system is the means by which all tissues other than skeletal muscle are innervated (Fig. 5.12).

The axons of the autonomic nervous system leave their cell body, which is located in the CNS, as preganglionic fibres, synapse in the appropriate ganglion, and leave as postganglionic fibres. These postganglionic fibres reach the effector cells.

The neurotransmitter released by preganglionic fibres at autonomic ganglia, regardless of whether sympathetic or parasympathetic, is ACh.

The ACh receptors located on postganglionic fibres are of the nicotinic type.

In general, the sympathetic and parasympathetic systems mediate opposite effects (Fig. 5.20).

Autonomic ganglia

Fig. 5.13 summarizes the differences between ganglionic nicAChR and those found on skeletal muscle at the NMJ.

Ganglion-stimulating drugs
Nicotinic agonists

There are few agonists that act selectively on the nicAChR without affecting muscarinic receptors. Carbachol is the best example of a drug that shows preference for the nicotinic receptor, but its action is not selective. Nicotine and lobeline both show preference for ganglionic nicotinic receptors, but at slightly higher concentrations than those needed to affect

Fig. 5.12 Somatic and autonomic nervous systems: organization and neurotransmitters. (ACh, acetylcholine; CNS, central nervous sytem; DA, dopamine; NA, noradrenaline.)

Distinguishing features of nicotinic acetylcholine receptors		
	Skeletal muscle	Neurons
Structure	2α 1β 1γ or ε 1δ	2α 3β
Specific agonists	Suxamethonium	DMPP
Specific antagonists	Gallamine Tubocurarine α-bungarotoxin	Hexamethonium Mecamylamine κ-bungarotoxin
Function	End-plate region depolarization at NMJ	Neuronal depolarization in ganglia and CNS

Fig. 5.13 Distinguishing features of the ganglionic nicotinic acetylcholine receptors and those found on skeletal muscle at the neuromuscular junction. (DMPP, dimethylphenylpiperazinium.)

ganglionic transmission. Nicotine and lobeline are able to stimulate the NMJ.

These drugs have no clinical use, since their range of effects is vast, affecting both sympathetic and parasympathetic transmission:

- Sympathetic effects include tachycardia and vasoconstriction leading to hypertension.
- Parasympathetic effects include increased gastrointestinal motility and glandular secretions.

Ganglion-blocking drugs

Autonomic ganglia can be blocked presynaptically by inhibiting ACh synthesis, vesicular packaging, or release (p. 85), or postsynaptically by blocking the nicotinic receptors.

Non-depolarizing ganglion blockers

A few of these drugs act solely as competitive antagonists, blocking receptors without depolarizing the ganglion. Most block the ion channel, as well as the associated receptor, and they produce their action through this former mechanism. For example:

- Some ganglion blockers, such as tubocurarine, are not antagonists at the ganglionic nicotinic receptor; they produce ganglion block through channel blockade.
- Tubocurarine also blocks transmission at the NMJ, but it does this through receptor antagonism.
- Hexamethonium was initially developed for use in treating hypertension, but it is no longer in clinical use.

- Trimetaphan is the only clinically useful ganglion blocker. It is used where controlled hypotension is needed, such as in anaesthesia. It has a short duration of action, and it can be administered intravenously.

Ganglion-blocking drugs have a wide range of complex effects, although the sympathetic and parasympathetic systems tend to oppose one another. The effects of ganglion-blocking drugs include:

- Arteriolar vasodilatation leading to a marked reduction in blood pressure (block of sympathetic ganglia).
- Postural and postexercise hypotension (loss of cardiac reflexes).
- Slight reduction in cardiac output.
- Inhibition of gastrointestinal secretions and motility, leading to constipation, urinary retention, impotence, and failure of ejaculation.

Sympathetic nervous system

The fibres of the sympathetic nervous system leave the CNS from the thoracolumbar regions of the spinal cord (T1–L3). They synapse in ganglia located close to the spinal cord. These ganglia form a chain along each side of the spinal cord, which is known as sympathetic trunk.

The major transmitter released by postganglionic fibres at the junction with effector cells is noradrenaline (NA).

Adrenal medulla

Some postganglionic neurons in the sympathetic division do not have axons, but instead they release their transmitters directly into the bloodstream. These neurons are located in the adrenal medulla.

On stimulation by preganglionic fibres, the adrenal medulla acts as an endocrine gland, releasing its hormones/transmitters into the systemic circulation which consist of ~80% adrenaline, ~20% noradrenaline, as well as small amounts of dopamine, neuropeptides, and ATP.

Adrenoceptors

In 1913 Henry Dale observed that adrenaline constricted some blood vessels but relaxed others, while in 1948 Ahlquist defined two receptor subtypes based on the rank order of potency of three agonists, namely isoprenaline, adrenaline, and noradrenaline. The two receptor subtypes were α and β. Potency at:

- α-receptors is noradrenaline > adrenaline > isoprenaline.

- β-receptors is isoprenaline > adrenaline > noradrenaline.

Effects mediated by α-adrenoreceptors
Alpha$_1$-receptors
Alpha$_1$-receptors are located postsynaptically. Their activation causes smooth muscle contraction (except for the non-sphincter part of the gastrointestinal tract, where activation causes relaxation), glycogenolysis in the liver, and potassium release from the liver and salivary glands. Transduction is via G-proteins and an increase in the second messengers inositol (1,4,5) triphosphate (IP$_3$) and diacylglycerol (DAG).

Alpha$_2$-receptors
Alpha$_2$-receptors are located mainly presynaptically, but also postsynaptically on liver cells, platelets, and the smooth muscle of blood vessels. The activation of presynaptic α$_2$-receptors inhibits noradrenaline release and, therefore, provides a means of end-product negative feedback. Activation of postsynaptic α$_2$-receptors causes blood vessel constriction and platelet aggregation. Transduction is via G-proteins and a decrease in the second messenger cyclic adenosine monophosphate (cAMP).

Effects mediated by β-adrenoceptors
Beta$_1$-receptors
Beta$_1$-receptors are mainly postsynaptic and located in the heart, platelets, and non-sphincter part of the gastrointestinal tract. They can, however, be found presynaptically. Activation causes an increase in the rate and force of contraction of the heart, relaxation of the non-sphincter part of the gastrointestinal tract, aggregation of platelets, an increase in the release of noradrenaline, lipolysis in fat, and amylase secretion from the salivary glands. Presynaptically, their activation causes an increase in noradrenaline release. Transduction is via G-proteins and an increase in the second messenger cAMP.

Beta$_2$-receptors
Beta$_2$-receptors are located postsynaptically. Their activation causes smooth muscle relaxation, glycogenolysis in the liver, inhibition of histamine release from mast cells, and tremor in skeletal muscle. Transduction is via G-proteins and an increase in the second messenger cAMP.

Many of the adrenoceptor agonists and antagonists are not entirely specific for just the α- or the β-adrenoceptors, so side effects are common, and they should be remembered.

Drugs acting on the sympathetic system
Fig. 5.14 summarizes the drugs acting on the sympathetic system.

Presynaptic agents
Noradrenaline synthesis: The precursor to noradrenaline is L-tyrosine, which is taken up by adrenergic neurons.

Drugs decreasing noradrenaline synthesis: The rate-limiting step (RLS) is the conversion of tyrosine to dihydroxyphenylalanine (dopa), which is catalysed by tyrosine hydroxylase and inhibited by a methyltyrosine. Noradrenaline provides a negative feedback upon this step. Carbidopa inhibits dopa decarboxylase and is used in Parkinson's disease to increase dopamine levels. Because this is not the RLS, drugs that inhibit dopa decarboxylase do not greatly affect noradrenaline synthesis. Administering α-methyldopa (used in hypertension) results in the formation of a false transmitter, α-methylnoradrenaline.

Drugs increasing noradrenaline synthesis: Levodopa (L-dopa) administration bypasses the RLS and is used in Parkinson's disease. Noradrenaline is stored in vesicles as a complex with ATP and a protein called chromogranin A.

Drugs inhibiting noradrenaline storage: Reserpine is a drug used in the treatment of hypertension and schizophrenia. It reduces stores of noradrenaline by preventing the accumulation of noradrenaline in vesicles. Its action is effectively irreversible since it has a very high affinity for the noradrenaline storage site. The displaced noradrenaline is immediately broken down by monoamine oxygenase (MAO) and is therefore unable to exert sympathetic effects.

Drugs inhibiting the breakdown of leaked noradrenaline stores: These include monoamine oxidase inhibitors (MAOIs) and catechol-O-methyltransferase (COMT) inhibitors. They prevent the breakdown of leaked catecholamines so that

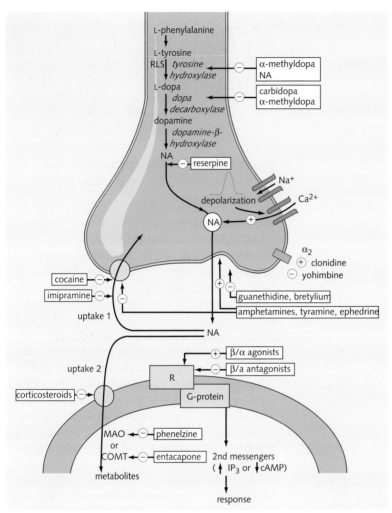

Fig. 5.14 Drugs affecting adrenergic transmission. (cAMP, cyclic adenosine monophosphate; COMT, catechol-*O*-methyltransferase; IP$_3$, inositol triphosphate; MAO, monoamine oxidase; NA, noradrenaline; RLS, rate-limiting step.)

noradrenaline that leaves the vesicles is protected and eventually leaks out from the nerve ending.

Drugs inhibiting noradrenaline release: These include guanethidine and bretylium. These are adrenergic neuron-blocking drugs that prevent the exocytosis of noradrenaline from nerve terminals; they are used as hypotensive drugs. They are taken up by uptake 1 and concentrated in nerve terminals where they have a local anaesthetic effect on impulse conduction. The tricyclic antidepressants, which inhibit uptake 1, prevent these drugs from exerting their effects. Clonidine is an α$_2$-receptor agonist and, therefore, inhibits noradrenaline release.

Drugs promoting noradrenaline release: These include: amphetamines, tyramine, and ephedrine, which are sympathomimetic drugs that act indirectly. They are taken up by uptake 1 and displace noradrenaline from the vesicles. Because they also inhibit MAO, the displaced noradrenaline is not broken down, and it is able to exert sympathetic effects. These drugs act in part through a direct agonist effect on adrenoceptors. Yohimbine is an α$_2$-receptor antagonist and it, therefore, prevents noradrenaline from exerting a negative feedback effect on noradrenaline release.

Postsynaptic agents

Adrenoceptor agonists: These are termed 'sympathomimetics'. They activate postsynaptic receptors, eliciting a response (Fig. 5.15).
Adrenoceptor antagonists: These are termed 'sympatholytics'. They block postsynaptic receptors (Fig. 5.16).

Inactivation

Uptake 1: This is located on neuronal terminals, and it is the main mechanism for noradrenaline inactivation. Uptake 1 has a high affinity for the

Adrenoceptor agonists				
Drug	Receptor	Uses	Side effects	Phamacokinetics
Noradrenaline	α/β	No use clinically	Hypertension, tachycardia, ventricular arrhythmias	Poor oral absorption, metabolized by MAO and COMT, $t_{1/2} \sim 2$ min
Adrenaline	α/β	Anaphylactic shock Cardiac resuscitation with local anaesthetics	Hypertension, tachycardia, ventricular arrhythmias	Poor oral absorption, metabolized by MAO and COMT, $t_{1/2} \sim 2$ min given intravenously or intramuscularly
Oxymetazoline	α	Nasal decongestant	Rebound congestion	Given intranasally
Phenylephrine	$α_1$	Hypotension Nasal decongestant	Hypertension Reflex bradycardia	Metabolized by MAO $t_{1/2} < 1$ min, given intramuscularly or intranasally
Clonidine	$α_2$	Hypertension Migraine	Drowsiness, hypotension	Good oral absorption, $t_{1/2} \sim 12$ h
Isoprenaline	β	Asthma Cardiac resuscitation	Arrhythmias, tachycardia	Metabolized by COMT, given sublingually or as aerosol $t_{1/2} \sim 2$ h
Dobutamine	$β_1$	Heart failure	Tachycardia	
Salbutamol	$β_2$	Asthma Premature labour	Arrhythmias, tachycardia, vasodilatation	Given by aerosol $t_{1/2} \sim 4$ h

Fig. 5.15 Adrenoceptor agonists and their clinical uses. (COMT, catechol-O-methyltransferase; MAO, monoamine oxidase.)

Adrenoceptor antagonists				
Drug	Receptor	Uses	Side effects	Pharmacokinetics
Labetalol	α/β	Hypertension	Postural hypotension	Oral absorption $t_{1/2} \sim 4$ h
Phentolamine	α	No clinical use	Hypotension Tachycardia Nasal congestion	Metabolized by the liver, given intravenously $t_{1/2} \sim 2$ h
Prazosin	$α_1$	Hypertension	Hypotension Tachycardia Nasal congestion Drowsiness	Oral absorption, metabolized by the liver $t_{1/2} \sim 4$ h
Yohimbine	$α_2$	No clinical use	Hypertension Excitement	Oral absorption, metabolized by the liver $t_{1/2} \sim 4$ h
Propranolol	β	Hypertension Angina Arrhythmias	Bronchoconstriction Heart failure	Oral absorption, first-pass metabolism, 90% plasma-protein-bound $t_{1/2} \sim 4$ h
Practolol	$β_1$	Hypertension Angina Arrhythmias	Bronchoconstriction Heart failure	Oral absorption $t_{1/2} \sim 4$ h
Butoxamine	$β_2$	No clinical use		

Fig. 5.16 Adrenoceptor antagonists and their clinical uses. (COMT, catechol-O-methyltransferase; MAO, monoamine oxidase.)

uptake of noradrenaline (K = 0.3 mmol/L in the rat) but the maximum rate of uptake is low (V_{max} = 1.2 nmol/g per minute in the rat). It has a specificity rank of noradrenaline > adrenaline > isoprenaline; it is blocked by cocaine, amphetamines, and tricyclic antidepressants (e.g. imipramine), which therefore potentiate the actions of noradrenaline.

Uptake 2: This is located outside neurons (e.g. in smooth muscle, cardiac muscle, and endothelium), and it is the main mechanism for the removal of circulating adrenaline from the bloodstream. It has a low affinity for the uptake of noradrenaline (K = 250 mmol/L in the rat) but a high maximum rate of uptake (V_{max} = 100 nmol/g per minute in the rat). Uptake 2 has a specificity rank of adrenaline > noradrenaline > isoprenaline, and it is blocked by corticosteroids.

Metabolism of catecholamines by monoamine oxidase: MAO is found on the surface of mitochondria, principally within adrenergic nerve terminals but also in other cells, such as those of the liver and intestines. MAO metabolizes catecholamines into their corresponding aldehydes. It comprises two major forms: MAO_A and MAO_B. Noradrenaline is mainly broken down by MAO_A in nerve terminals. Inhibitors of MAO increase the releasable store of noradrenaline, but they do not greatly potentiate sympathetic transmission, since catecholamines are mainly inactivated by reuptake. MAOIs include the antidepressant drugs phenelzine and tranylcypromine.

Metabolism of catecholamines by catechol-O-methyltransferase: Catechol-O-methyltransferase (COMT) is found in all tissues and breaks down most catecholamines and the byproducts of the actions of MAO. COMT metabolizes catecholamines to give a methoxy derivative. Entacapone is a drug used clinically for parkinsonism, and a COMT inhibitor.

Parasympathetic nervous system

The fibres of the parasympathetic nervous system leave the CNS from the sacral region (S3 and S4) of the spinal cord and via cranial nerves III, VII, IX, and X. The fibres synapse in ganglia, which, unlike the sympathetic system, are located within the innervated organs themselves.

The major transmitter released by postganglionic fibres at the junction with effector cells is ACh.

Parasympathetic receptors

The ACh released by postganglionic nerve fibres acts on muscarinic (M) receptors, of which between three and five subtypes exist.

'Neuroparietal' M_1 receptors

M_1 'neuroparietal' receptors are principally found in the CNS, peripheral neurons, and gastric parietal cells. Their effects tend to be excitatory, depolarizing membranes through a decrease in potassium conductance. Activation causes central excitation and gastric acid secretion, while transduction is via G-proteins and an increase in the second messengers IP_3 and DAG through stimulation of phospholipase C.

'Neurocardiac' M_2 receptors

M_2 'neurocardiac' receptors are found in the heart and on peripheral neurons. Their effects are inhibitory, increasing potassium conductance and inhibiting calcium channels. In the heart, their activation causes a decrease in the rate (via potassium) and force of contraction (via calcium). Transduction is via G-proteins and a decrease in the second messenger cAMP through inhibition of adenylyl cyclase.

'Smooth muscle–glandular' M_3 receptors

M_3 'smooth muscle–glandular' receptors are found in smooth muscle and glands. Their effects tend to be excitatory, increasing sodium conductance. Activation causes glandular secretions such as saliva and sweat, and smooth muscle contraction. Transduction is via G-proteins and an increase in the second messengers IP_3 and DAG. M_3 receptors are also located on vascular endothelium, activation of which causes vasodilatation, through the release of endothelium-derived relaxing factor (EDRF).

'Eye' M_4 receptors

M_4 'eye' receptors are believed to be exclusive to the eye. Their activation causes constriction of the pupil and accommodation for near vision. Transduction is via G-proteins and a decrease in the second messenger cAMP through inhibition of adenylyl cyclase.

Drugs acting on the parasympathetic system

Fig. 5.17 summarizes the drugs that act on the parasympathetic system.

Presynaptic agents

For information regarding presynaptic agents, see p. 77.

Anticholinesterases

For information regarding anticholinesterases, see p. 78.

Postsynaptic agents

Muscarinic-receptor agonists: These are termed 'parasympathomimetic', they activate postsynaptic receptors (Fig. 5.18).

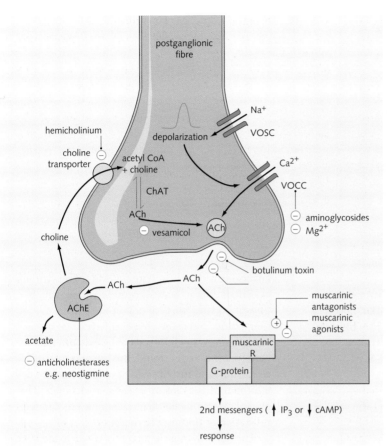

Drugs acting on the parasympathetic nervous system

Drug	Muscarinic receptors	Nicotinic receptors	Uses
Carbachol	++	+	Gut and bladder stimulation postoperatively
Methacholine	+++	+	
Bethanechol	+++	—	Gut and bladder stimulation postoperatively
Muscarine	+++	—	
Pilocarpine	++	—	To decrease intraocular pressure in glaucoma

Fig. 5.18 Muscarinic agonists and their clinical uses.

Muscarinic-receptor antagonists: These are termed 'parasympatholytic' and block postsynaptic receptors (Fig. 5.19).

Non-selective antagonists can be used in anaesthesia to prevent bronchial secretions and vagal slowing of heart rate.

Different tissues respond differently to muscarinic antagonists (Fig. 5.20). Salivary, sweat, and bronchial glands are the most sensitive and can be blocked by very low doses of atropine. In contrast, the parietal cells are the most resistant, and the block of gastric acid secretion requires high doses of atropine.

The side effects of muscarinic antagonists include:

- Dry mouth and skin, and increased body temperature (inhibition of salivary and sweat glands).
- Blurred vision and pupil no longer responsive to light (dilatation of pupil).
- Paralysis of accommodation: cycloplegia (relaxation of ciliary muscle).
- Urinary retention.
- Central excitation: irritability and hyperactivity.
- Sedation (hyoscine).

Muscarinic antagonists		
Drug	**Muscarinic receptor**	**Specific uses**
Atropine	Non-selective	Reduces gastrointestinal motility Cardiac arrest
Hyoscine	Non-selective	Motion sickness
Ipratropium	Non-selective	Bronchodilator
Cyclopentolate	M_4	Dilation of pupil
Tropicamide	M_4	Dilation of pupil
Pirenzepine	M_1	Reduces gastric acid secretion
Trihexyphenidyl (benzhexol)	M_1	Parkinson's disease

Fig. 5.19 Muscarinic antagonists and their clinical uses.

Sympathetic transmission is enhanced under conditions of stress, known as the 'fight-or-flight response'.

Nitrergic nervous system

Nitric oxide is now well recognized as a neurotransmitter in the CNS, and more recently it has been attributed to have numerous roles to play in the peripheral nervous system too.

Nitric oxide is generated by the action of the enzyme nitric oxide synthase (NOS), of which constitutive and inducible isoforms exist. L-arginine is the amino acid precursor of nitric oxide synthesis.

Nitric oxide activates the guanylyl cyclase enzyme, which is responsible for generating cyclic guanosine monophosphate (cGMP). The synthesis of cGMP in turn activates a protein kinase, which phosphorylates ion channels in the plasma membrane, and causes hyperpolarization of the smooth muscle cell. Intracellular calcium ions are consequently sequestered into the endoplasmic reticulum, and further calcium influx into the cell inhibited by the closure of calcium channels. The overall effect of a fall in intracellular calcium is a relaxation of the smooth muscle.

The smooth muscle effects of nitric oxide in the peripheral nervous system are now recognized to be important in the gastrointestinal system, and in sexual arousal in both sexes, particularly in the male.

Therapeutic manipulation of the nitrergic nervous system is confined to the male reproductive system at present, and the agents currently used in the management of erectile dysfunction (e.g. sildenafil, or Viagra®) are discussed in Chapter 9.

Effects of sympathetic and parasympathetic nerve stimulation

Target tissue	Sympathetic		Parasympathetic		Overall effect
Nerve terminals	α_2	Decreased release	M_2	Decreased release	Decreased transmission
Smooth muscle					
Blood vessels	$\alpha_{1/2}$ b_2	Contraction Relaxation	M_3	Relaxation (via EDRF)	Vasoconstriction Vasodilatation
Bronchi	β_2 α_1	Relaxation Contraction	M_3 M_3	Contraction Secretion	Bronchodilatation Bronchoconstriction Bronchosecretion
Gastrointestinal tract: non-sphincter sphincter secretions	β_1/α_1 α_1	Relaxation Contraction	M_3 M_3 M_3	Contraction Relaxation Secretion	Increased/decreased motility and tone GI secretions
Parietal cells			M_1	Contraction	Gastric acid secretion
Pancreas			M_3	Contraction	Increased secretions
Uterus	α_1 β_2	Contraction Relaxation	M_3 M_3		
Bladder: detrusor sphincter	β_2 α_1	Relaxation Contraction	M_3 M_3	Contraction Relaxation	Micturition Urine retention
Seminal tract Vas deferens Penis venous sphincter	α_1 β_2 α_1	Contraction Relaxation Contraction	M_3	Vasodilatation	Ejaculation Ejaculation Erection
Radial muscle (iris) Ciliary muscle Lacrimal gland	α_1 β_2	Contraction Relaxation	M_4 M_4 M_4	Relaxation Contraction Contraction	Pupil relaxation/constriction Accommodation Tear secretion
Heart	β_1	Increased rate and force	M_2	Decreased rate and force	
Liver	α_1/β_2	Glycogenolysis			
Fat	β_1	Lipolysis			
Salivary glands	α_1/β_1	Secretion of thick saliva	M_3	Abundant secretion of watery saliva	
Platelets	α_2	Platelet aggregation			
Mast cells	β_2	Inhibition of histamine release			

Fig. 5.20 Summary table of the opposing effects of sympathetic and parasympathetic nerve stimulation on body tissues.

- How does the size of a nerve fibre affect its potential to be blocked?
- Summarize the mechanism of action of local anaesthetics, the importance of pH, and the two routes by which block occurs.
- Describe how presynaptic agents can be used to block transmission at the neuromuscular junction. Give examples and describe their clinical use.
- By which routes can local anaesthetics be administered? Give a clinical use for each example given.
- What are the distinguishing characteristics between non-depolarizing and polarizing postsynaptic blocking drugs? Give examples and describe their clinical use.
- What are the clinical features of the adverse reactions to local anaesthetics. Why are local anaesthetic drugs not used in end arteries?
- Discuss, and give examples of, the effects of anticholinesterases, and how these are used clinically.
- Describe the events that occur during transmission across the neuromuscular junction.
- How do nicotinic and muscarinic acetylcholine receptors differ in the location and mechanism of action?
- Describe the function and divisions of the autonomic nervous system.
- Summarize the action and counter-actions of the sympathetic and parasympathetic nervous systems on the major organs of the body.
- Name the mediators involved in presynaptic and postsynaptic transmission, and the receptors involved in the sympathetic nervous system.
- Name the mediators involved in presynaptic and postsynaptic transmission, and the receptors involved in the parasympathetic nervous system.
- What is the role of the adrenal gland in promoting a systemic response other than its synthesis and release of steroids? What innervates this?
- List the main classes of adrenoceptors, their subdivisions, and the tissues in which they predominate.
- For each of the class of adrenoceptor, name their naturally occurring agonist(s), and physiological role in the human.
- List the common adrenoceptor agonist and antagonist drugs, their route of administration, adverse effects, and clinical uses.
- By what mechanisms is acetylcholine cleared from the synaptic cleft and from the synaptic terminal? Name the drugs which inhibit these pathways.
- Outline the mechanism of action of the different classes of muscarinic receptors, and their likely physiological roles.
- What are the side effects most commonly reported by patient taking anticholinergic drugs?

6. Central Nervous System

Parkinsonism

Parkinson's disease and parkinsonism
Definitions
Parkinson's disease is a progressive neurological disorder of the basal ganglia that occurs most commonly in the elderly.

Parkinsonism is most commonly caused by Parkinson's disease, though numerous other causes do exist. Parkinsonism is characterized by a resting tremor, slow initiation of movements (bradykinesia), and muscle rigidity known collectively as the 'parkinsonian triad'. A patient with parkinsonism will present with characteristic signs including:

- A shuffling gait.
- A blank 'mask-like' facial expression.
- Speech impairment.
- An inability to perform skilled tasks.

Pathogenesis
Analysis of brains of parkinsonian patients post mortem shows a substantially reduced concentration of dopamine (less than 10% of normal) in the basal ganglia. The basal ganglia exert an extrapyramidal neural influence that normally acts to maintain smooth voluntary movement.

The main pathology in Parkinson's disease is a progressive degeneration of the dopaminergic neurons of the substantia nigra, which project in the nigrostriatal pathway to the corpus striatum (Fig. 6.1). The inhibitory dopaminergic activity of the nigrostriatal pathway is, therefore, considerably reduced (by 20–40%) in people with Parkinson's disease.

The reduction in the inhibitory dopaminergic activity of the nigrostriatal pathway results in unopposed cholinergic neuron hyperactivity from the corpus striatum, which contributes to the pathological features of parkinsonism. Frank symptoms of parkinsonism appear only when more than 80% of the dopaminergic neurons of the substantia nigra have degenerated.

Parkinson's disease is progressive, with continued loss of dopaminergic neurons in the substantia nigra correlating well with worsening of clinical symptoms.

Untreated Parkinson's eventually results in dementia and death.

Aetiology
The cause of Parkinson's disease is unknown in most cases ('idiopathic') although both endogenous and environmental neurotoxins are known to be responsible in causing parkinsonism (Fig. 6.2).

The possibility of a neurotoxic cause has been strengthened by the finding that 1-methyl-4-phenyl-1,2,3,6-tetrahydropyridine (MPTP), a chemical contaminant of heroin, causes irreversible damage to the nigrostriatal dopaminergic pathway. This damage can lead to the development of symptoms similar to those of idiopathic Parkinson's disease; it has been seen in Californian drug users and induced in experimental primates.

Drugs that block dopamine receptors can also induce parkinsonism. Neuroleptic drugs (pp. 102–105) used

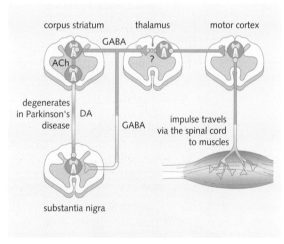

Fig. 6.1 Basal ganglia systems involved in Parkinson's disease. (ACh, acetylcholine; DA, dopamine; GABA, γ-aminobutyric acid.) (Redrawn from Page et al, 2002.)

Aetiology of parkinsonism

- Mostly unknown (idiopathic Parkinson's disease)
- Toxin induced: MPTP; carbon monoxide, manganese
- Drug induced: neuroleptics (dopamine antagonists)
- Rare causes: cerebral ischaemia; viral encephalitis and others?

Fig. 6.2 Aetiological mechanisms in the development of parkinsonism. (MPTP, methyl-4-phenyl-1,2,3,6-tetrahydropyridine.)

in the treatment of schizophrenia can produce parkinsonian symptoms as an adverse effect.

Rare causes of parkinsonism are cerebral ischaemia (progressive atherosclerosis or stroke), viral encephalitis, or other pathological damage.

Treatment of parkinsonism

The treatment of parkinsonism is based on correcting the imbalance between the dopaminergic and cholinergic systems at the basal ganglia (Fig. 6.3). Two major groups of drugs are used: drugs that increase dopaminergic activity between the substantia nigra and the corpus striatum, and anticholinergic drugs that inhibit striatal cholinergic activity.

Drugs that increase dopaminergic activity
Dopamine precursors

An example of a dopamine precursor is levodopa (L-dopa).

Mechanism of action: L-dopa is the immediate precursor of dopamine and is able to penetrate the blood–brain barrier to replenish the dopamine content of the corpus striatum. L-dopa is decarboxylated to dopamine in the brain by dopa decarboxylase, and it has beneficial effects produced through the actions of dopamine on D_2 receptors (Fig. 6.3). Dopamine itself is not used, owing to its inability to cross the blood–brain barrier.

Route of administration: L-dopa is administered orally. It reaches peak plasma concentrations after 1–2 hours and only 1% reaches the brain, owing to peripheral metabolism.

Indications: L-dopa is used in the treatment of parkinsonism (excluding drug-induced extrapyramidal symptoms).

Contraindications: Closed-angle glaucoma.

Adverse effects: The extensive peripheral metabolism of L-dopa means that large doses have to be given to

Fig. 6.3 Drugs used to treat parkinsonism and their site of action. (ACh, acetylcholine; L-dopa, levodopa; MAO_B, monoamine oxidase B; COMT, catechol-O-methyl transferase; DA, dopamine.)

produce therapeutic effects in the brain. Large doses are more likely to produce adverse effects. These include:

- Nausea and vomiting.
- Psychiatric side effects (schizophrenia-like symptoms).
- Cardiovascular effects (hypotension).
- Dyskinesias.

Nausea and vomiting are caused by stimulation of dopamine receptors in the chemoreceptor trigger zone in the area postrema (p. 173), which lies outside the blood–brain barrier.

Psychiatric side effects are common limiting factors in L-dopa treatment; these include vivid dreams, confusion, and psychotic symptoms more commonly seen in schizophrenia. These effects are probably a result of increased dopaminergic activity in the mesolimbic area of the brain, possibly similar to that found pathologically in schizophrenia (dopaminergic overactivity is implicated in schizophrenia, p. 101).

Hypotension is common but usually asymptomatic. Cardiac arrhythmias are due to increased catecholamine stimulation following the excessive peripheral metabolism of L-dopa.

Dyskinesias can often develop and tend to involve the face and limbs. They usually reflect over-treatment and respond to simple dose reduction.

Three strategies have been developed to optimize L-dopa treatment, to maximize the central effects of L-dopa within the brain, and minimize its unwanted peripheral effects. These strategies involve co-administration of:

- Carbidopa, an inhibitor of dopa decarboxylase in the periphery, that cannot penetrate the blood–brain barrier. Hence, extracerebral conversion of L-dopa to dopamine is inhibited.
- Domperidone, a dopamine antagonist, that does not penetrate the blood–brain barrier and can, therefore, block the stimulation of dopamine receptors in the periphery.
- Selegiline and entacapone, MAO_B and COMT inhibitors, respectively, which inhibit dopamine degradation in the central nervous system (CNS).

Therapeutic notes: Initially, treatment with L-dopa is effective in 80% of patients with possible restoration of near-normal motor function, but although L-dopa restores dopamine levels in the short term, therapy has no effect on the underlying degenerative disease process.

As progressive neuronal degeneration continues, the capacity of the corpus striatum to covert L-dopa to dopamine diminishes. This affects the majority of patients within 5 years and manifests itself as 'end of dose deterioration' (a shortening of duration of each dose of L-dopa), and the 'on–off effect' (rapid fluctuations in clinical state, varying from increased mobility and a general improvement to increased rigidity and hypokinesia). The latter effect occurs suddenly and for short periods from a few minutes to a few hours, tending to worsen with length of treatment.

Dopamine agonists

Examples of dopamine agonists include bromocriptine, ropinirole, pergolide, lisuride, and apomorphine.

Mechanism of action: Bromocriptine, ropinirole, pergolide, lisuride, and apomorphine are dopamine agonists selective for the D_2 receptor (Fig. 6.3). Apomorphine also has agonist action at D_1 receptors.

Route of administration: Oral. Apomorphine is given by the subcutaneous route.

Indications: Dopamine agonists are used in combination with L-dopa in an attempt to reduce the late adverse effects of L-dopa therapy ('end of dose deterioration' and 'on–off effect') or when L-dopa alone does not adequately control the symptoms.

Adverse effects: The adverse effects of dopamine agonists are essentially similar to those of L-dopa (i.e. nausea, postural hypotension, psychiatric symptoms), but they tend to be more common and more severe. Apomorphine produces profound nausea and vomiting.

Therapeutic notes: Currently, bromocriptine is the most clinically used of the dopamine agonists in the treatment of Parkinson's disease.

Drugs stimulating release of dopamine

Amantadine is an example of a drug that stimulates the release of dopamine (Fig. 6.3).

Mechanism of action: Facilitation of neuronal dopamine release and inhibition of its reuptake into nerves, and additional muscarinic blocking actions.

Route of administration: Oral.

Indications: Amantidine has a synergistic effect when used in conjunction with L-dopa therapy in Parkinson's disease.

Adverse effects: Anorexia, nausea, and hallucinations.

Therapeutic notes: Amantadine has modest antiparkinsonian effects, but it is only of short-term benefit, since most of its effectiveness is lost within 6 months of initiating treatment.

Monoamine oxidase B inhibitors

Selegiline is an example of a MAO_B inhibitor.

Mechanism of action: Selegiline selectively inhibits the MAO_B enzyme in the brain that is normally responsible for the degradation of dopamine (Fig. 6.3). By reducing the catabolism of dopamine, the actions of L-dopa are potentiated, thus allowing the dose to be reduced by up to one third. There is evidence to suggest that selegiline may slow the progression of the underlying neuronal degeneration in Parkinson's disease.

Route of administration: Oral.

Indications: MAO_B inhibitors can be used on their own in mild cases of parkinsonism or in conjunction with L-dopa to reduce 'end-of-dose' deterioration in severe parkinsonism.

Adverse effects: The adverse effects of MAO_B inhibitors are those that might be expected by potentiation of L-dopa.

Catechol-*O*-methyl transferase inhibitors

Entacapone has recently been introduced as a catechol-O-methyl transferase (COMT) inhibitor.

Mechanism of action: Dopamine is broken down by a second pathway, in addition to that of MAO_B. The enzyme COMT is responsible for the degradation of dopamine to inactive methylated metabolites. COMT inhibitors specifically inhibit this enzyme.

Route of administration: Oral.

Indications: As an adjunct to L-dopa preparations when 'end-of-dose' is problematic.

Contraindications: Phaeochromocytoma.

Adverse effects: Nausea, vomiting, abdominal pain, and diarrhoea.

Therapeutic notes: An earlier COMT inhibitor was withdrawn due to hepatotoxicity, and so liver monitoring with serum enzymes is recommended.

Drugs that inhibit striatal cholinergic activity
Anticholinergic agents

Benzatropine, procyclidine, and orphenadrine are examples of anticholinergic (antimuscarinic) agents.

Mechanism of action: Benzatropine, procyclidine and orphenadrine are antagonists at the muscarinic receptors that mediate striatal cholinergic excitation (Fig. 6.3). Their major action in the treatment of Parkinson's disease is to reduce the excessive striatal cholinergic activity that characterizes the disease.

Route of administration: Oral.

Adverse effects: Typical peripheral anticholinergic effects, such as a dry mouth and blurred vision, are less common. More often, patients experience a variety of CNS effects, ranging from mild memory loss to acute confusional states.

Therapeutic notes: Termination of anticholinergic treatment should be gradual, as parkinsonism can worsen when these drugs are withdrawn. Anticholinergic drugs are most effective in controlling tremor rather than other symptoms of Parkinson's disease.

Transplantation

The transplantation of cells from the substantia nigra of human fetuses into the putamen of patients with Parkinson's disease has shown some success in controlling parkinsonian symptoms.

Transplantation in the treatment of Parkinson's disease is still experimental, and its role is highly controversial.

Note that with the possible exception of selegiline, none of the drugs used in Parkinson's disease affect the inevitable progressive degeneration of nigrostriatal dopaminergic neurons. The disease process is unaffected, just compensated for by drug therapy.

Dementia

Alzheimer's disease is a specific process that results in dementia, and is unrelated to the dementias associated with stroke, brain trauma, and alcohol. Alzheimer's disease is very common in the elderly, and its prevalence increases markedly with age.

Alzheimer's disease is progressive, and it is associated with shrinkage of the brain substance, loss of neuronal tissue, and deposition of so-called amyloid plaques. The clinical features include deterioration in cognitive function, disorientation, and generalized confusion.

Neuropharmacological studies have shown that despite widespread shrinkage of the brain, loss of neurons in the forebrain is most marked, and a relative selective loss of cholinergic neurons most likely accounts for the features of this dementia.

The obvious therapeutic target is, therefore, restoration of cholinergic function.

Certain cholinesterase inhibitors appear to improve cognitive functioning in as many as 50% of patients, and delay subsequent deterioration in mental capacity.

Cholinesterase inhibitors

Donepezil, galantamine, and rivastigmine are cholinesterase inhibitors, licensed for use in dementia in the UK.

Mechanism of action: The cholinesterase inhibitors prevent the breakdown of acetylcholine within the synaptic cleft, and they enhance endogenous cholinogenic activity within the CNS and peripheral tissues.

Route of administration: Oral.

Indications: Mild to moderate dementia in Alzheimer's disease.

Contraindications: Pregnancy, breastfeeding, hepatic and renal impairment.

Adverse effects: Nausea, vomiting, diarrhoea, anorexia, and agitation.

Anxiety and sleep disorders

Anxiety and anxiolytics

Anxiety is a state characterized by psychological symptoms such as a diffuse, unpleasant, and vague feeling of apprehension, often accompanied by physical symptoms of autonomic arousal such as palpitations, light-headedness, perspiration, 'butterflies', and, in some people, restlessness.

While occasional anxiety is perfectly normal, it is a common and disabling symptom in a variety of mental illnesses including phobias, panic disorders, and obsessive compulsive disorders. Drugs used to treat such anxiety disorders are called anxiolytics.

Sleep disorders and hypnotics

Insomnia is a common and non-specific disorder that may be reported by 40–50% of people at any given time.

Causes of insomnia include medical illness, alcohol or drugs, periodic limb movement disorder, sleep apnoea, and psychiatric illness. Without an obvious underlying cause, it is known as primary or psycho-physiological.

Hypnotics are drugs used to treat psycho-physiological (primary) insomnia. The distinction between the treatment of anxiety and that of sleep disorders is not clear-cut, particularly if anxiety is the main impediment to sleep.

Gamma-aminobutyric acid (GABA) receptor

The γ-aminobutyric (GABA) receptors of the GABA$_A$ type are involved in the actions of some classes of hypnotic/anxiolytic drugs, notably:

- The benzodiazepines (BDZs), which are currently the most commonly used clinically.
- Newer non-benzodiazepine hypnotics, e.g. zopiclone.
- The now obsolete barbiturates.

The GABA$_A$ receptor belongs to the superfamily of ligand-gated ion channels. It consists of several subunits—α, β, γ, and δ—which form the GABA/Cl$^-$ channel complex, as well as containing benzodiazepine and barbiturate modulatory receptor sites. The GABA site appears to be located on the α- and β-subunits while the benzodiazepine modulatory site is distinct and located on the γ-subunit.

GABA released from nerve terminals binds to postsynaptic GABA$_A$ receptors, the activation of which increases the Cl$^-$ conductance of the neuron.

Occupation of the benzodiazepine sites by benzodiazepine receptor agonists enhances the actions of GABA on the Cl$^-$ conductance of the neuronal membrane. The barbiturates similarly enhance the action of GABA, but by occupying a distinct modulatory site (Fig. 6.4).

Anxiolytic and hypnotic drugs

The pharmacotherapy of anxiety and sleep disorders involves several different classes of drug, as shown in Fig. 6.5, and non-pharmacological management relying upon cognitive and behaviour psychotherapy.

Benzodiazepines

Benzodiazepines are drugs with anxiolytic, hypnotic, muscle relaxant, and anticonvulsant actions that are used in the treatment of both anxiety states and insomnia.

Different benzodiazepines are marked as hypnotics and anxiolytics. It is mainly the duration of action that determines the choice of drug (see below).

Mechanism of action: Benzodiazepines potentiate the action of GABA, the primary inhibitory neurotransmitter in the CNS. They do this by binding to a site on GABA$_A$ receptors, increasing their affinity for GABA. This results in an increased opening frequency of these ligand-gated Cl$^-$ channels, thus potentiating the effect of GABA release in terms of inhibitory effects on the postsynaptic cell (Fig. 6.4).

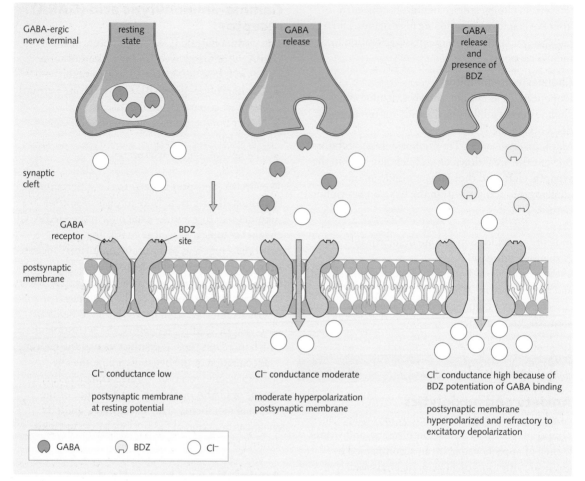

Fig. 6.4 Diagrammatic representation of the GABA$_A$ receptor and how its activity is enhanced by benzodiazepines and similarly by barbiturates. (BDZ, benzodiazepine; GABA γ-aminobutyric acid; Cl⁻, chloride ion.) (Redrawn from Page et al, 2002.)

Indications: Benzodiazepines are used clinically in the short-term relief of severe anxiety and severe insomnia, preoperative sedation, status epilepticus, and acute alcohol withdrawal.

Route of administration: Oral is the usual route. Intravenous, intramuscular and rectal preparations are available.

Contraindications: Benzodiazepines should not be given to people with bronchopulmonary disease, and they have additive or synergistic effects with other central depressants such as alcohol, barbiturates, and antihistamines.

Adverse effects: Benzodiazepines have several adverse effects:

- Drowsiness, ataxia, and reduced psychomotor performance are common; therefore, care is necessary when driving or operating machinery.
- Dependence becomes apparent after 4–6 weeks, and is both physical and psychological. The

withdrawal syndrome (in 30% of patients) comprises rebound anxiety and insomnia, tremulousness, and twitching.

Although in overdose benzodiazepines alone are relatively safe when compared with other sedatives (e.g. barbiturates), if benzodiazepines are taken in combination with alcohol the CNS-depressant effects are potentiated and fatal respiratory depression can result. Treatment is with the benzodiazepine antagonist flumazenil.

Therapeutic notes: Benzodiazepines are active orally, and they differ mainly in respect of their duration of action (Fig. 6.6). Short-acting agents (e.g. lorazepam and temazepam) are metabolized to inactive compounds, and these are used mainly as sleeping pills because of the relative lack of 'hangover' effects in the morning. Some long-acting agents (e.g. diazepam) are converted to long-lasting active

Anxiolytics and hypnotics	
Anxiolytics	**Hypnotics**
Benzodiazepines (act on GABA$_A$ receptors) e.g. diazepam, lorazepam	Benzodiazepines (act on GABA$_A$ receptors) e.g. triazolam, temazepam, lormetazepam, nitrazepam
Acting on serotonergic receptors (act on 5-HT$_{1A}$ or 5-HT$_3$ receptors) e.g. buspirone	Non-benzodiazepine hypnotics (act on GABA$_A$ receptors) e.g. zopiclone and zolpidem
Other drugs e.g. propranolol antidepressants	Other drugs e.g. choral hydrate chlormethiazole barbiturates (obsolete) sedative antidepressants sedative antihistamines

Fig. 6.5 Drugs used to treat anxiety and sleep disorders. (GABA, γ-aminobutyric acid; 5-HT, 5-hydroxytryptamine.)

Approximate elimination half-lives of benzodiazepines	
Benzodiazepine	**Approximate half-life (hours)**
Midazolam	2 – 4
Temazepam	8 – 12
Lormetazepam	10
Lorazepam	12
Nitrazepam	24
Diazepam	32 (one metabolite is active for up to 200 hours)

Fig. 6.6 Approximate elimination half-lives of the benzodiazepines.

metabolites with half-lives longer than the administered parent drug. With others (e.g. nitrazepam) it is the parent drug itself that is metabolized slowly. Such drugs are more suitable for an anxiolytic effect maintained all day long, or when early morning waking is the problem.

Non-benzodiazepine hypnotics

Zopiclone, zolpidem, and zaleplon are new-generation hypnotics that have a short duration of action with little or no hangover effect.

Although these drugs are not benzodiazepines, they act in a comparable manner to benzodiazepines on the GABA$_A$ receptor, although (it is thought) at a different site.

Anxiolytic drugs acting at serotonergic receptors

The serotonergic theory of anxiety suggests that serotonergic transmission is involved in anxiety as, in

general, stimulation of this system causes anxiety while a reduction in serotonergic neuronal activity reduces anxiety.

The serotonergic theory prompted the development of anxiolytic drugs that act to moderate serotonergic neurotransmission while not causing sedation and incoordination.

5-hydroxytryptamine 1A agonists

Buspirone is a serotonergic (5-hydroxytryptamine 1A; 5-HT$_{1A}$) agonist.

Mechanism of action: In the raphe nucleus the dendrites of serotonergic neurons possess inhibitory presynaptic autoreceptors of the 5-HT$_{1A}$ subtype that, when stimulated, decrease the firing of 5-HT neurons. This class of anxiolytic agents called the azapirones are thought to reduce 5-HT transmission by acting as partial agonists at these 5-HT$_{1A}$ receptors. Buspirone is the first of this new class of anxiolytics. Sumatriptan is similar.

Route of administration: Oral.

Indications: Buspirone is indicated for the short-term relief of generalized anxiety disorder.

Contraindications: 5-HT$_{1A}$ agonists should not be used in people with epilepsy.

Adverse effects: The adverse effects of 5-HT$_{1A}$ agonists include nervousness, dizziness, headache, and light-headedness.

In contrast to benzodiazepines, buspirone does not cause significant sedation or cognitive impairment, and it carries only a minimal risk of dependence and withdrawal. It does not potentiate the effects of alcohol.

Therapeutic notes: The anxiolytic effect of buspirone gradually evolve over 1–3 weeks.

5-hydroxytryptamine 3 antagonists

Ondansetron is a 5-HT$_3$ receptor antagonist that is well established for use as an antiemetic drug.

Ondansetron also has anxiolytic properties by virtue of its antagonism at the excitatory postsynaptic 5-HT$_3$ receptor.

Beta-adrenoreceptor blockers

Beta-adrenoreceptor blockers or β-blockers, e.g. propranolol, can be very effective in alleviating the somatic manifestations of anxiety caused by marked sympathetic arousal, such as palpitations, tremor, sweating, and diarrhoea.

Mechanism of action: β-blockers act by antagonism at β-adrenoreceptors so that excessive catecholamine release does not produce the sympathetic responses of tachycardia, sweating, etc. β-blockers are also used in cardiovascular disease (p. 132).

Route of administration: Oral.

Indications: β-blockers are indicated in patients with predominantly somatic symptoms; this, in turn, may prevent the onset of worry and fear. Patients with predominantly psychological symptoms may obtain no benefit. β-blockers can be useful in social phobias and to reduce performance anxiety in musicians, for whom fine motor control may be critical.

Contraindications: β-blockers should not be used in people with asthma or heart failure.

Adverse effects: β-blockers can cause bradycardia, heart failure, bronchospasm, and peripheral vasoconstriction.

Barbiturates

Barbiturates are non-selective CNS depressants that produce effects ranging from sedation and reduction of anxiety to unconsciousness and death from respiratory and cardiovascular failure. Barbiturates increase GABA-mediated inhibition by acting on the same receptor as benzodiazepines, though at a different site.

At low doses, barbiturates prolong the duration of individual Cl^- channel openings triggered by a given GABA stimulus (benzodiazepines increase the frequency of Cl^- channel openings). At high doses, they are far more depressant than benzodiazepines because they start to increase Cl^- conductance directly, thus decreasing the sensitivity of the postsynaptic membrane to excitatory transmitters.

While very popular until the 1960s as sedative/hypnotic agents, they are now obsolete since they readily lead to psychological and physical dependence, and a relatively small overdose can be fatal. Conversely, benzodiazepines, which have largely replaced barbiturates as sedative/hypnotics, have been taken in huge overdoses without serious long-term effects.

Barbiturates are still important in anaesthesia (p. 112) and to a lesser extent in the treatment of epilepsy (p. 105).

Miscellaneous agents

There are a number of miscellaneous hypnotic agents that have been used historically, and which are still prescribed under certain circumstances.

Chloral hydrate and derivatives

Chloral hydrate is metabolized to trichloroethanol, which is an effective hypnotic. It is cheap, but it causes gastric irritation and there is no convincing evidence that it has any advantage over the newer benzodiazepines.

Chloral hydrate and its derivatives were previously popular hypnotics for children. Current thinking does not justify the use of hypnotics in children, and these drugs now have very limited uses.

Clomethiazole (chlormethiazole)

Clomethiazole may be a useful hypnotic in the elderly because of the relative freedom from hangover effects. It has no advantage over benzodiazepines in younger adults.

Clomethiazole was once indicated to attenuate the symptoms of acute alcohol withdrawal, though it has been largely replaced by the benzodiazepine chlordiazepoxide.

Antidepressants

If the underlying cause of insomnia is associated with depression, or particularly in depressed patients exhibiting anxiety and agitation, then tricyclic antidepressants (TCAs) with sedative actions (p. 98), e.g. amitriptyline, may be useful, as they act as a hypnotic when given at bedtime. Alternatively, selective serotonin reuptake inhibitors (SSRIs, p. 98) may correct the mood disorder, and lessen the symptoms of anxiety or insomnia.

Sedative antihistamines

The older antihistamine drugs, e.g. diphenhydramine, have antimuscarinic actions and pass the blood–brain barrier, commonly causing drowsiness and psychomotor impairment.

Proprietary brands of diphenhydramine are on sale to the public to relieve temporary sleep disturbances, as these drugs are relatively safe.

 An understanding of the $GABA_A/Cl^-$ channel complex is central to the mechanism of action of several classes of hypnotic/anxiolytic drugs. You should be aware which these are.

Affective disorders

Affective disorders

Affective disorders involve a disturbance of mood (cognitive/emotional symptoms) associated with changes in behaviour, energy, appetite, and sleep (biological symptoms).

Affective disorders can be thought of as pathological extremes of the normal continuum of human moods, from extreme excitement and elation (mania) to severe depressive states.

There are two types of affective disorder, unipolar affective disorders and bipolar affective disorders.

Unipolar affective disorders

Unipolar affective disorder is characterized by misery, malaise, despair, guilt, apathy, indecisiveness, low energy and fatigue, changes in sleeping pattern, loss of appetite, and suicidal thoughts.

Attempts have been made to classify types of depression as either 'reactive' or 'endogenous' in origin.

Reactive depression is where there is a clear psychological cause, e.g. bereavement. It involves less-severe symptoms and less likelihood of biological disturbance. It affects 3–10% of the population, with the incidence increasing with age, and it is more common in females.

Endogenous depression is where there is no clear cause and more severe symptoms, e.g. suicidal thoughts, and a greater likelihood of biological disturbance, e.g. insomnia, anorexia. It affects 1% of the population, usually starting in early adulthood, and affecting both sexes equally.

The distinction between reactive and endogenous depression is of importance since there is some evidence that depressions with endogenous features tend to respond better to drug therapy.

Bipolar affective disorders

Bipolar affective disorder (BPAD) presents with mood and behaviour oscillating between depression and mania, and it is, therefore, also known as manic–depressive disorder.

Bipolar affective disorder develops earlier in life than unipolar depressive disorders, and it tends to be inherited. It affects 1% of the population, and it can have associated elements of psychotic phenomena.

Monoamine theory of depression

The aetiology of major depressive disorders is not clear. Genetic, environmental, and neurochemical influences have all been examined as possible aetiological factors.

The most widely accepted neurochemical explanation of endogenous depression involves the monoamines (noradrenaline, NA; serotonin, 5-HT; dopamine, DA). The original hypothesis of depression, 'the monoamine theory', stated that depression resulted from a functional deficit of these transmitter amines, while conversely mania was caused by an excess.

The monoamine theory explains why:
- Drugs that deplete monoamines are depressant, e.g. reserpine and methyldopa.
- A wide range of drugs that increase the functional availability of monoamine neurotransmitters improve mood in depressed patients, e.g. TCAs and monoamine oxidase inhibitors (MAOIs).
- The concentration of monoamines and their metabolites is reduced in the cerebrospinal fluid (CSF) of depressed patients.
- In some post mortem studies the most consistent finding is an elevation in cortical 5-HT$_2$ binding.

The monoamine theory cannot explain why:
- A number of compounds that increase the functional availability of monoamines, e.g. amphetamines, cocaine, and L-dopa, have no effect on the mood of depressed patients.
- Some older, atypical antidepressants e.g. iprindole, worked without manipulating monoaminergic systems.
- There is a 'therapeutic delay' of 2 weeks between the full neurochemical effects of antidepressants and the start of their therapeutic effect.

It is unlikely, therefore, that monoamine mechanisms alone are responsible for the symptoms of depression. Other systems that may be involved in depression include:
- The GABA system.
- The neuropeptide systems, particularly vasopressin and the endogenous opiates.
- Secondary-messenger systems also appear to have a crucial role in some treatments.

Treatment of unipolar depressive disorders

The major classes of drug that are used to treat depression, and their mechanisms of action, are summarized in Fig. 6.7.

Although almost certainly flawed and incomplete, the monoamine theory is probably the best way to rationalize your thinking about affective disorders, and to understand the mechanism of action of the drugs used in their treatment.

Major classes of antidepressant drug and mechanism of action		
Class of antidepressant drug	Examples	Mode of action
Tricyclic antidepressants (TCAs)	Amitriptyline Imipramine Lofepramine	Non-specific blockers of monoamine uptake
Specific serotonin reuptake inhibitors (SSRIs)	Fluoxetine Paroxetine Sertraline	Selective blockers of 5-HT reuptake
Serotonin–noradrenaline reuptake inhibitors (SNRIs)	Venlafaxine	Selective blockers of 5-HT and noradrenaline uptake
Monoamine oxidase inhibitors (MAOIs)	Phenelzine Tranylcypromine	Non-competitive, non-selective irreversible blockers of MAO_A and MAO_B
Reversible inhibitors of MAO_A (RIMAs)	Moclobemide	Reversibly inhibit MAO_A selectively
Atypical	Reboxetine Mirtazapine	Act by various mechanisms that are poorly understood

Fig. 6.7 Major classes of antidepressant drug and their mechanism of action. (5-HT, 5-hydroxytryptamine; MAO, monoamine oxidase.)

Tricyclic antidepressants and related drugs

Examples of TCAs and related drugs include amitriptyline, imipramine, dosulepin(dothiepin), and lofepramine.

Mechanism of action: TCAs act by blocking 5-HT and noradrenaline uptake into the presynaptic terminal from the synaptic cleft (Fig. 6.8). They have a certain affinity for H_1 and muscarinic receptors, and for α_1- and α_2-receptors.

Contraindications: TCAs and related drugs should not be used in:

- Recent myocardial infarction or arrhythmias (especially heart block) since TCAs increase the risk of conduction abnormalities.
- Manic phase.
- Severe liver disease.
- Epilepsy, where TCAs lower the seizure threshold.
- Patients taking other anticholinergic drugs, alcohol, and adrenaline as TCAs potentiate the effects of these. Lidocaine (lignocaine) is contraindicated in combination with TCAs, owing to a potentially fatal drug interaction.

Adverse effects: While TCAs are an effective therapy for depression, the adverse effects can reduce patient compliance and acceptability. Side effects include:

- Muscarinic blocking effects such as a dry mouth, blurred vision, and constipation.
- Alpha-adrenergic blocking effects causing postural hypotension.
- Noradrenaline uptake block in the heart, increasing the risk of arrhythmias.
- Histamine-blocking effects leading to sedation.
- Weight gain.

TCAs are relatively dangerous in overdose. Patients present with confusion, mania, and potentially fatal arrhythmias due to the cardiotoxic nature of the drug.

Therapeutic notes: No individual TCA has superior antidepressant activity, and the choice of drug is usually determined by the most acceptable or desired side effects. For example, drugs with sedative actions, such as amitriptyline or trimipramine, are the TCAs of choice for patients in agitated or anxious states. The most recent TCA is lofepramine, which causes fewer antimuscarinic side effects, and is less dangerous if taken in overdose.

Therapeutic effects take 2–3 weeks to develop. TCA-related antidepressants should be withdrawn slowly.

Specific serotonin reuptake inhibitors

Specific serotonin (5-HT) reuptake inhibitors (SSRIs) are the most recently introduced class of antidepressant agent. Fluoxetine (Prozac®) is an SSRI. Other examples include citalopram, fluvoxamine, paroxetine, and sertraline.

Mechanism of action: SSRIs act with a high specificity for potent inhibition of serotonin reuptake into nerve terminals from the synaptic cleft, while having only minimal effects on noradrenaline uptake (Fig. 6.8). They block serotonin transporters, which belong to a class of Na^+/Cl^--coupled transporters.

Contraindications: Contraindications with SSRIs are few. They should not be used with MAOIs as the combination can cause a potentially fatal serotonergic syndrome of hyperthermia and cardiovascular collapse.

Adverse effects: The side effect profile of SSRIs is much better than that of TCAs and MAOIs as there are no amine interactions, anticholinergic actions, adrenergic blockade, or toxic effects in overdose. Adverse effects, however, caused by their effect on serotonergic nerves throughout the body, include nausea, diarrhoea, insomnia, anxiety,

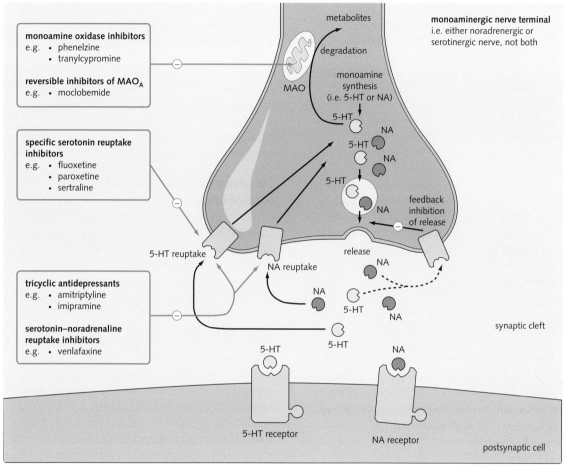

Fig. 6.8 Site of action of the major classes of drug used to treat unipolar depression. (5-HT, 5-hydroxytryptamine (serotonin); MAO, monoamine oxidase; NA, noradrenaline.)

and agitation. Sexual dysfunction is sometimes a problem.

Therapeutic notes: SSRIs have a similar efficacy to that of TCAs. It is their clinical advantages and lack of side effects that have led to their popularity. These include no anticholinergic effects, no toxicity in overdose, and no cardiotoxic effects. SSRIs are now the most widely prescribed antidepressants.

Serotonin–noradrenaline reuptake inhibitors

The only drug currently in the serotonin–noradrenaline reuptake inhibitor (SNRIs) new class of antidepressants is venlafaxine.

Mechanism of action: SNRIs cause potentiation of neurotransmitter activity in the CNS, probably by inhibiting reuptake of both serotonin and noradrenaline (Fig. 6.8).

Contraindications: The drug interactions of SNRIs are much like those of SSRIs; however, extra care must be taken with hypertensive patients as venlafaxine raises blood pressure.

Adverse effects: The adverse effects of SNRIs are similar to those of SSRIs, but they occur with lower frequency.

Therapeutic notes: The pharmacological effects of venlafaxine are similar to those of the TCAs, but adverse effects are reduced because it has little affinity for cholinergic and histaminergic receptors or α-adrenoreceptors.

Monoamine oxidase inhibitors

Examples of irreversible monoamine oxidase inhibitors (MAOIs) include phenelzine, tranylcypromine, and isocarboxazid, and examples of reversible inhibitors of MAO_A (RIMAs) include moclobemide.

Mechanism of action: MAOIs block the action of MAO_A and MAO_B, which are neuron enzymes that metabolize (degrade) the monoamines (noradrenaline, 5-HT, and dopamine) (Fig. 6.8). MAO has two main isoforms, MAO_A and MAO_B, which differ in terms of substrate preference; inhibition of the MAO_A form correlates best with antidepressant efficacy. Both non-selective irreversible blockers of MAO_A and MAO_B, and drugs that reversibly inhibit MAO_A are available.

Adverse effects: Dietary interactions may occur, such as the 'cheese reaction'. MAO in the gut wall and liver normally breaks down ingested tyramine. When the enzyme is inhibited, tyramine reaches the circulation and this causes the release of noradrenaline from sympathetic nerve terminals; this can lead to a severe and potentially fatal rise in blood pressure. Patients on MAOIs must, therefore, avoid foods rich in tyramine, which include cheese, game, and alcoholic drinks. Preparations containing sympathomimetic amines (e.g. cough mixtures and nasal decongestants) should also be avoided. MAOIs are not specific, and they reduce the metabolism of barbiturates, opioids, and alcohol. Side effects include CNS stimulation causing excitement and tremor, sympathetic blockade causing postural hypotension, and muscarinic blockade causing a dry mouth and blurred vision. Phenelzine can be hepatotoxic.

Therapeutic notes: Response to treatment with MAOIs may be delayed for 3 weeks or more. Phobic and depressed patients with atypical, hypochondriacal, or hysterical features are said to respond best to MAOIs. Because of the dietary and drug restrictions outlined above, MAOIs are largely reserved for depression refractory to other antidepressants and treatment.

Atypical antidepressants

Examples of atypical antidepressants include reboxetine and mirtazapine.

Mechanism of action: Reboxetine is a selective inhibitor of noradrenaline reuptake, increasing the concentration of this mediator in the synaptic cleft. Mirtazapine has α_2-adrenoreceptor-blocking activity, which, by acting on inhibitory α_2-autoreceptors on central noradrenergic nerve endings, may increase the amount of noradrenaline in the synaptic cleft.

Contraindications: The contraindications for atypical antidepressants are similar to those for TCAs.

Adverse effects: Atypical antidepressants generally cause less autonomic side effects and are less dangerous in overdose, owing to their lower cardiotoxicity compared with TCAs. Mirtazapine may cause agranulocytosis.

Therapeutic notes: Mirtazapine is sedative, and it is, therefore, used in depression when a degree of sedation is desirable. Neither reboxetine nor mirtazapine are currently first-line drugs for the treatment of depression.

Treatment of bipolar affective disorders

Bipolar affective disorder (BPAD) is treated with a combination of mood stabilizers and antidepressants, and sometimes antipsychotics (p. 102). Mood stabilizers include lithium and carbamazepine.

Lithium

Lithium is administered as lithium carbonate, and it is the most widely used mood stabilizer, with antimanic and antidepressant activity.

Mechanism of action: The mechanism of action of lithium is unclear, but it probably involves modulation of secondary-messenger pathways of cAMP and inositol triphosphate (IP_3). It is known that lithium inhibits the pathway for recapturing inositol for the resynthesis of polyphosphoinositides. It may exert its effect by reducing the concentrations of lipids important in secondary signal transduction in the brain.

Indications: Lithium salts are mainly used in the prophylaxis and treatment of BPAD, but also in the prophylaxis and treatment of acute mania and in the prophylaxis of resistant recurrent depression.

Contraindications: Some drugs may interact, causing a rise in plasma lithium concentration and so should be avoided. Such drugs include antipsychotics, non-steroidal anti-inflammatory drugs (NSAIDs), diuretics, and cardioactive drugs. Lithium is excreted via the kidney, and caution should be employed in patients with renal impairment.

Adverse effects: Lithium has a long plasma half-life and a narrow therapeutic window; therefore, side effects are common and plasma concentration monitoring is essential. Early side effects include thirst, nausea, diarrhoea, tremor, and polyuria; late side effects include weight gain, oedema, acne, nephrogenic diabetes insipidus, and hypothyroidism. Toxicity/overdose (serum level >2–3 mmol/L) effects include vomiting, diarrhoea, tremor, ataxia, confusion, and coma.

Therapeutic notes: The decision to give prophylactic lithium requires specialist advice, and careful monitoring after initiation of treatment is essential.

Carbamazepine
Carbamazepine is as effective as lithium in the prophylaxis of BPAD and acute mania, particularly in rapidly alternating BPAD.

Mechanism of action: Carbamazepine is a GABA agonist, and this may be the basis of its antimanic properties. The relevance of its effect in stabilizing neuronal sodium, and on calcium channels, is unclear.

Adverse effects: Drowsiness, diplopia, nausea, ataxia, rashes, and headache; blood disorders such as agranulocytosis and leucopenia; and drug interactions with lithium, antipsychotics, TCAs, and MAOIs. Many other drugs can be affected by the effect of carbamazepine on inducing hepatic enzymes. Diplopia, ataxia, clonus, tremor, and sedation are associated with acute carbamazepine toxicity.

Therapeutic notes: At the start of treatment with carbamazepine, plasma concentrations should be monitored to establish a maintenance dose.

Mania hardly ever exists in isolation from depression, which is why it is referred to as bipolar affective disorder, as it has two faces.

Psychotic disorders

Basic concepts
Psychotic disorders are characterized by a mental state that is out of touch with reality, involving a variety of abnormalities of perception, thought, and ideas.
Psychotic illnesses include:
- Schizophrenia.
- Schizoaffective disorder.
- Delusional disorders.
- Some depressive and manic illnesses.

Schizophrenia is the most important of these psychotic illnesses, because of its prevalence, young age of onset, and chronic and disabling nature.

Neuroleptics, or antipsychotics, are drugs used in the treatment of psychotic disorders.

Schizophrenia
Epidemiology
Schizophrenia characteristically develops in people aged 15–45 years; it has a relatively stable cross-cultural incidence affecting 1% of the population; 64% of cases are male.

Symptoms and signs
Schizophrenia is a psychotic illness characterized by multiple symptoms affecting thought, perceptions, emotion, and volition.

Symptoms fall into two groups (positive and negative) that may have different underlying causes.
Positive symptoms include:
- Delusions, which are false personal beliefs held with absolute conviction.
- Hallucinations, which are false perceptions in the absence of a real external stimulus; most commonly, these are auditory (hearing voices) and occur in 60–70% of schizophrenics, but they can be visual, tactile, or olfactory.
- Thought alienation and disordered thought, which is the belief that one's thoughts are under the control of an outside agency (e.g. aliens, MI5). This type of belief is common, and thought processes are often incomprehensible.

Negative symptoms include:
- Poverty of speech, which is a restriction in the amount of spontaneous speech.
- Flattening of affect, which is a loss of normal experience and expression of emotion.
- Social withdrawal.
- Anhedonia, which is an inability to experience pleasure.
- Apathy, involving reduced drive, energy, and interest.
- Attention deficit, manifested by inattentiveness at work or on interview.

The distinction between the positive and negative symptoms found in schizophrenia is of importance as neuroleptic drugs tend to have most effect on positive symptoms, while negative symptoms are fairly refractory to treatment and carry a worse prognosis.

Theories of schizophrenia
The cause of schizophrenia remains mysterious. Any theory of the cause of schizophrenia must take into

account the strong, though not invariable, hereditary tendency (50% concurrence in monozygotic twins), as well as the environmental factors known to predispose towards its development.

Many hypotheses have been suggested to explain the manifestations of schizophrenia at the level of neurotransmitters in the brain. The potential role of excessive dopaminergic activity, in particular, has attracted considerable attention. Evidence for this theory includes the following:

- Most antipsychotic drugs block dopamine receptors, the clinical dose being proportional to the ability to block D_2 receptors.
- Single positive electron tomography ligand scans show that there are increased D_2 receptors in the nucleus accumbens of schizophrenic patients.
- Psychotic symptoms can be induced by drugs that increase dopaminergic activity, such as some of the anti-parkinsonian agents.

However, there is much evidence that the dopaminergic theory fails to explain. Current research indicates a likely role for other neurotransmitters in schizophrenia, including 5-HT, GABA, and glutamate. Although the dopamine theory cannot explain many of the features and findings in schizophrenia, most current pharmacological treatment (typical neuroleptics) is aimed at dopaminergic transmission (Fig. 6.9).

Neuroleptic drugs

The treatment of schizophrenia and all other psychotic illnesses involves the use of antipsychotic medication, the neuroleptic drugs. Neuroleptic drugs produce a general improvement in all the acute positive symptoms of schizophrenia, but it is less clear how effective they are in the treatment of chronic schizophrenia and negative symptoms.

Mechanism of action: Antipsychotic drugs have a variety of structures and fall into various classes (Fig. 6.10). There is a strong correlation between clinical potency and affinity for D_2 receptors among the typical neuroleptics.

Neuroleptics take days or weeks to work, suggesting that secondary effects (e.g. increase in number of D_2 receptors in limbic structure) may be more important than a direct effect of D_2 receptor block. It was once thought, therefore, that neuroleptics exerted their antipsychotic effect by interfering with dopamine transmission at D_2 receptors in the mesocortical and mesolimbic systems. The development of newer atypical

Dopamine receptors		
Type	**2nd messengers + cellular effects**	**Location in CNS and postulated function**
D_1	cAMP increase	• Mainly postsynaptic inhibition • Functions unclear
D_2	cAMP decrease K^+ conductance up Ca^{2+} conductance down	• Mainly presynaptic inhibition of dopamine synthesis/release in nigrostriatal, mesolimbic, and tuberoinfundibular systems • Affinity of neuroleptics for D_2 receptors correlates with antipsychotic potency
D_3	Unknown	• Localized mainly in limbic and cortical structures concerned with cognitive functions and emotional behaviour • Not clear whether antipsychotic effects of neuroleptics are mediated by the D_3 type
D_4	Unknown	• Similar to D_3 type; clozapine has particular affinity for D_4 receptors

Fig. 6.9 Classes of dopamine receptor. (CNS, central nervous system.)

neuroleptics that are not very active at the D_2 receptor but which are still clinically effective has challenged this hypothesis.

Most neuroleptics also block other monoamine receptors, and this is often the cause of some of the side effects of these drugs.

The distinction between typical and atypical groups is not clearly defined, but it rests partly on the incidence of extrapyramidal motor side effects and partly on receptor specificity. Atypical neuroleptics are less prone to producing motor disorders than other drugs, and they tend to have different pharmacological profiles with respect to dopamine and other receptor specificity.

Route of administration: All the neuroleptic drugs can be given orally, though some of the typical drugs can be given by the intramuscular route, which prolongs their release, and aids drug compliance.

Typical neuroleptics
Phenothiazines

This class of compounds is subdivided into three groups by the type of side chain attached to the mother structure (phenothiazine ring) (Fig. 6.10). Side-effect patterns vary with the different side chains:

- Propylamine side chains, e.g. in chlorpromazine, produce strong sedation, a moderate muscarinic

Neuroleptic drugs		
Class	**Chemical classification**	**Examples**
Typical anti-psychotics	Phenothiazines: • propylamine side chains • piperidine side chains • piperazine side chains	Chlorpromazine Thioridazine Fluphenazine
	Butyrophenones	Haloperidol
	Thioxanthines	Flupentixol
Atypical anti-psychotics	Dibenzodiazepines	Clozapine, olanzapine
	Dopamine/5-HT blockers: • diphenylbutylpiperidines • substituted benzamides • benzixasoles	Pimozide Sulpiride Risperidone

Fig. 6.10 Classes of neuroleptic drugs. (5-HT, 5-hydroxytryptamine.)

block, and moderate motor disturbance. Indicated for violent patients, owing to their sedative effect.
• Piperidine side chains, e.g. in thioridazine, produce moderate sedation, strong muscarinic block, and low motor disturbance. Favoured for use in the elderly.
• Piperazine side chains, e.g. in fluphenazine, produce low sedation, low muscarinic block, and strong motor disturbance. Contraindicated for use in the elderly, owing to the motor effects.

Butyrophenones and thioxanthenes

The butyrophenone and thioxanthene groups of compounds have the same profile of low sedation, low muscarinic block, and high incidence of motor disturbance.

An example of a butyrophenone compound is haloperidol; flupentixol is an example of the thioxanthenes.

Atypical neuroleptics
Dibenzodiazepines

Dibenzodiazepines such as clozapine and olanzapine have a low affinity for the D_2 receptor and a higher affinity for D_1 and D_4 receptors.
Indications: In the UK and US, atypical neuroleptics are indicated only in chronic cases refractory to other drugs, or with severe motor disturbance. This is because of a 1% risk of potentially fatal neutropenia in those patients on these agents.
Adverse effects: Clozapine has a low incidence of adverse motor effects because of its low affinity for the D_2 receptor. Side effects of dibenzodiazepines

include hypersalivation, sedation, weight gain, tachycardia, and hypotension.
Therapeutic notes: Olanzapine is similar to clozapine, though carries less risk of agranulocytosis.

Dopamine/5-HT blockers

Examples of dopamine/5-HT blockers include the diphenylbutylpiperidines and the benzixasoles. Examples of the former include pimozide and substituted benzamides (e.g. sulpiride); examples of the latter include risperidone.

Sulpiride, and the newer agent pimozide, show high selectivity for D_2 receptors compared with D_1 or other neurotransmitter receptors. Both drugs are effective in treating schizophrenia but, sulpiride is claimed to have less tendency to cause adverse motor effects. Pimozide appears to be similar to conventional neuroleptic agents, but it has a longer duration of action, allowing once-daily medication.

Benzixasoles such as risperidone show a high affinity for 5-HT receptors and a lower affinity for D_2 receptors. With this class of drugs, extrapyramidal motor side effects occur with less frequency than with 'classic' neuroleptics.

Adverse effects of neuroleptics

Neuroleptic drugs cause a variety of adverse effects (Fig. 6.11).

The majority of the unwanted effects of neuroleptics can be inferred from their pharmacological actions, such as the disruption of dopaminergic pathways (the major action of most neuroleptics) and the blockade of monoamine and other receptors, including muscarinic receptors, α-adrenoreceptors, and histamine receptors.

Adverse effects of neuroleptics
• Acute neurological effects: acute dystonia, akathisia, parkinsonism • Chronic neurological effects: tardive dyskinesia, tardive dystonia • Neuroendocrine effects: amenorrhoea, galactorrhoea, infertility • Idiosyncratic: neuroleptic malignant syndrome • Anticholinergic: dry mouth, blurred vision, constipation, urinary retention, ejaculatory failure • Antihistaminergic: sedation • Antiadrenergic: hypotension, arrhythmia • Miscellaneous: photosensitivity, heat sensitivity, cholestatic jaundice, retinal pigmentation

Fig. 6.11 Adverse effects of the neuroleptics. (Redrawn from Page et al, 2002.)

In addition, individual drugs may cause immunological reactions or have their own characteristic side-effect profile.

Adverse effects on the dopaminergic pathways

There are three main dopaminergic pathways in the brain (Fig. 6.12):

- Mesolimbic and/or mesocortical dopamine pathways running from groups of cells in the midbrain to the nucleus accumbens and amygdala. This pathway affects thoughts and motivation.
- Nigrostriatal dopamine pathways running from the midbrain to the caudate nuclei. This pathway is important in smooth motor control.

- Tuberoinfundibular neurons running from the hypothalamus to the pituitary gland, the secretions of which they regulate.

Antagonism of dopamine receptors leads to interference with the normal functioning of these pathways, brining about unwanted side effects as well as the desired antipsychotic effect. This antagonism is the cause of the most serious side effects associated with neuroleptic use, which include:

- Psychological effects due to D_2 receptor blockade of the mesolimbic/mesocortical pathway.
- Movement disorders due to D_2 receptor blockade of the nigrostriatal pathways.

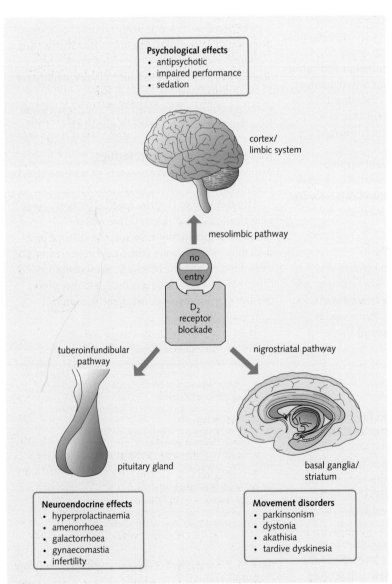

Fig. 6.12 Effect of D_2 dopamine receptor blockade on the dopaminergic pathways in the brain.

Psychological effects
- antipsychotic
- impaired performance
- sedation

cortex/limbic system

mesolimbic pathway

no entry

D_2 receptor blockade

tuberoinfundibular pathway

nigrostriatal pathway

pituitary gland

basal ganglia/striatum

Neuroendocrine effects
- hyperprolactinaemia
- amenorrhoea
- galactorrhoea
- gynaecomastia
- infertility

Movement disorders
- parkinsonism
- dystonia
- akathisia
- tardive dyskinesia

- Neuroendocrine disorders due to D_2 receptor blockade of the tuberoinfundibular pathway.

It is by dopaminergic antagonism of the mesolimbic mesocortical pathway that it is thought that typical neuroleptics exert their antipsychotic effects. However, as a side effect of mesolimbic and mesocortical dopaminergic inhibition, sedation and impaired performance are common.

Blocking of dopamine receptors in the basal ganglia (corpus striatum) frequently results in distressing and disabling movement disorders. Two main types of movement disorder occur. Acute reversible parkinsonian-like symptoms (tremor, rigidity, and akinesia) are treated by dose reduction, anticholinergic drugs, or switching to an atypical neuroleptic. Slowly developing tardive dyskinesia, often irreversible, and manifesting as involuntary movements of the face, trunk, and limbs, appears months or years after the start of neuroleptic treatment. It may be a result of proliferation or sensitization of dopamine receptors. Incidence is unpredictable, and it affects approximatley 20% of long-term users of neuroleptics. Treatment is generally unsuccessful. The newer atypical neuroleptics may be less likely to induce tardive dyskinesia.

By reducing the negative feedback on the anterior pituitary, over-secretion of prolactin can result (hyperprolactinaemia). This can lead to gynaecomastia, galactorrhoea, menstrual irregularities, impotence, and weight gain in some patients (Fig. 6.12).

Adverse effects from non-selective receptor blockade

The adverse effects of neuroleptics from non-selective receptor blockade include:

- Anticholinergic effects due to muscarinic-receptor blockade, such as dry mouth, urinary retention, constipation, blurred vision, etc.
- Adverse effects due to α-adrenoreceptor blockade. Many neuroleptics have the capacity to block α-adrenoreceptors and cause postural hypotension.
- Adverse effects due to histamine-receptor blockade. Antagonism of central histamine H_1 receptors may contribute to sedation.

Adverse effects due to individual drugs or immune reactions

The neuroleptic drug clozapine can cause neutropenia due to toxic bone marrow suppression, while pimozide can cause sudden death secondary to cardiac arrhythmia.

Immune reactions to neuroleptic drugs can include dermatitis, rashes, photosensitivity, and urticaria. Such reactions are more common with the phenothiazines, which can also cause deposits in the cornea and lens.

Neuroleptic malignant syndrome:

Neuroleptic malignant syndrome is the most lethal adverse effect of neuroleptic use. It is an idiosyncratic reaction of unknown pathophysiology. Symptoms include fever, extrapyramidal motor disturbance, muscle rigidity, and coma. Urgent treatment is indicated.

Neuroleptics have many side effects, some related to their principal mechanism of action (dopamine receptor antagonism) and some unrelated to this. Learn these well as they are a popular examination topic.

Nausea and vertigo

Nausea and vertigo are common clinical problems, and they may represent a whole array of pathologies. The use of antiemetic drugs can be very effective at alleviating these symptoms, though caution must be taken to ensure the underlying mechanism for the symptoms is investigated.

Antiemetic drugs are discussed in the gastrointestinal chapter (Ch. 10, p. 173).

Epilepsy

Definitions

Epilepsy is a chronic disease, in which seizures result from the abnormal discharge of cerebral neurons.

A seizure is a particular behaviour produced by an abnormal high-frequency discharge of a group of neurons, starting focally and spreading to a varying extent to affect other parts of the brain. According to the focus and spread of discharges, seizures may be classified as:

- Partial (focal), which originate at a specific focus and do not spread to involve other cortical areas.

- Generalized, which usually have a focus (often in the temporal lobe) and then spread to other areas.

Different epileptic syndromes can be classified on the basis of seizure type and pattern, with other clinical features (such as age of onset), anatomical location of focus, and aetiology taken into account.

Common types of epileptic syndromes

Epileptic syndromes result from either generalized seizures or focal seizures (Fig. 6.13).

Generalized seizure involves loss of consciousness, and it may be convulsive or non-convulsive:
- Tonic–clonic or grand-mal epilepsy, is a convulsive generalized seizure characterized by periods of tonic muscle rigidity followed later by massive jerking of the body (clonus).
- Absence, or petit-mal, seizures are generalized seizures characterized by changes in consciousness lasting less than 10 seconds. They occur most commonly in children, where they can be confused with day-dreaming.

The effect on the body of focal seizures depends on the location of the abnormal signal focus: e.g. involvement of the motor cortex will produce convulsions whereas involvement of the brainstem can produce unconsciousness. Psychomotor or temporal lobe epilepsy results from a partial seizure with cortical activity localized to the temporal lobe. Such seizures are characterized by features including impaired consciousness or confusion, amnesia, emotional instability, atypical behaviour, and outbursts.

Partial motor seizures have their focus in cortical motor regions and they present with convulsive or tonic activity corresponding to the neurons involved, e.g. the left arm.

Another type of epileptic syndrome is status epilepticus. This is a state in which fits follow each other without consciousness being regained. Status epilepticus constitutes a medical emergency because of possible exhaustion of vital centres.

Causes of epilepsy

The aetiology of epilepsy is unknown in 60–70% of cases, but heredity is an important factor.

Damage to the brain—for example, by tumours, head injury, infections, or cerebrovascular accident—may subsequently cause epilepsy.

The neurochemical basis of the abnormal discharges in epilepsy are not known, but it may involve altered GABA metabolism.

Treatment of epilepsy

Drugs used to treat epilepsy are termed antiepileptics; the term anticonvulsant is also used.

The aim of pharmacological treatment of epilepsy is to minimize seizure activity/frequency, without producing adverse drug effects.

Mechanisms of action of antiepileptics

Antiepileptic drugs act generically to inhibit the rapid, repetitive neuronal firing that characterizes seizures. There are three established mechanisms of action by which the antiepileptic drugs achieve this (Fig. 6.14).

Inhibition of ionic channels involved in neuronal excitability

Drugs such as phenytoin, carbamazepine, and valproate inhibit the 'fast' sodium current. These drugs bind preferentially to inactivated (closed) sodium channels, preventing them from opening. The high-frequency repetitive depolarization of neurons during a seizure increases the proportion of sodium channels in the inactivated state susceptible to blockade. Eventually, sufficient sodium channels become blocked so that the 'fast' neuronal sodium current is insufficient to cause a depolarization. Note that neuronal transmission at normal frequencies is relatively unaffected because a much smaller proportion of the sodium channels are in the inactivated state.

Ethosuximide inhibits 'T-type' low-threshold, fast-inactivating calcium. Absence seizures involve oscillatory neuronal activity between the thalamus and the cerebral cortex. The oscillation involves 'T-type' calcium channels, which produce low-threshold spikes, thus allowing groups of cells to fire in bursts. It appears that the anti-absence drug ethosuximide reduces this fast-inactivating calcium current, dampening the thalamocortical oscillations

Classification of common epileptic syndromes	
Partial (local, focal) seizures	**Generalized seizures**
• Psychomotor (temporal lobe) epilepsy	• Tonic–clonic seizure or grand-mal epilepsy
• Partial motor epilepsy	• Absence seizure or petit-mal epilepsy

Fig. 6.13 Classification of common epileptic syndromes.

Fig. 6.14 Mechanism and site of action of antiepileptic drugs. (BARB, barbiturates; GABA, γ-aminobutyric acid; GAD, glutamic acid decarboxylase; Glu, glutamate.)

that are critical in the generation of such absence seizures.

Inhibition of excitatory transmission

Drugs that block excitatory amino acid receptors (*N*-methyl-D-aspartate (NMDA) antagonists) have been shown to be antiepileptic in animal models. Such drugs may prove useful in the clinical treatment of epilepsy in the future. Lamotrigine, one of the newer antiepileptic agents, inhibits the release of glutamate as one of its actions, and this may contribute to its antiepileptic activity.

Enhancement of GABA-mediated inhibition

This can take any of the following forms:

- Enhancement by direct GABA agonist properties, e.g. by gabapentin, another of the newer antiepileptics, agent which has been designed to mimic GABA in the CNS.
- Potentiation of chloride currents through the $GABA_A/Cl^-$ channel complex, e.g. by benzodiazepines and barbiturates. The increased postsynaptic inhibitory chloride current at $GABA_A$ receptors, hyperpolarizes neurons and makes them refractory to excitation (Fig. 6.4).
- Inhibition of GABA degradation in the CNS, e.g. by vigabatrin, which is an irreversible inhibitor of GABA transaminase ($GABA_T$), the enzyme normally responsible for metabolism of GABA in the neuron. Inhibition of $GABA_T$, therefore, leads to an increase in synaptic levels of GABA and so enhances GABA-mediated inhibition.

 Remember that epilepsy is simply aberrant electrical activity spreading throughout an area of, or the whole of, the brain. Antiepileptic medications limit the propagation of this spread, and inhibit symptoms developing.

Antiepileptic drugs (anticonvulsants)

Antiepileptic drugs can be classified according to their mechanism of action, but in clinical practice it is useful to think of the drugs according to their use (Figs 6.14 and 6.15).

Phenytoin

Mechanism of action: This involves use-dependent block of voltage-gated sodium channels.

Drugs used for epilepsy classified by clinical use		
Seizure type	**Primary drugs**	**Secondary drugs**
Partial and/or generalized tonic–clonic seizures	• Sodium valproate • Carbamazepine	• Phenytoin • Vigabatrin • Gabapentin • Lamotrigine • Phenobarbital
Absence seizures	• Ethosuximide • Sodium valproate	• Phenobarbital • Lamotrigine
Status epilepticus	• Lorazepam	• Diazepam • Clonazepam

Fig. 6.15 Drugs used for epilepsy, classified by clinical use.

Phenytoin reduces the spread of a seizure. Electroencephalographic (EEG) recordings show that phenytoin does not stop the 'spiking' at a focus (i.e. it does not prevent the ignition of an epileptic discharge), but it does stop it spreading and causing overt clinical symptoms.

Route of administration: Oral, intravenous.

Indications: Phenytoin is indicated in all forms of epilepsy except absence seizures. Neuralgic pain (p. 66).

Contraindications: Phenytoin has many contraindications, mainly because it induces the hepatic cytochrome P_{450} oxidase system, increasing the metabolism of oral contraceptives, anticoagulants, dexamethasone, and pethidine.

Adverse effects: The adverse effects of phenytoin may be dosage- or non-dosage-related. The dosage-related effects of phenytoin affect the cerebellovestibular system, leading to ataxia, blurred vision, and hyperactivity. Acute toxicity causes sedation and confusion. The non-dosage-related effects include collagen effects such as gum hypertrophy and coarsening of facial features; allergic reactions, e.g. rash, hepatitis, and lymphadenopathy; haematological effects, e.g. megaloblastic anaemia; endocrine effects, e.g. hirsutism (hair growth); and teratogenic effects (it may cause congenital malformations).

Therapeutic notes: The use of phenytoin is complicated by its zero-order pharmacokinetics, characteristic toxicities, and necessity for long-term administration. Phenytoin has a narrow therapeutic index, and the relationship between dose and plasma concentration is non-linear. This is because phenytoin is metabolized by a hepatic enzyme system that is saturated at therapeutic levels. Small dosage increases may, therefore, produce large rises in plasma concentrations with acute side effects. Monitoring of plasma concentration greatly assists dosage adjustment. Because of its adverse effects and narrow therapeutic window, phenytoin is no longer a first-line treatment for any of the seizure syndromes.

Sodium valproate

Mechanism of action: Sodium valproate has two mechanisms of action: like phenytoin, it causes use-dependent block of voltage-gated sodium channels; it also increases the GABA content of the brain when given over a prolonged period.

Route of administration: Oral, intravenous.

Indications: Sodium valproate is useful in all forms of epilepsy.

Contraindications: Sodium valproate should not be given to people with acute liver disease or a history of hepatic dysfunction.

Adverse effects: Sodium valproate has many fewer side effects than other antiepileptics; the main problems are gastrointestinal upset and, more importantly, liver failure. Hepatic toxicity appears to be more common when sodium valproate is used in combination with other antiepileptics.

Therapeutic notes: Sodium valproate is well absorbed orally and has a half-life of 10–15 hours. Sodium valproate is now the first line drug for most types of seizure syndromes.

Carbamazepine

Mechanism of action: Like phenytoin, carbamazepine causes use-dependent block of voltage-gated sodium channels.

Route of administration: Oral, rectal.

Indications: Carbamazepine can be used in all forms of epilepsy except absence seizures. Neuralgic pain (p. 66).

Contraindications: Like phenytoin, carbamazepine is a strong enzyme inducer and so causes similar drug interactions.

Adverse effects: The adverse effects of carbamazepine are really limited to the nervous system—ataxia, nystagmus, dysarthria, vertigo, and sedation.

Therapeutic notes: Carbamazepine is well absorbed orally with a long half-life (25–60 hours) when first given. Enzyme induction subsequently reduces this half-life.

Ethosuximide

Mechanism of action: Ethosuximide exerts its effects by inhibition of low-threshold calcium currents ('T-currents').

Route of administration: Oral.

Indications: Ethosuximide is the drug of choice in simple absence seizures and is particularly well-tolerated in children.

Contraindications: Ethosuximide may make tonic–clonic attacks worse.

Adverse effects: The adverse effects of ethosuximide include gastrointestinal upset, drowsiness, mood swings, and skin rashes. Rarely, it causes serious bone marrow depression.

Vigabatrin

Mechanism of action: Vigabatrin exerts its effects by irreversible inhibition of GABA transaminase.

Route of administration: Oral.

Indications: Vigabatrin is indicated in epilepsy not satisfactorily controlled by other drugs.

Contraindications: Vigabatrin should not be used in people with a history of psychosis because of the side effect of hallucinations.

Adverse effects: Drowsiness, dizziness, depression, and visual hallucinations.

Therapeutic notes: Vigabatrin is a new drug, used as an adjunct to other therapies.

Lamotrigine

Mechanism of action: Lamotrigine appears to act via an effect on sodium channels, and inhibiting the release of excitatory amino acids.

Route of administration: Oral.

Indications: Monotherapy and adjunctive treatment of partial seizures and generalized tonic–clonic seizures. Neuralgic pain (p. 66).

Contraindications: Hepatic impairment.

Adverse effects: Rashes, fever, malaise, drowsiness, and, rarely, hepatic dysfunction.

Therapeutic notes: Lamotrigine is one of the newer classes of antiepileptic agents, and its use in practice is gradually increasing.

Gabapentin

Mechanism of action: Gabapentin is a lipophilic drug that was designed to act like GABA in the CNS (agonist), though it does not appear to have GABA-mimetic actions. Its mechanism of action remains elusive.

Route of administration: Oral.

Indications: As an adjunct to therapy in partial epilepsy with or without secondary generalization.

Contraindications: Caution to avoid sudden withdrawal, in the elderly and in those with renal impairment.

Adverse effects: Somnolence, dizziness, ataxia, fatigue, and, rarely, cerebellar signs.

Therapeutic notes: Like lamotrigine, gabapentin is a relatively new drug, and it is not as widely used as other, more traditional agents.

Barbiturates

Examples of barbiturates include phenobarbital and primidone.

Mechanism of action: Barbiturates cause potentiation of chloride currents through the $GABA_A/Cl^-$ channel complex.

Route of administration: Oral, intravenous.

Indications: Barbiturates are used in all forms of epilepsy, including status epilepticus.

Contraindications: Barbiturates should not be used in children, the elderly, and people with respiratory depression.

Adverse effects: The main side effect of barbiturates is sedation, which limits their use clinically, along with the danger of potentially fatal CNS depression in overdose. Phenobarbital is a good inducer of cytochrome P_{450}, and so it can be involved in drug interactions.

Therapeutic notes: Only the long-acting barbiturates are antiepileptic. Phenobarbital has a plasma half-life of 10 hours. The strong sedating nature of these drugs now limits their use in the management of epilepsy.

Benzodiazepines

Examples of benzodiazepines include clonazepam and clobazam.

Mechanism of action: Benzodiazepines cause potentiation of chloride currents through the $GABA_A/Cl^-$ channel complex (Fig. 6.4).

Route of administration: Oral, intravenously.

Indications: Clonazepam is useful for tonic–clonic and partial seizures. Lorazepam and diazepam are effective in the management of status epilepticus.

Contraindications: Benzodiazepines should not be used in people with respiratory depression.

Adverse effects: The most common adverse effect of the benzodiazepines is sedation. Intravenous lorazepam and diazepam can depress respiration.

Therapeutic notes: The repeated seizures of status epilepticus can damage the brain and be potentially life threatening, so they should be controlled by administration of intravenous diazepam. Lorazepam has a longer half-life than diazepam.

Other anticonvulsants

Other agents used as antiepileptics include levetiracetam, tiagabine, topiramate, acetazolamide, and piracetam. Their indications and side effect profiles can be obtained from the *British National Formulary* (BNF).

Status epilepticus

Intravenous benzodiazepines (lorazepam or diazepam) are first line drugs in status epilepticus. If these fail to bring an end to seizure activity, intravenous sodium valproate or phenytoin, or carbamazepine via a nasogastric tube should be attempted, ideally in an intensive care setting. Final options include intravenous clomethiazole (p. 96), and thiopental (p. 112).

General anaesthetics

Concepts of general anaesthesia

General anaesthesia is the absence of sensation associated with a reversible loss of consciousness.

General anaesthetics are used as an adjunct to surgical procedures in order to render the patient unaware of, and unresponsive to, painful stimuli. Modern anaesthesia is characterized by the so-called balanced technique, in which drugs and anaesthetic agents are used specifically to produce:

- Analgesia.
- Sleep/sedation.
- Muscle relaxation and abolition of reflexes.

No one drug or anaesthetic agent can produce all these effects, and so a combination of agents is used in the three clinical stages of surgical general anaesthesia. The three stages are:

- Premedication.
- Induction.
- Maintenance.

Some may argue that a fourth stage exists, in which drugs are used to reverse the action of agents given in the previous three stages.

Premedication

Premedication is often given on the ward before the patient is taken to the operating theatre (Fig. 6.16), and it has four component aims:

- Relief from anxiety.
- Reduction of parasympathetic bradycardia and secretions.
- Analgesia.
- Prevention of postoperative emesis.

Relief from anxiety

Oral benzodiazepines, e.g. diazepam and lorazepam (p. 93), are most effective and they perform three useful functions:

- To relieve apprehension and anxiety before anaesthesia.
- To lessen the amount of general anaesthetic required to achieve and to maintain unconsciousness.
- Possibly, to sedate postoperatively.

Reduction of parasympathetic bradycardia and secretions

Muscarinic antagonists, e.g. atropine and hyoscine (Ch. 5), are used to prevent salivation and bronchial secretions, and more importantly to protect the heart from arrhythmias, particularly bradycardia caused by some inhalation agents and neuromuscular blockers.

Analgesia

Opioid analgesics, e.g. fentanyl (Ch. 4), are often given prior to an operation: although the patient is unconscious during surgery, adequate analgesia is important to stop physiological stress reactions to pain. Non-steroidal anti-inflammatory drugs are useful alternatives and adjuncts to opiates, though are likely to be inadequate for severe postoperative pain used alone.

Postoperative antiemesis

Drugs that provide postoperative antiemesis include metoclopramide and prochlorperazine. Nausea and vomiting are common after general anaesthesia, often because of the administration of opioid drugs peri- and postoperatively. Antiemetic drugs can be given with the premedication to inhibit this.

Induction

Intravenous agents are used to produce a rapid induction of unconsciousness. Intravenous agents are preferred by patients, since injection lacks the menacing quality of having a mask placed over the face (Fig. 6.16).

Prevention of acid aspiration in emergency and obstetric operations is crucial, and it relies on the administration of either an H_2-receptor antagonist or a proton pump inhibitor prior to induction (Ch. 10).

Maintenance

Inhalation anaesthetic agents are used to maintain a state of general anaesthesia after induction in most patients, though intravenous agents can be used via a continuous pump (Fig. 6.16).

Anaesthetic agents

Anaesthetic agents depress all excitable tissues including central neurons, cardiac muscle, and smooth and striated muscle. Different parts of the CNS have different sensitivities to anaesthetics, and the reticular activating system, which is responsible for consciousness, is among the most sensitive. Hence, it is possible to use anaesthetics at a concentration that produces unconsciousness without unduly depressing the cardiovascular or respiratory centres of the brain, or the myocardium. However, for the majority of anaesthetics the margin of safety is small.

Intravenous anaesthetics

Intravenous anaesthetics, e.g. thiopental, propofol, and ketamine, are all CNS depressants. They produce anaesthesia by relatively selective depression of the reticular activating system of the brain. They may be used alone for short surgical procedures, but they are used mainly for the induction of anaesthesia, and, therefore, it is rapidity of onset that is the desirable feature.

Intravenous anaesthetics are all highly lipid-soluble agents and cross the blood–brain barrier

Fig. 6.16 General anaesthetic agents.

General anaesthetics		
Premedication	**Induction/ intravenous agents**	**Maintenance/ inhalation agents**
• Relief from anxiety e.g. diazepam, lorazepam • Reduction of parasympathetic bradycardia and secretions e.g. atropine, hyoscine • Analgesia e.g. NSAIDs, fentanyl • Postoperative antiemesis e.g. metoclopramide, prochlorperazine	• Barbiturates e.g. thiopental • Non-barbiturates e.g. propofol, ketamine	Nitrous oxide Halothane Enflurane Isoflurane

rapidly; their rapid onset (<30 seconds) results from this rapid transfer into the brain, and high cerebral blood flow. Duration of action is short (minutes) and terminated by redistribution of the drug from the CNS into less-well-perfused tissues (Fig. 6.17); drug metabolism is irrelevant to recovery.

Thiopental

Mechanism of action: Thiopental is a highly lipophilic member of the barbiturate group of CNS depressants that act to potentiate the inhibitory effect of GABA on the $GABA_A/Cl^-$ receptor channel complex.

Route of administration: Intravenous.

Indications: Rapid induction of general anaesthesia.

Contraindications: Thiopental should not be given to a patient with a previous allergy to it. Porphyria.

Adverse effects: Respiratory depression, myocardial depression (bradycardia), vasodilatation, and anaphylaxis. There is a risk of severe vasospasm if it is accidentally injected into an artery.

Therapeutic notes: Thiopental is a widely used induction agent, but it has no analgesic properties. It provides smooth and rapid (<30 seconds) induction but, owing to its narrow therapeutic margin, overdosage with consequent cardiorespiratory depression can occur. Thiopental is given as the

Fig. 6.17 Graph illustrating how redistribution of intravenous anaesthetic agents causes a short central duration of action. (Adapted from *Pharmacology* by H Rang, M Dale, J Ritter,1995. By permission of Churchill Livingstone.)

sodium salt, which is unstable in solution and so it must be made up immediately before use.

Propofol

Mechanism of action: Propofol is similar to thiopental in its mechanism of action.

Route of administration: Intravenous.

Indications: Rapid induction of general anaesthesia.

Contraindications: Propofol should not be given to patients with a previous allergy to it.

Adverse effects: Convulsions, anaphylaxis, and delayed recovery from anaesthesia have occasionally been reported as side effects.

Therapeutic notes: Propofol is associated with rapid recovery without nausea or hangover, and it is very widely used. Propofol is the drug of choice if an intravenous agent is to be used to maintain anaesthesia by a continuous infusion.

Etomidate

Mechanism of action: The mechanism of action of etomidate is similar to that of thiopental.

Route of administration: Intravenous.

Indications: Rapid induction of general anaesthesia.

Contraindications: Etomidate should not be given to patients with a previous allergy to it.

Adverse effects: Extraneous muscle movement and pain on injection, and possible adrenocortical suppression.

Therapeutic notes: Etomidate is an induction agent that gained favour over thiopental because of its larger therapeutic margin and faster metabolism leading to fewer hangover effects. Etomidate is more prone to causing extraneous muscle movement and pain on injection compared with other agents.

Ketamine

Mechanism of action: Ketamine produces full surgical anaesthesia but the form of the anaesthesia is known as dissociative anaesthesia, as the patient may remain conscious though amnesic and insensitive to pain. This effect is probably related to an action on NMDA-type glutamate receptors.

Ketamine is a derivative of the street drug phencyclidine (PCP/'angel dust').

Route of administration: Intravenous, intramuscular.

Indications: Ketamine is used in the induction and maintenance of anaesthesia, especially in children.

Contraindications: Ketamine should not be given to people with hypertension or psychosis.

Adverse effects: These include cardiovascular stimulation, tachycardia, and raised arterial blood pressure, as well as transient psychotic sequelae such as vivid dreams and hallucinations.

Therapeutic notes: Ketamine is not often used as an induction agent, owing to the high incidence of dysphoria and hallucinations during recovery in adults. These effects are much less marked in children, and ketamine, in conjunction with a benzodiazepine, is often used for minor procedures in paediatrics.

Like the benzodiazepines and the barbiturates, thiopental and propofol act via the GABA$_A$/Cl$^-$ receptor in causing CNS depression.

Inhalation anaesthetics

Examples of inhalation anaesthetics include halothane, enflurane, isoflurane, sevoflurane and desflurane. Nitrous oxide also has anaesthetic properties.

Inhalation anaesthetics may be gases or volatile liquids. They are commonly used for the maintenance of anaesthesia after induction with an intravenous agent.

Mechanism of action: It is not known exactly how inhalation anaesthetic agents produce their effects. Unlike most drugs, inhalation anaesthetics do not all belong to one recognizable chemical class. The shape and electronic configuration of the molecule are evidently unimportant. A distinct anaesthetic 'receptor' is, therefore, unlikely; it would seem that the pharmacological action of inhalation anaesthetics is dependent on the physicochemical properties of the molecule.

Three theories of anaesthesia have received the most attention—the lipid, hydrate, and protein theories.

The lipid theory arose because a close correlation was noticed between anaesthetic potency and lipid solubility. It has been suggested that anaesthetics dissolve in membrane lipid and affect its physical state by two possible mechanisms. These are:

- Volume expansion, which is supported by pressure reversal of anaesthesia, but qualitative inconsistencies exist.

- Membrane fluidization, although the high concentrations required and weak effect of temperature make this difficult to accept.

The hydrate theory arose because anaesthetic molecules stabilize water molecules in their vicinity. It has been suggested that this alteration of the membrane accounts for the effects of anaesthetics.

While there is some correlation between potency and the ability to form hydrates, anomalous compounds such as sulphur hexafluoride do not form hydrates, but they do have anaesthetic properties.

The protein theory arose because there is increasing evidence that anaesthetics may act by binding to discrete hydrophobic domains of membrane proteins. This would explain the 'cut-off' phenomenon and the stereoselectivity of anaesthetics. The protein theory is currently popular, but the nature of the target protein(s) in the CNS has not been identified. Possible targets include voltage-operated channels, receptor-operated channels, or secondary-messenger systems.

Pharmacokinetic aspects: The depth of anaesthesia produced by inhalation anaesthetics is directly related to the partial pressure (tension) of the agent in the arterial blood, as this determines the concentration of agent in the CNS. The concentration of anaesthetic in the blood is in turn determined by:

- The concentration of anaesthetic in the inspired gas (alveolar concentration).
- The solubility of the anaesthetic in blood (blood/gas partition coefficient).
- Cardiac output.
- Alveolar ventilation.

Rapid induction and recovery are important properties of an anaesthetic agent, allowing flexible control over the arterial tension (and hence brain tension) and, therefore, the depth of anaesthesia. The speed at which induction of anaesthesia occurs is determined by two properties of the anaesthetic: its solubility in blood (blood/gas partition coefficient) and its solubility in fat (lipid solubility). Therefore:

- Agents of low blood solubility (e.g. nitrous oxide, enflurane) produce rapid induction and recovery because relatively small amounts are required to saturate the blood, and so the arterial tension (and hence brain tension) rises and falls quickly (Fig. 6.18).
- Agents of high blood solubility (e.g. halothane) have much slower induction and recovery times

Fig. 6.18 Rate of equilibration of inhalation anaesthetics in humans. (*, blood gas coefficient—larger numbers indicate higher solubility and are associated with longer induction and recovery times.) (Adapted from *Uptake and Distribution of Anaesthetic Agents*, by EM Papper and R Kitz, McGraw Hill, 1963.)

because much more anaesthetic solution is required before the arterial anaesthetic tension approaches that of the inspired gas (Fig. 6.18).

- Agents with high lipid solubility (e.g. ether) accumulate gradually in the body fat during prolonged anaesthesia, and so may produce a prolonged hangover if used for a long operation (Fig. 6.18).

Nitrous oxide

Mechanism of action: See above.
Route of administration: Inhalation.
Indications: Nitrous oxide is used in the maintenance of anaesthesia (in combination with other agents), and for analgesia (50% mixture in oxygen: Entonox®).
Contraindications: Pneumothorax: nitrous oxide diffuses into air containing closed spaces resulting in an increased pressure, in the case of pneumothorax, this may compromise breathing.
Adverse effects: Nitrous oxide was thought to be relatively free of side effects—it has little effect on cardiovascular and respiratory systems—but the risk of bone marrow suppression is now a known factor.
Therapeutic notes: Nitrous oxide cannot produce surgical anaesthesia when administered alone, because of a lack of potency. It is commonly used as

a non-flammable carrier gas for volatile agents, allowing their concentration to be reduced. As a 50% mixture in oxygen, nitrous oxide is a good analgesic, and it is used in childbirth and by paramedics.

Halothane

Mechanism of action: See above.
Route of administration: Inhalation.
Indications: Halothane is used in the maintenance of anaesthesia.
Contraindications: Halothane should not be given to people with a previous reaction to halothane or exposure to halothane in the previous 3 months.
Adverse effects: Like most volatile anaesthetics, halothane causes cardiorespiratory depression. Respiratory depression results in elevated pCO_2 and perhaps ventricular arrhythmias. Halothane also depresses cardiac muscle fibres and may cause bradycardia. The result of this is a concentration-dependent hypotension.

The most significant toxic effect of halothane is severe hepatic necrosis, which occurs in 1 in 35 000 cases. Lesser degrees of liver damage may occur more frequently. The damage is caused by metabolites of the 20% of administered halothane that is biotransformed in the liver (80% of an administered dose is excreted by the lungs).
Therapeutic notes: Halothane is a halogenated hydrocarbon, and it is probably the most widely used inhalation agent.

Enflurane

Mechanism of action: See above.
Route of administration: Inhalation.
Indications: Enflurane is used in the maintenance of anaesthesia.
Contraindications: Enflurane should not be given to people with epilepsy.
Adverse effects: Enflurane causes cardiorespiratory depression similar to that with halothane, although the incidence of arrhythmias is much lower than with halothane.

Enflurane undergoes only 2% metabolism in the liver, so it is much less likely than halothane to cause hepatotoxicity. The disadvantage of enflurane is that it may cause electroencephalogram (EEG) changes and muscle twitching, and special caution is needed in epileptic subjects.
Therapeutic notes: Enflurane is a volatile anaesthetic similar to, but less potent than, halothane, about twice the concentration being necessary for

maintenance. Induction and recovery times are faster than for halothane.

Isoflurane

Mechanism of action: See above.

Route of administration: Inhalation.

Indications: It is used in the maintenance of anaesthesia.

Contraindications: Susceptibility to malignant hyperthermia.

Adverse effects: Isoflurane has actions similar to those of halothane, but it has less effects upon the cardiorespiratory system. Hypotension is caused by a dose-related decrease in systemic vascular resistance rather than a marked fall in cardiac output. Less hepatic metabolism (0.2%) occurs than with enflurane, so hepatotoxicity is even rarer.

Therapeutic notes: Isoflurane is an isomer of enflurane. It has a potency intermediate between that of halothane and enflurane.

Nitrous oxide is used as an adjunct to other inhaled anaesthetic agents, as it reduces the dose required to maintain a steady state of anaesthesia, thus limiting side effects, and allowing more rapid recovery.

Use of neuromuscular blockers in anaesthesia

For some operations, e.g. intra-abdominal, complete relaxation of skeletal muscle is essential. Some general anaesthetic agents have significant neuromuscular blocking actions, but drugs that specifically block the neuromuscular junction are frequently employed, e.g. suxamethonium, rocuronium, vecuronium, and atracurium (Ch. 5).

Drug misuse

Concepts of drug misuse

Historically there has been a long relationship between humans and the non-therapeutic use of drugs that act on the mind and body. Virtually all cultures have used drugs for non-therapeutic purposes: for instance, the Incas used psychoactive fungi and the ancient Egyptians (and many other cultures since) used alcohol.

It is important to realize that the misuse of drugs is a socially defined concept that has as much to do with the legal, religious, moral, and cultural framework of a society as the pharmacological properties of the drug itself. Drugs now banned in the UK, e.g. opium, were once popular and legal in nineteenth century England, while attitudes to alcohol vary both historically and geographically from total prohibition to deep entrenchment in the culture.

Humans show great ingenuity in creating, harvesting, obtaining, and taking drugs for non-therapeutic reasons, and they go to great lengths to do so. The sheer prevalence and associated co-morbidity makes drug misuse an important medical subject.

Definitions

Drug misuse

Drug misuse is defined as the use of drugs that causes actual physical or mental harm to an individual or to society, or that is illegal. Therefore, drug misuse includes alcohol, nicotine, and the damaging overprescription of tranquillizers, as well as the more obvious illicit drugs such as ecstasy or amphetamines.

The term 'drug abuse' is synonymous with 'drug misuse' but it is currently less in vogue owing to its negative connotations.

Drug dependence

Drug dependence is defined as the compulsion to take a drug repeatedly, with distress being caused if this is prevented.

Drugs of dependence all have rewarding effects (this is why they are taken), but they also have unpleasant (aversive) effects, often as the drug leaves the brain.

Dependence involves psychological factors as well as physical aspects. These are not exclusive and there is a mixture of both in most people who are dependent upon drugs.

Psychological dependence is when the rewarding effects (positive reinforcement) predominate to cause a compulsion to continue taking the drug.

Physical dependence is when the distress on stopping the drug (negative reinforcement) is the main reason for continuing to take it, i.e. avoidance of the 'withdrawal syndrome'.

Drug tolerance

Drug tolerance is the necessity to increase the dose of an administered drug progressively in order to maintain the effect that was produced by the (smaller) original doses. Drug tolerance is a phenomenon that develops with chronic administration of a drug.

Many different mechanisms can give rise to drug tolerance, though they are rather poorly understood. These include:

- Downregulation of receptors.
- Changes in receptors.
- Exhaustion of biological mediators or transmitters.
- Increased metabolic degradation (enzyme induction).
- Physiological adaptation.

Withdrawal

Withdrawal is the term used to describe the syndrome of effects caused by stopping administration of a drug. It results from the change of (neuro)physiological equilibrium induced by the presence of the drug (Fig. 6.19).

Legal aspects of drug misuse (UK)
Misuse of Drugs Act 1971

The Misuse of Drugs Act 1971 prohibits certain activities in relation to 'controlled drugs', in particular their manufacture, supply, and possession. The Act is primarily a legal document for use by the police and judiciary. The penalties applicable to offences involving the different drugs are graded broadly according to the harmfulness attributable to a drug when it is misused, and for this purpose the drugs are categorized into three classes (Fig. 6.20).

Misuse of Drugs Regulations 1985

The Misuse of Drugs Regulations 1985 are a set of working regulations that define the classes of persons who are authorized to supply and possess controlled drugs while acting in their professional capacities, and lay down the conditions under which these activities may be carried out.

In these regulations, drugs of addiction or high misuse potential are divided into five schedules, each specifying the requirements governing such aspects as import, export, production, supply, possession, prescription, and record keeping that apply to them (Fig. 6.21).

These regulations are more relevant than the 1971 Act to the clinical practice of health professionals (Fig. 6.21).

Classes of controlled drugs		
Class A drugs	**Class B drugs**	**Class C drugs**
Cocaine	Amphetamines	Benzodiazepines
MDMA ('ecstasy')	Cannabis	Androgenic and
Diamorphine (heroin)	Barbiturates	anabolic steroids
and other strong	Some weak	Human chorionic
opioids	opioids	gonadotrophin
Lysergic acid	Others	Others
diethylamide class B		
(LSD) substances		
when prepared for		
injection		
Others		

Fig. 6.20 Classes of controlled drugs. (MDMA, methylenedioxymethamfetamine.)

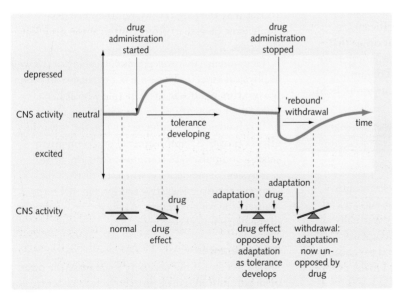

Fig. 6.19 Tolerance to, and withdrawal from central nervous system (CNS) depressant drugs, e.g. alcohol. The graph for tolerance of and withdrawal from CNS stimulant drugs, e.g. cocaine, would be a mirror image in the x-axis of what is shown.

Misuse of drugs regulations 1985	
Classification and example	**Controlled drug requirements**
Schedule 1 • drugs that have no medicinal use e.g. cannabis, LSD	Possession and supply prohibited without Home Office authority (given e.g. for research)
Schedule 2 • medicinal drugs with high misuse potential e.g. heroin, morphine, pethidine, cocaine	Drugs subject to full controlled drug requirements, e.g. special prescription requirements, safe custody, register keeping
Schedule 3 • medicinal drugs of lesser misuse potential e.g. minor stimulants, barbiturates, some analgesics	Drugs subject to some controlled drug requirements, e.g. special prescription requirements, but not safe custody or register keeping
Schedule 4 • mainly benzodiazepines with abuse potential e.g. benzodiazepines, anabolic steroids	Minimal requirements
Schedule 5 • high-strength preparations of non-controlled drugs	Virtually no controlled drug requirements other than the retention of invoices for 2 years

Fig. 6.21 Misuse of drugs regulations 1985. (LSD, lysergic acid diethylamide.)

Notification and Supply to Addicts Regulations 1973

The Notification and Supply to Addicts Regulations 1973 require that any doctor who attends to a person who he or she suspects is addicted to a notifiable drug is legally required to furnish details, in writing, of that person's particulars to the Chief Medical Officer. The idea of this is to maintain a confidential 'index of addicts' that can be checked, to safeguard against addicts obtaining supplies simultaneously from two or more doctors.

Drugs of misuse

Drugs with a high potential for misuse fall into many distinct pharmacological categories. They may or may not be used therapeutically, and they may be illegal or legal (Fig. 6.22).

Central stimulants
Amphetamines

Street names: Speed, Whizz, Billy, Uppers.
Mechanism of action: Amphetamines cause the release of monoamines and the inhibition of monoamine reuptake, especially of dopamine and noradrenaline in neurons.
Route of administration: Amphetamines are administered orally, or 'snorted' as a powder nasally; sometimes used intravenously.
Effects: The effects of amphetamines include the following: increased motor activity; euphoria and

Summary table of drugs with a high misuse potential	
Drug class	**Examples**
Central stimulants	Cocaine Amphetamines MDMA (ecstasy) Nicotine
Central depressants	Alcohol Benzodiazepines Barbiturates
Opioid analgesics	Morphine Heroin (diamorphine) Methadone
Cannabinoids	Cannabis Tetrahydrocannabinoids (THCs)
Hallucinogens	LSD Mescaline Psilocybin
Dissociative anaesthetics	Ketamine Phencyclidine

Fig. 6.22 Drugs with high potential for misuse. (LSD, lysergic acid diethylamide; MDMA, methylenedioxy-methamfetamine.)

excitement; anorexia and insomnia; peripheral sympathomimetic effects, such as hypertension and inhibition of gut motility; and stereotyped behaviour and psychosis, which develop with prolonged usage.
Clinical uses: The (very few) clinical uses of amphetamines are for narcolepsy and for

hyperkinesis in children. They are no longer recommended as appetite suppressants, owing to their adverse effects.

Tolerance, dependence, and withdrawal: Tolerance to the peripheral sympathomimetic stimulant effects of amphetamines develops rapidly, but it develops much more slowly to other effects such as locomotor stimulation. Amphetamines cause strong psychological dependence but no real physical dependence. After stopping chronic use, the individual will usually enter a deep, long sleep ('REM rebound') and awake feeling tired, depressed, and hungry. This state may reflect the depletion of the normal monoamine stores.

Adverse effects: Acute amphetamine toxicity causes cardiac arrhythmias, hypertension, and stroke. Chronic toxicity causes paranoid psychosis, vasoconstriction, tissue anoxia at sites of injection or snorting, and damage to the fetal brain *in utero*.

Try to use the correct chemical name when describing drugs of misuse, rather than a street name or personal favourite—i.e. amphetamines rather than Whizz or Speed—it tends to go down better with examiners!

Cocaine

Street names: Coke, Charlie, Snow, Crack (free base).

Mechanism of action: Cocaine strongly inhibits the reuptake of catecholamines at noradrenergic neurons, and thus strongly enhances sympathetic activity.

Route of administration: Cocaine hydrochloride is usually snorted nasally. 'Crack' is the free base, which is more volatile and which does not decompose on heating. It can, therefore, be smoked, producing a brief intense 'rush'.

Effects: The behavioural effects produced by cocaine are similar to those produced by amphetamines, such as euphoria. The euphoric effects may be greater, and there is less of a tendency for stereotypical behaviour and paranoid delusions.

The effects of cocaine hydrochloride (lasting about an hour) are not as long lasting as those of amphetamine, while those obtained from crack are brief (minutes).

Clinical uses: Cocaine is occasionally used as a topical anaesthetic by ear, nose, and throat specialists.

Tolerance, dependence, and withdrawal: Cocaine causes strong psychological dependence but no real physical dependence. Withdrawal causes a marked deterioration in motor performance, which is restorable on provision of the drug.

Adverse effects: Acute cocaine toxicity causes toxic psychosis, cardiac arrhythmias, hypertension, and stroke. Chronic toxicity causes paranoid psychosis, vasoconstriction, tissue anoxia at sites of injection or snorting, and damage to the fetal brain.

Methylenedioxymethamfetamine

Street names: Ecstasy, E, Disco Biscuits, Pills.

Mechanism of action:

Methylenedioxymethamfetamine (MDMA) is an amphetamine derivative that has a mechanism of action similar to that of amphetamines (release of monoamines, inhibition of monoamine reuptake). MDMA especially has actions on serotonergic neurons, potentiating 5-HT.

Route of administration: MDMA is usually taken as a pill containing other psychoactive drugs, such as amphetamine or ketamine.

Effects: MDMA has mixed stimulant and hallucinogenic properties, especially in its pure form. Euphoria, arousal, and perceptual disturbances are common. Uniquely, MDMA has the effect of creating a feeling of euphoric empathy, so that social barriers are reduced.

Clinical uses: MDMA has no clinical use. Trials have been licensed in the USA for its evaluation as a treatment for people with social avoidant personality disorders.

Tolerance, dependence, and withdrawal: It is not currently known to what extent tolerance and dependence occur with MDMA. The withdrawal syndrome is similar to that with amphetamines.

Adverse effects: The most serious acute consequences of acute MDMA toxicity appear to be hyperthermia, exhaustion, and dehydration caused indirectly by the repetitive locomotor behaviour induced (dancing!). Very rarely this results in fatality. Chronic MDMA toxicity causes neurodegeneration of serotonergic nerves in the brains of experimental primates. The correlation to humans is not known.

Nicotine

Nicotine is found in cigarettes, cigars, pipes, and chewing tobacco. Various therapeutic products are available which contain nicotine as part of nicotine replacement therapy for those wishing to withdraw from their nicotine addiction. These are discussed at the end of the chapter.

Mechanism of action: Nicotine exerts its effects by causing nicotinic acetylcholine receptor (nicAChR) excitation leading to neurotransmitter release and nicAChR desensitization.

Route of administration: Nicotine is usually inhaled, although it can be chewed.

Effects: Nicotine has both stimulant and relaxant properties. Physiologically, nicotine increases alertness, decreases irritability, and relaxes skeletal muscle tone.

Peripheral effects due to ganglionic stimulation include tachycardia, increased blood pressure, and decreased gastrointestinal motility.

Clinical uses: Nicotine has no clinical use.

Tolerance, dependence, and withdrawal: Tolerance to nicotine occurs rapidly, first to peripheral effects but later to central effects.

Nicotine is highly addictive, causing both physical and psychological dependence.

Withdrawal from tobacco often leads to a syndrome of craving, irritability, anxiety, and increased appetite for approximately 2–3 weeks.

Adverse effects: Acute nicotine toxicity causes nausea and vomiting. Chronic toxicity caused by smoking leads to more morbidity in the UK than all other drugs combined, predisposing to all of the following diseases, often greatly so:
- Cardiovascular diseases, including atherosclerosis, hypertension, and coronary heart disease.
- Cancer of the lung, bladder, and mouth.
- Respiratory diseases such as bronchitis, emphysema, and asthma.
- Fetal growth retardation.

Central depressants
Ethanol
Mechanism of action: Ethanol, or alcohol, acts in a similar way to volatile anaesthetic agents, as a general CNS depressant. The cellular mechanisms involved may include inhibition of calcium entry, hence reduction in transmitter release, as well as potentiation of inhibitory GABA transmission.

Route of administration: Ethanol is administered orally.

Effects: The familiar effects of ethanol intoxication range from increased self-confidence and motor incoordination through to unconsciousness and coma. Peripheral effects include a self-limiting diuresis and vasodilatation.

Clinical uses: Ethanol is used as an antidote to methanol poisoning.

Tolerance, dependence, and withdrawal: Tolerance, and physical and psychological dependence all occur with ethanol, such that 15 000 people a year are admitted to psychiatric hospital for alcohol dependence and psychosis, and up to 20% of males on a medical ward have alcohol-related disabilities.

The alcohol withdrawal syndrome is a rebound of the nervous system after adaptation to the depression caused by alcohol. This syndrome occurs in two stages:
- Early stage ('hangover'), which is common and starts 6–8 hours after cessation of drinking. It involves tremulousness, nausea, retching, and sweating.
- Late stage (delirium tremens), which is much less common and starts 48–72 hours after cessation of drinking. It involves delirium, tremor, hallucinations, and confusion.

Management of these late withdrawal symptoms involves sedation with clomethiazole or benzodiazepines; clonidine may be useful.

Adverse effects: Acute ethanol toxicity causes ataxia, nystagmus, coma, respiratory depression, and death. Chronic ethanol toxicity causes neurodegeneration (potentiated by vitamin deficiency), dementia, liver damage, pancreatitis, etc., and accompanying psychiatric illness—depression/psychosis is common.

Benzodiazepines
Mechanism of action: Benzodiazepines exert their effects by potentiation of inhibitory GABA transmission (p. 93)

Route of administration: Benzodiazepines are administered orally.

Effects: The effects of benzodiazepines include sedation, agitation, and ataxia.

Clinical uses: Benzodiazepines are heavily prescribed as anxiolytics and hypnotics.

Tolerance, dependence, and withdrawal: Benzodiazepines have a potential for misuse—tolerance and dependence are common.

A physical withdrawal syndrome can occur in patients given benzodiazepines, even for short periods. Symptoms include rebound anxiety and insomnia with depression, nausea, and perceptual changes that may last from weeks to months.

Adverse effects: The adverse effects of acute benzodiazepine toxicity include hypotension and confusion. Cognitive impairment occurs in chronic benzodiazepine toxicity.

Opioid analgesics
Diamorphine (heroin) and other opioids
Street names: Smack, Dragon, Brown.

Mechanism of action: Opioids, e.g. diamorphine, show agonist action at opioid receptors (p. 62).

Note that the sense of euphoria and well-being produced by strong opioids undoubtedly contributes to their analgesic activity by helping to reduce the anxiety and stress associated with pain. This effect also accounts for the illicit use of these drugs by addicts.

Route of administration: Opioids are generally taken intravenously by misusers as this produces the most intense sense of euphoria ('rush').

Effects: Opioids produce feelings of euphoria and well-being. Other effects are mentioned on p. 64.

Clinical uses: Opioids are used in analgesia for moderate to severe pain.

Tolerance, dependence, and withdrawal: Tolerance to opioid analgesics develops quickly in addicts and results in larger and larger doses of the drug being needed to achieve the same effect.

Dependence involves both psychological factors and physical factors. Psychological dependence is based on the positive reinforcement provided by euphoria.

There is a definite physical withdrawal syndrome in addicts following cessation of drug treatment with opioids. This syndrome comprises a complex mixture of irritable and sometimes aggressive behaviour, combined with extremely unpleasant autonomic symptoms such as fever, sweating, yawning, pupillary dilatation, and piloerection that gives the state its colloquial name of 'cold turkey'. Patients are extremely distressed and restless and strongly crave the drug. Symptoms are maximal at 2 days and largely disappear in 7–10 days.

Treatment of withdrawal: Methadone is a long-acting opiate, active orally, that is used to wean addicts from their addiction. The withdrawal symptoms from this longer-acting compound are more prolonged, but less intense than, for example, those of heroin. Treatment usually involves substitution of methadone followed by a slow reduction in dose over time.

Clonidine, an α_2-adrenoreceptor agonist, inhibits firing of locus ceruleus neurons, and it is effective in suppressing some components of the opioid withdrawal syndrome, especially the nausea, vomiting, and diarrhoea.

Adverse effects: Acute opioid toxicity causes the following:
- Confusion, drowsiness, and sedation. Initial excitement is followed by sedation and finally coma on overdose.
- Shallow and slow respiration, due to reduction of sensitivity of the respiratory centre to CO_2.
- Vomiting, due to stimulation of the chemoreceptor trigger zone.
- Autonomic effects such as tremor and pupillary constriction.
- Bronchospasm, flushing, and arteriolar dilatation due to histamine release.

Acute toxicity may be countered by use of an opioid antagonist such as naloxone.

The adverse effects of direct chronic toxicity are minor (p. 64).

Heroin addicts are able to tolerate 300–600 mg doses several times per day. This is 30–60 times the normal dose needed to produce an analgesic effect. A non-addict given this would die of respiratory depression.

Cannabinoids
Cannabis
Street names: Puff, Weed, Pot, Dope, Gear, Grass, Resin, Ganja, Blow.

There are two forms of cannabis: marijuana is the dried leaves and flowers of the cannabis plant, and hashish is the extracted resin of the cannabis plant.

Mechanism of action: How cannabis exerts its effects is not clearly defined, but it includes both depressant, stimulant, and psychomimetic effects.

The active constituent of cannabis is D^9-tetrahydrocannabinol (THC), though metabolites that also have activity may be important.

Route of administration: Cannabis is usually smoked, although it may be eaten.

Effects: Cannabis has several effects:
- Subjectively, users feel relaxed and mildly euphoric.
- Perception is altered, with apparent sharpening of sensory experience.
- Appetite is enhanced.

- Peripheral actions include vasodilatation and bronchodilatation, and a reduction in intraocular pressure.

Clinical uses: Cannabis is not currently licensed for use in the UK. It is being evaluated for palliative or symptomatic relief use in certain conditions in the USA, e.g. for the antiemetic effect of THC, and a possible role in treatment of multiple sclerosis and glaucoma.

Tolerance, dependence, and withdrawal: Tolerance to cannabis occurs to a minor degree. It is not dangerously addictive, with only moderate physical and psychological withdrawal effects noted, such as mild anxiety/dysphoria and sleep disturbances.

Adverse effects: Acute cannabis toxicity causes confusion and hallucinations. Chronic toxicity may cause flashbacks, memory loss, and 'de-motivational syndrome'.

Psychotomimetic drugs or hallucinogens

Street names: Acid, Trips, Magic mushrooms.

Examples of psychotomimetic drugs include LSD, mescaline, and psilocybin.

Mechanism of action: How LSD, mescaline, and psilocybin produce changes in perception is not well understood, but it seems to involve serotonin. LSD appears to affect serotonergic systems by acting on 5-HT_2 inhibitory autoreceptors on serotonergic neurons to reduce their firing. Whether LSD is an agonist, an antagonist, or both is not clear.

Route of administration: Psychotomimetic drugs are administered orally as a liquid, pills, or paper stamps.

Effects: Psychotomimetic drugs cause a dramatically altered state of perception—vivid and unusual sensory experiences combined with euphoric sensations. Hallucinations, delusions, and panic can occur; this is known as a 'bad trip' and it can be terrifying.

Clinical uses: Psychotomimetic drugs have no clinical uses.

Tolerance, dependence, and withdrawal: Tolerance to, dependence on, and withdrawal from psychotomimetic drugs are not significant.

Adverse effects: Acute toxicity from psychotomimetic drugs causes frightening delusions or hallucinations that can lead to accidents or violence. In chronic toxicity, 'flashbacks' (a recurrence of hallucination) may occur long after the 'trip'. Other psychotic symptoms may also occur.

Smoking cessation

The most successful smoking-cures combine psychological and pharmacological treatments.

Pharmacological options largely rely on nicotine-replacement, once the patient has stopped smoking, with gradual reduction in nicotine. The latest drug to be used to help cigarette smokers is amfebutamone (Zyban®), which is derived from an antidepressant.

Nicotine products

Mechanism of action: Measured doses of nicotine are used to replace nicotine derived from cigarettes once the patient has stopped smoking, meeting the physical nicotine needs. The dose of nicotine is gradually reduced over 10–12 weeks.

Route of administration: Oral (chewing gum, sublingual tablets), transdermal (patches), nasal (spray), inhalation.

Indications: Adjunct to smoking cessation.

Contraindications: Severe cardiovascular disease, recent cerebrovascular accident, pregnancy, and breastfeeding.

Adverse effects: Nausea, dizziness, headache and cold and influenza-like symptoms, palpitations.

Therapeutic notes: Nicotine products are not generally available on the National Health Service.

Amfebutamone (Zyban®)

Mechanism of action: Amfebutamone is a selective inhibitor of the neuronal uptake of noradrenaline and dopamine. This is believed to reduce nicotine craving and withdrawal symptoms.

Route of administration: Oral.

Indications: Adjunct to smoking cessation.

Contraindications: History of epilepsy and eating disorders, pregnancy, and breastfeeding.

Adverse effects: Dry mouth, gastrointestinal disturbances, insomnia, tremor, and impaired concentration.

Therapeutic notes: Amfebutamone is available on the National Health Service.

While smoking may be more socially acceptable than say taking heroin, the difficulties faced by those wishing to stop their habit can be enormous, which is why psychological intervention has a role to play alongside pharmacological methods.

- Describe the signs and symptoms of parkinsonism, and the aetiological factors in its pathogenesis.
- List the more common classes of drugs used to treat Parkinson's disease, their route of administration, mechanism of action, and adverse effects.
- What mechanisms are available to optimize L-dopa treatment, without enhancing its adverse effects?
- What are the psychological and somatic symptoms of anxiety? Name the classes of drugs used in its management.
- By what mechanism do anxiolytics exert their effect? What are their routes of administration and adverse effects?
- What classes of drugs are used to treat insomnia, and under what circumstances should hypnotic drugs be prescribed?
- What are the affective disorders, and what are their proposed biochemical abnormalities?
- List the main classes of drugs used in the management of mood disorders, their mechanisms of action, and adverse effects.
- What are the advantages of the selective serotonin reuptake inhibitors over the tricyclic antidepressants?
- Outline the concept of psychotic disorders and give examples of two positive and two negative symptoms.
- Explain the underlying pathophysiology of psychotic disease, and the rationale for drug treatment.
- List the more common typical and atypical drugs used in psychotic disease. What are their mechanisms of action, and adverse effects?
- What is epilepsy, and what are the biochemical/structural causes for its clinical features?
- List the more common antiepileptic drugs, their routes of administration, and major adverse effects. Summarize their general mechanism of action.
- Outline the principles, and drugs used in the management of status epilepticus.
- What are the components needed for adequate general anaesthesia prior to surgery?
- Name one drug used in each stage of anaesthesia, from premedication, induction, and maintenance. What are their routes of administration, general mechanisms of action, and adverse effects?
- What is the role of nitrous oxide as an anaesthetic gas?
- Which drugs are commonly misused? What forms of classification exist for drugs of misuse?
- What treatment options are available to people who wish to stop smoking, but who suffer from nicotine withdrawal? How do these agents act, and what are their main adverse effects?

7. Cardiovascular System

Heart

Cardiac anatomy and physiology

The heart as a pump

The heart functions as a pump that, together with the vascular system, supplies the tissues with blood containing oxygen and nutrients as well as removing waste products.

The flow of blood around the body is as follows (Fig. 7.1):

- Deoxygenated blood from body tissues reaches the right atrium through the systemic veins (the superior and inferior venae cavae).
- Blood flows into the right ventricle, which then pumps the deoxygenated blood via the pulmonary circulation to the lungs, where the blood becomes oxygenated before reaching the left atrium.
- Blood flows from the left atrium into the left ventricle, where it is pumped into the systemic circulation, via the aorta, to supply the tissues of the body.

Cardiac rate and rhythm

The sinoatrial node (SAN), located in the roof of the right atrium near the entrance of the superior vena cava, and the atrioventricular node (AVN), located at the base of the right atrium, possess a spontaneous intrinsic rhythm.

Since the SAN discharges at a frequency higher than other regions of the heart (80 impulses/minute), it is the pacemaker for the heart, and as such it determines the heart rate.

The action potential generated by the SAN spreads throughout both atria, reaching the AVN, from which it enters the interventricular septum by means of the bundle of His. The bundle of His splits into left and right branches making contact with the Purkinje fibres, which conduct the impulse throughout the ventricles, causing the ventricles to contract (Fig. 7.2).

Cardiac action potential

The shape of the action potential is characteristic of the location of its origin (i.e. whether from nodal tissue, the atria, or the ventricles) (Fig. 7.2).

Non-nodal cells

The resting membrane potential across the ventricular cell membrane is approximately -85 mV; this is because the resting membrane is more permeable to potassium than to other ions. Four

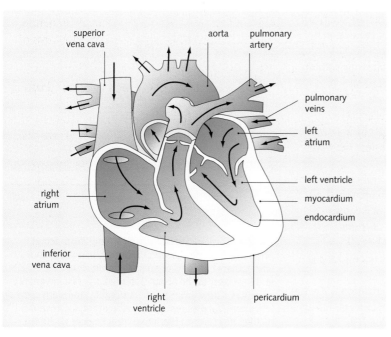

Fig. 7.1 Blood flow through the heart chambers. (Redrawn from Page et al, 2002.)

superior vena cava

aorta

pulmonary artery

pulmonary veins

left atrium

left ventricle

myocardium

endocardium

right atrium

inferior vena cava

right ventricle

pericardium

123

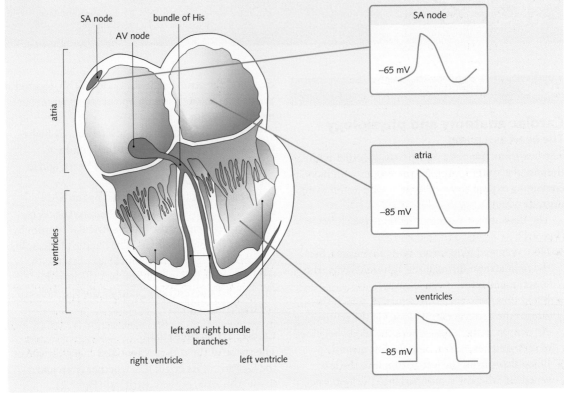

Fig. 7.2 Regional variation in action potential configuration throughout the heart. (AV, atrioventricular; SA, sinoatrial.) (Redrawn from Page et al, 2002.)

phases occurring at the ventricular cell membrane are:

- Phase 0 or depolarization. Depolarization occurs when the membrane potential reaches a critical value of –60 mV. The upstroke of the action potential is due to the transient opening of voltage-gated sodium channels, allowing sodium ions into the cell. In addition, potassium conductance falls to very low levels.
- Phase 1 or partial repolarization. Partial repolarization occurs as a result of the inactivation of the sodium current, and a transient outward potassium current.
- Phase 2 or plateau phase. The membrane remains depolarized at a plateau of approximately 0 mV. This is because of the activation of a voltage-dependent slow inward calcium current, conducting positive charge into the cell, and a delayed rectifier potassium current conducting positive charge out of the cell.
- Phase 3 or repolarization. Repolarization is a result of the inactivation of the calcium current and an increase in potassium conductance (Fig. 7.3).

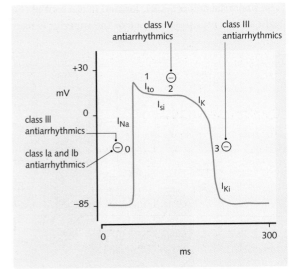

Fig. 7.3 Configuration of a typical ventricular action potential showing the ionic currents, the phases, and where Class I, III, and IV antiarrhythmic drugs act. (1, 2, and 3, phases of the action potential; I_{Na}, fast inward Na^+ current; I_{si}, slow inward Ca^{2+} current; I_{to}, transient outward K^+ current; I_K, delayed rectifier K^+ current; I_{Ki}, inward rectifier K^+ current.) (Redrawn from Page et al, 2002)

Nodal cells

The resting membrane potential of nodal cells is approximately –60 mV.

In nodal cells, there is no fast sodium current. Instead, the action potential is initiated by an inward calcium current, and because calcium spikes conduct slowly, there is a delay of approximately 0.1 seconds between atrial and ventricular contraction.

Nodal cells have a phase known as phase 4 or the pacemaker potential. This phase involves a gradual depolarization that occurs during diastole and is known as the f current (I_f, funny). The f current is activated by hyperpolarization at –45 mV, and consists of sodium and calcium ions entering the cell (Fig. 7.4).

Autonomic control of the heart

Both the parasympathetic and sympathetic nervous systems influence the heart, though parasympathetic activity predominates, which explains why the heart rate is lower than the inherent firing frequency of the SAN.

The sympathetic nervous system mediates its effects through the cardiac nerve, and activation of β_1-adrenoceptors. These are linked to adenylyl cyclase, and their activation causes increased levels of cyclic adenosine monophosphate (cAMP), and a subsequent increase in intracellular calcium levels.

The parasympathetic nervous system mediates its effects through the vagus nerve, and activation of M_2-receptors. These are also linked to adenylyl cyclase, but their activation causes decreased levels of cAMP, and a subsequent decrease in intracellular calcium levels.

The effects of the sympathetic and parasympathetic nervous systems on the heart are summarized in Fig. 7.5.

Cardiac contractility

Myocardial contraction is the result of calcium entry through L-type channels, giving rise to an increase in cytosolic calcium (Fig. 7.6).

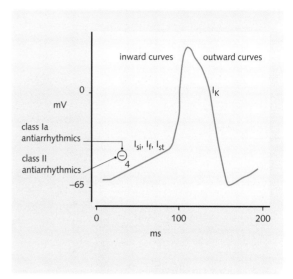

Fig. 7.4 Configuration of a typical sinoatrial node action potential showing the ionic currents, the phases, and where class Ia and II antiarrhythmic drugs act. (4, phase of the action potential; I_{si}, an inward current carried by Ca^{2+} ions; I_f, a 'funny' current carried by Na^+ and Ca^{2+} ions; I_{st}, the sustained inward Na^+ current; I_K, the delayed rectifier current which is an outward K^+ current.) (Redrawn from Page et al, 2002.)

The calcium is derived from two sources: the sarcoplasmic reticulum within the cell, and the extracellular medium.

Extracellular calcium enters the cell, triggering larger amounts of calcium to be released from the sarcoplasmic reticulum, a process known as calcium-induced calcium release.

During contraction, the intracellular levels of calcium rise to levels 10 000 times greater than those at rest. Calcium binds to troponin C, thus modifying the position of actin and myosin filaments, and allowing the cell to contract.

Contraction ceases only once calcium has been removed from the cytoplasm. This occurs through two mechanisms:

Fig. 7.5 Effects of the sympathetic and parasympathetic system on the heart. (AV, atrioventricular.)

Effects of the sympathetic and parasympathetic systems on the heart		
	Sympathetic	Parasympathetic
Heart rate	Increased	Decreased
Force of contraction	Increased	Decreased
Automaticity	Increased	Reduced
AV node conduction	Facilitated	Inhibited
Cardiac efficiency	Reduced	Increased

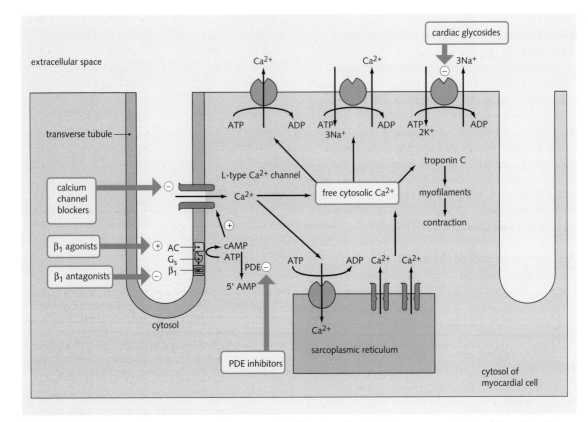

Fig. 7.6 Effects of drugs on cardiac contractility. (AC, adenylyl cyclase; β1, β1-adrenoceptor; G_s, stimulatory G-protein; PDE, phosphodiesterase.)

- Calcium is pumped out of the cell via the electrogenic Na^+/Ca^{2+} exchanger, which pumps one calcium ion out for every three sodium ions in.
- Calcium is re-sequestered into sarcoplasmic reticulum stores by a Ca^{2+} ATPase pump.

Cardiac dysfunction
Congestive cardiac failure
Congestive cardiac failure (CCF) is the combined failure of both the left and right sides of the heart.

The incidence of cardiac failure in the United Kingdom is between 1–5 per 1000 per year, and this doubles for each decade of life after the age of 45; over 100 000 hospital admissions annually are directly related to cardiac failure.

CCF occurs when the cardiac output does not meet the needs of the tissues. This is thought to result from defective excitation–contraction coupling, with progressive systolic and diastolic ventricular dysfunction.

Some of the causes and symptoms and signs of acute and chronic cardiac failure are listed in Fig. 7.7.

The characteristics of left and right ventricular failure are listed in Fig. 7.8.

The body attempts to compensate for the effects of CCF by two processes—extrinsic and intrinsic.

Fig. 7.7 Causes and symptoms/signs of acute and cardiac failure (CF).

Causes and symptoms/signs of acute and chronic cardiac failure			
Causes		Symptoms/signs	
Acute CF	Chronic CF	Acute CF	Chronic CF
Myocardial infarction Acute valvular lesion	Systemic hypertension Myocardial infarction Valvular lesions Cardiomyopathies	Tachycardia Hypotension Dyspnoea Pulmonary oedema Systemic oedema	Exertional dyspnoea Systemic oedema Cardiomegaly Fatigue Orthopnoea

Characteristics of right and left ventricular failure	
Right ventricular failure	**Left ventricular failure**
Reduced cardiac output	Reduced cardiac output
Hypotension	Hypotension
Peripheral oedema	Pulmonary oedema
Raised jugular venous pressure	Dyspnoea
Hepatomegaly	Fatigue
Ascites	

Fig. 7.8 Characteristics of right and left ventricular failure.

Extrinsic neurohumoral reflexes: Extrinsic neurohumoral reflexes aim to maintain cardiac output and blood pressure such that hypotension → activation of baroreceptors (receptors responding to changes in pressure) → increased sympathetic activity → increased heart rate and vasoconstriction → increased cardiac contractility and vascular tone → increased arterial pressure.

However, the greater the resistance (arterial pressure) against which the heart must pump reduces both the ejection fraction and the perfusion of the tissues.

The reduced perfusion of the kidneys activates the renin–angiotensin system, leading to renin secretion and subsequent elevation of plasma angiotensin II and aldosterone levels (see Fig. 7.14).

Angiotensin II causes peripheral vasoconstriction and aldosterone increases sodium retention, leading to increased water retention, oedema, and an increased preload.

Intrinsic cardiac compensation: The increased cardiac preload leads to incomplete emptying of the ventricles and an increase in end-diastolic pressure.

The heart eventually fails, owing to the massive increase in myocardial energy requirements.

Arrhythmias

Sudden death as a result of arrhythmias is the most common cause of death in developed countries, and it usually results from underlying cardiovascular pathology such as atherosclerosis.

Myocardial ischaemia is one of the most important causes of arrhythmias, and it occurs when a coronary artery becomes occluded, thus preventing sufficient blood from reaching the myocardium. Accumulation of endogenous biological mediators, including potassium, cAMP, thromboxane A_2, and free radicals, are believed to initiate arrhythmias.

Reperfusion after coronary occlusion is necessary for tissue recovery and prevention of myocardial necrosis, but spontaneous resumption of coronary flow is often itself a cause of arrhythmias.

Arrhythmias have been defined according to their appearance on the electrocardiogram (ECG) by the Lambeth Conventions. These include:
- Ventricular: premature beats, tachycardia, fibrillation, and torsade de pointes.
- Atrial: premature beats, tachycardia, flutter, and fibrillation.

The two main mechanisms by which cardiac rhythm becomes dysfunctional are abnormal impulse generation (automatic or triggered) and abnormal impulse conduction.

Abnormal impulse generation

Automatic: Automatic abnormal impulse generation is likely to cause sinus and atrial tachycardia, and ventricular premature beats. It can be:
- Enhanced: pathological conditions, such as ischaemia, may effect nodal and conducting tissue so that their inherent pacemaker frequency is greater than that of the SAN. Ischaemia causes partial depolarization of tissues (owing to a decrease in the activity of the electrogenic sodium pump) and catecholamine release, thus enhancing the automaticity of the slow pacemakers (AVN, Purkinje fibres, bundle of His) and often giving rise to an ectopic focus triggering the development of a premature beat.
- Abnormal: a premature beat may also develop in atrial or ventricular tissue, which is not normally automatic.

Triggered: Forms of triggered abnormal impulse generation are:
- Early after-depolarizations (EADs), which are likely to cause torsade de points and reperfusion-induced arrhythmias. EADs are triggered during repolarization, i.e. phase 2 or 3, of a previously normal impulse. They may result from a decrease in the delayed rectifier K^+ current, and they are associated with abnormally long action potentials. They are, therefore, more likely to occur during bradycardia and class III antiarrhythmic drug treatment.
- Delayed after-depolarizations (DADs) are triggered once the action potential has ended, i.e. during phase 4, of a previously normal impulse. DADs usually result from cellular calcium

overload, associated with ischaemia, reperfusion, and cardiac glycoside intoxication.

Abnormal impulse conduction

Heart block: Heart block is likely to cause ventricular premature beats, and it results from damage to nodal tissue (most commonly the AVN) caused by conditions such as infarction. AV block may be first, second, or third degree, manifesting itself from slowed conduction to complete block of conduction, where the atria and ventricles beat independently.

Re-entry: Re-entry is likely to cause ventricular and atrial tachycardia and fibrillation, atrial flutter, and Wolff–Parkinson–White syndrome. Re-entry is of two types: circus movement and reflection.

In circus movement, an impulse re-excites an area of the myocardium, recently excited, after the refractory period has ended. This usually occurs in a ring of tissue in which a unidirectional block is present, preventing anterograde conduction of the impulse, but allowing retrograde conduction of the same impulse. This results in its continuous circulation, termed circus movement. The time taken for the impulse to propagate around the ring must exceed the refractory period; therefore, administration of drugs that prolong the refractory period will interrupt the circuit and terminate re-entry.

Reflection occurs in non-branching bundles within which electrical dissociation has taken place. Owing to this electrical dissociation, an impulse can return over the same bundle.

 Don't panic. Arrhythmias are difficult to fully understand. Aim to know the more common arrhythmias, their causes and presentations, and their immediate and subsequent long-term management. If you master that, then try to add in the cellular events and mechanism of drug action.

Angina pectoris

Angina is associated with acute myocardial ischaemia, and results from underlying cardiovascular pathology. When coronary flow does not meet the metabolic needs of the heart, a radiating chest pain results; this is angina pectoris.

Stable or classical angina is due to fixed stenosis of the coronary arteries, and it is brought on by exercise and stress.

Unstable angina or crescendo angina can occur suddenly at rest, and it becomes progressively worse, with an increase in the number and severity of attacks. The following conditions can all cause unstable angina:

- Coronary atherosclerosis.
- Coronary artery spasm.
- Transient platelet aggregation and coronary thrombosis.
- Endothelial injury causing the accumulation of vasoconstrictor substances.
- Coronary vasoconstriction following adrenergic stimulation.

Variant angina or Prinzmetal's angina occurs at rest, at the same time each day, and it is usually due to coronary artery spasm. It is characterized by an elevated ST segment on the ECG during chest pain, and it may be accompanied by ventricular arrhythmias.

Treatment of cardiac dysfunction
Drugs used in heart failure
Cardiac glycosides

Examples of cardiac glycosides include digoxin and digitoxin.

Cardiac glycosides possess an aglycone steroid nucleus, conveying the pharmacological activity of these compounds; an unsaturated lactone ring, conveying cardiotonic activity; and sugar moieties, able to modulate potency and pharmacokinetic distribution.

Although the positive inotropic actions of cardiac glycosides shift the Frank–Starling ventricular function curve to a more favourable position (Fig. 7.9), thus improving the symptoms of CCF, there is no evidence that they have a beneficial effect on the long-term prognosis of patients with CCF.

Mechanism of action: Cardiac glycosides act by inhibiting the membrane Na^+/K^+ ATPase pump (Fig. 7.6). This increases intracellular Na^+ concentration, thus reducing the sodium gradient across the membrane and decreasing the amount of calcium pumped out of the cell by the Na^+/Ca^{2+} exchanger during diastole. Consequently, the intracellular calcium concentration rises, leading to an increase in the force of cardiac contraction and maintaining normal blood pressure.

Positive inotropes and congestive cardiac failure (CCF)

Fig. 7.9 The Frank–Starling curve, positive inotropes, and congestive cardiac failure (CCF). Normal cardiac output is determined by the pressure in the left ventricle at end-diastole. In CCF, the set point for cardiac output is reduced and cardiac output falls (1). Compensatory neurohumoral responses become activated which increase end-diastolic pressure and improve cardiac output; however, this can give rise to backward failure (2). Positive inotropic agents increase cardiac output (3). The improved cardiac output reduces the drive for a high end-diastolic pressure, and decompensation occurs to a new set point (4).

In addition, cardiac glycosides alter the electrical activity of the heart, both directly and indirectly. At therapeutic doses they indirectly decrease the heart rate, slow atrioventricular (AV) conductance and shorten the atrial action potential by stimulating vagal activity. This is useful in atrial fibrillation. At toxic doses they indirectly increase the sympathetic activity of the heart, and cause arrhythmias, including heart block. The direct effects are mainly due to loss of intracellular potassium, and they are most pronounced at high doses. The resting membrane potential is reduced, causing enhanced automaticity, slowed cardiac conduction, and increased AVN refractory period.

The increased cytosolic calcium concentration may reach toxic levels, thereby saturating the sarcoplasmic reticulum sequestration mechanism and causing oscillations in calcium owing to calcium-induced calcium release. This results in oscillatory after-potentials and subsequent arrhythmias.

In addition, cardiac glycosides have a direct effect on α-adrenoceptors, causing vasoconstriction and a consequent increase in peripheral vascular resistance, which is further enhanced by a centrally mediated increase in sympathetic tone.

Route of administration: Oral.

Indications: Heart failure and supraventricular arrhythmias.

Contraindications: Heart block, hypokalaemia associated with the use of diuretics (the lack of competition from potassium potentiates the effects of cardiac glycosides on the Na^+/K^+ ATPase pump).

Adverse effects: Arrhythmias, anorexia, nausea and vomiting, visual disturbances, and abdominal pain and diarrhoea.

Therapeutic notes: The cardiac glycosides have a very narrow therapeutic window, and toxicity is, therefore, relatively common. If this occurs, the drug should be withdrawn and, if necessary, potassium supplements and antiarrhythmic drugs administered. For severe intoxication, antibodies specific to cardiac glycosides are available.

Phosphodiesterase inhibitors

Examples of phosphodiesterase (PDE) inhibitors include enoximone and milrinone. These have been developed as a result of the many adverse effects and problems associated with cardiac glycosides. There is no evidence that these improve the mortality rate.

Mechanism of action: The type III PDE isoenzyme is found in myocardial and vascular smooth muscle.

Phosphodiesterase is responsible for the degradation of cAMP; therefore, inhibiting this enzyme raises cAMP levels and this causes an increase in myocardial contractility and vasodilatation (Fig. 7.6). Cardiac output is increased, and pulmonary wedge pressure and total peripheral resistance are reduced, without much change in heart rate or blood pressure.

Route of administration: Intravenous.

Indications: PDE inhibitors are given for severe acute heart failure that is resistant to other drugs.

Adverse effects: Nausea and vomiting, arrhythmias, liver dysfunction, abdominal pain, and hypersensitivity.

Beta-adrenoceptor agonists

Examples of β-adrenoceptor agonists (p. 140) include dobutamine and dopamine. They are used intravenously in CCF emergencies (Fig. 7.6).

Drugs with proven mortality benefits in cardiac failure should be remembered. They are β-adrenoceptor antagonists, ACE inhibitors, nitrates with hydralazine, and spironolactone.

Diuretics

The diuretics used in CCF are thiazides, loop diuretics, and spironolactone.

Diuretics inhibit sodium and water retention by the kidneys, and so reduce oedema due to heart failure. Venous pressure and consequently cardiac preload are reduced, increasing the efficiency of the heart as a pump (Ch. 9). Spironolactone appears to have a beneficial effect in cardiac failure at doses lower than it would be expected to function as a diuretic.

Angiotensin-converting-enzyme inhibitors

For details of angiotensin-converting-enzyme (ACE) inhibitors see p. 135.

Nitrates

See antianginal drugs (p. 132).

Vasodilating drugs

Hydralazine is discussed on page 137.

Antiarrhythmic drugs

Antiarrhythmic drugs are classified according to a system devised by Vaughan Williams in 1970, and later modified by Harrison. A summary of the effects of the different classes of drug is given in Fig. 7.10.

Class I

All class I drugs block the voltage-dependent sodium channels in a dose-dependent manner. Their action resembles that of local anaesthetics (Ch. 5).

All class I drugs prolong the effective refractory period (terminate re-entry), and they convert unidirectional block to bidirectional block (prevent re-entry).

Class Ia

Examples of class Ia drugs include quinidine, procainamide, and disopyramide.

Class Ia drugs affect atrial muscle, ventricular muscle, the bundle of His, the Purkinje fibres, and the AVN.

Mechanism of action: Class Ia drugs block voltage-dependent sodium channels in their open (activated) or refractory (inactivated) state (Figs 7.3 and 7.4). Their effects are to slow phase 0 (increasing the effective refractory period), slow phase 4 (reducing automaticity), and to prolong action potential duration.

Route of administration: Oral, intravenous. Consult BNF.

Indications: Ventricular and supraventricular arrhythmias.

Contraindications: Heart block, sinus node dysfunction, cardiogenic shock, and severe uncompensated heart failure. Procainamide should not be given to patients with systemic lupus erythematosus.

Adverse effects: Arrhythmias, nausea and vomiting, hypersensitivity, thrombocytopenia, and agranulocytosis. Procainamide can cause a lupus-like syndrome, and disopyramide causes hypotension.

Class Ib

Examples of class Ib drugs include lidocaine (lignocaine), mexiletine, and phenytoin.

Mechanism of action: Class Ib drugs exert their effects in several ways (Fig. 7.3). These include:

	Effects of antiarrhythmic drugs				
Class	Example	Myocardial contractility	AV conduction	AP duration	Effective refractory period
Ia	Procainamide	↓	↓↓	↑	↑
Ib	Lignocaine	–	–	↓	↑↑
Ic	Flecainide	↓↓	↓↓	–	–
II	Propranolol	↓↓	–/↓	–	–
III	Amiodarone	–	↑	↑↑↑	↑↑↑
IV	Verapamil	↓↓↓	↓↓	↓↓	–

Fig. 7.10 Effects of the antiarrhythmic drugs. (AP, action potential; AV, atrioventricular.) The number of arrows indicates the degree of the effect caused.

- Blocking voltage-dependent sodium channels in their refractory (inactivated) state, i.e. when depolarized, as occurs in ischaemia.
- Binding to open channels during phase 0, and dissociating by the next beat if the rhythm is normal, but abolishing premature beats.
- Decreasing action potential duration.
- Increasing the effective refractory period.

Route of administration: Lidocaine (lignocaine) is administered intravenously, and mexiletine and phenytoin either orally or intravenously.
Indications: Ventricular arrhythmias following myocardial infarction. Phenytoin is used in epilepsy (Ch. 6).
Contraindications: Class Ib drugs should not be given to patients with sinoatrial disorders, AV block, and porphyria.
Adverse effects: Hypotension, bradycardia, drowsiness and confusion, convulsions, and paraesthesia (pins and needles).

Lidocaine (lignocaine) may cause dizziness and respiratory depression; mexiletine may cause nausea and vomiting, constipation, arrhythmias, and hepatitis; and phenytoin may cause nausea and vomiting, and peripheral neuropathy.

Class Ic
Flecainide is the only drug used from class Ic.
Mechanism of action: Flecainide blocks sodium channels in a fashion similar to the class Ia and Ib drugs, but it shows no preference for refractory channels. Class Ic drugs, therefore, result in a general reduction in the excitability of the myocardium.
Route of administration: Oral, intravenous.
Indications: Ventricular tachyarrhythmias.
Contraindications: Heart failure, history of myocardial infarction.
Adverse effects: Dizziness, visual disturbances, arrhythmias.

Class II
Examples of class II drugs include propranolol, atenolol, and pindolol (Figs 7.4 and 7.6).

Class II drugs are β-adrenoceptor antagonists (atenolol is β$_1$ selective) (p. 132). They have been shown to reduce sudden death after myocardial infarction by 50% (although this is believed to be due to prevention of cardiac rupture as opposed to prevention of ventricular fibrillation).

Class III
Examples of Class III drugs include bretylium, amiodarone, sotalol, and ibutilide.

Mechanism of action: All Class III drugs used clinically are potassium channel blockers. They prolong cardiac action potential duration (increased QT interval on the ECG), and they prolong the effective refractory period (Fig. 7.3).

Amiodarone also blocks sodium and calcium channels, i.e. slows phase 0 and 3, and blocks α- and β-adrenoceptors. Sotalol is a β-adrenoceptor antagonist with class III activity.
Route of administration: Bretylium is administered intravenously; amiodarone and sotalol are administered orally or intravenously.
Indications: Class III drugs are given for ventricular and supraventricular arrhythmias.
Contraindications: Bretylium should not be given to patients with phaeochromocytoma; amiodarone should not be given to those with AV block, sinus bradycardia, or thyroid dysfunction.

For contraindications regarding sotalol, see under β-blockers (p. 132).
Adverse effects: Class III drugs can cause arrhythmias, especially torsades de pointes.

Bretylium may cause hypotension, nausea and vomiting; amiodarone may cause thyroid dysfunction, liver damage, pulmonary disorders, photosensitivity, and neuropathy.

For adverse effects regarding sotalol see under β-blockers (p. 132).

Class IV
Examples of class IV drugs include verapamil and diltiazem (see Figs 7.3 and 7.6).

Class IV drugs are calcium antagonists that shorten phase 2 of the action potential, thus decreasing action potential duration. They are particularly effective in nodal cells, where calcium spikes initiate conduction.

Details of the drugs are given in the section on antianginal drugs (p. 132).

Other anti-arrhythmics
The cardiac glycosides (p. 128) and adenosine are agents used in arrhythmias, but which do not fit into the four classes described.

Adenosine
Adenosine is produced endogenously, and it acts upon many tissues, including the lungs, afferent nerves, and platelets.
Mechanism of action: Adenosine acts at A$_1$ receptors in cardiac conducting tissue and it causes myocyte hyperpolarization. This acts to slow the rate of rise of

an action potential, which brings about delay in conduction.

Route of administration: Intravenous.

Indications: Paroxysmal supraventricular tachycardia. Aid diagnosis of broad and narrow complex supraventricular tachycardia.

Contraindications: Second or third degree heart block, sick sinus syndrome.

Adverse effects: Transient facial flushing, chest pain, dyspnoea, and bronchospasm. Side effects are very short lived, often lasting less than 30 seconds.

Adrenaline

Adrenaline (epinephrine) is a sympathomimetic agent used in cardiac arrest and in the management of anaphylaxis. Adrenaline is discussed on p. 139.

 The drugs used in stable angina pectoris are β-adrenoceptor antagonists, nitrates, calcium antagonists, antiplatelets, and potassium channel activators.

Antianginal drugs

Acute attacks of angina are treated with sublingual nitrates or, in the hospital setting, with an opiate (Ch. 6).

Stable angina is treated with long-acting nitrates, antiplatelets, β-adrenoceptor antagonists, calcium antagonists, or potassium-channel activators.

Unstable angina is a medical emergency, and it requires hospital admission. Unstable angina is treated with:

- Antiplatelets (aspirin, clopidogrel, dipyridamole and the glycoprotein IIb/IIIa inhibitors, p. 146).
- Heparin/low-molecular weight heparin (p. 146).
- Standard antianginal drug regimen.

Organic nitrates

The organic nitrates glyceryl trinitrate (GTN), isosorbide mononitrate (ISMN), and isosorbide dinitrate (ISDN) can relieve angina within minutes.

Mechanism of action: Most nitrates are prodrugs, decomposing to form nitric oxide (NO), which activates guanylyl cyclase, thereby increasing the levels of cyclic guanosine monophosphate (cGMP). Protein kinase G is activated and contractile proteins are phosphorylated. Dilatation of the systemic veins decreases preload and, consequently, the oxygen demand of the heart, while dilatation of the coronary arteries increases blood flow and oxygen delivery to the myocardium.

Route of administration: Sublingual, oral (modified release), or from transcutaneous patches. GTN can be given by intravenous infusion.

Indications: Organic nitrates are given for the prophylaxis and treatment of angina, and in left ventricular failure.

Contraindications: Organic nitrates should not be given to patients with hypersensitivity to nitrates, or those with hypotension and hypovolaemia.

Adverse effects: Postural hypotension, tachycardia, headache, flushing, and dizziness.

Therapeutic notes: To avoid nitrate tolerance, a drug-free period of approximately 8 hours is needed.

Beta-adrenoceptor antagonists (β-blockers)

Examples of β-blockers include propranolol, atenolol, bisoprolol, and metoprolol.

Classes of drugs to treat angina, cardiac failure, and arrhythmias		
Angina	Heart failure	Arrhythmias
Organic nitrates	Cardiac glycosides	Na$^+$ channel blockers (Class I)
β$_1$-adrenoceptor antagonists	Phosphodiesterase inhibitors	β$_1$-adrenoceptor antagonists (Class II)
Ca^{2+} antagonists	β$_1$-adrenoceptor agonists	K$^+$ channel blockers (Class III)
Antiplatelets	Diuretics	Ca^{2+} antagonists (Class IV)
Potassium-channel activators	ACE inhibitors	Cardiac glycosides
	Nitrates	Adenosine
	Vasodilating drugs	

Fig. 7.11 Classes of drugs used to treat angina, cardiac failure, and arrhythmias.

Beta-adrenoceptors are found in many tissues, though the β_1-adrenoceptor is found predominantly in the heart, and the β_2-adrenoceptor found mainly in the smooth muscle of the vasculature (see p. 81). Some overlap does exist.

Different β-blockers have different affinity for the two types of adrenoceptor. Propranolol is non-selective, having equal affinity for both the β_1- and β_2-adrenoceptors. Atenolol, bisoprolol and metoprolol have greater affinity for the β_1-adrenoceptor, and are, therefore, more 'cardiac-specific'. Some β-blockers even appear to have partial agonistic effects at β-adrenoceptors, as well as antagonistic effects.

Mechanism of action: The aim of using β-adrenoceptor antagonists in cardiac disease is to block β-adrenoceptors in the heart. This has the effect of causing a fall in heart rate (slowing of phase 4, Fig. 7.4), in systolic blood pressure, in cardiac contractile activity, and in myocardial oxygen demand.

Route of administration: Oral, intravenous.

Indications: Angina, post-myocardial infarction, arrhythmias, hypertension, thyrotoxicosis, glaucoma, and anxiety.

Contraindications: Non-selective β-blockers (e.g. propranolol) must not be given to asthmatic patients. At high doses β_1-adrenoceptor antagonists lose their selectivity, and they should be used with caution in those with asthma. Other contraindications for β-blockers include bradycardia, hypotension, AV block, and CCF.

Adverse effects: Bronchospasm, fatigue and insomnia, dizziness, cold extremities (β_2-adrenoceptor effect), bradycardia, heart block, hypotension, and decreased glucose tolerance in diabetic patients.

Calcium-channel blockers

Examples of calcium-channel blockers include verapamil, diltiazem, and nifedipine.

Mechanism of action: Verapamil and diltiazem block L-type calcium channels found in the heart and in the vascular smooth muscle, thereby reducing calcium entry into cardiac and vascular cells (Figs 7.3, 7.6, and 7.12). This decrease in intracellular calcium reduces cardiac contractility and causes vasodilatation, which results in several effects: reduced preload due to the reduced venous pressure; reduced afterload due to the reduced arteriolar pressure; increased coronary blood flow; reduced cardiac contractility and thus reduced myocardial oxygen consumption; and a decreased heart rate. High doses of these drugs affect AV nodal conduction.

Nifedipine blocks L-type calcium-channels in vascular cells. It does not affect cardiac contractility, or AVN conduction, and its beneficial effects are due to increased coronary flow and peripheral vasodilatation.

Route of administration: Oral.

Indications: Calcium-channel blockers are used for the prophylaxis and treatment of angina and hypertension. Verapamil and diltiazem are given for supraventricular arrhythmias, and nifedipine for Raynaud's syndrome (peripheral vasoconstriction).

Contraindications: Calcium-channel blockers should not be given to patients in cardiogenic shock.

Nifedipine is contraindicated in advanced aortic stenosis; verapamil and diltiazem should not be given to patients in severe heart failure (owing to their negative inotropic action), to those taking β-blockers (risk of AV block and impaired cardiac output), and those with severe bradycardia.

Adverse effects: Verapamil and diltiazem may cause hypotension, rash, bradycardia, CCF, heart block, and constipation. Nifedipine may cause hypotension, rash, tachycardia, peripheral oedema, flushing, and dizziness.

 There are three classes of calcium-channel blockers. Two of them act mostly upon the heart (verapamil and diltiazem) and the other acts mostly upon peripheral vascular tone (nifedipine). Concurrent use of a β-adrenoceptor antagonist and a calcium-channel blocker could result in profound bradycardia.

Potassium-channel activators

Nicorandil is the only licensed drug in this class.

Mechanism of action: Nicorandil acts to activate the potassium channels of the vascular smooth muscle. Once activated, potassium flows out of the cells, causing hyperpolarization of the cell membrane. The hyperpolarized membrane inhibits the influx of calcium, and, therefore, inhibits contraction—the overall effect is relaxation of the smooth muscle, and vasodilatation (Fig. 7.12).

Route of administration: Oral.
Indications: Prophylaxis of angina.
Contraindications: Cardiogenic shock, left ventricular failure, hypotension.
Adverse effects: Headache, cutaneous vasodilatation, nausea, and vomiting.

Fig. 7.11 summarizes the main drug classes used in angina, cardiac failure, and arrhythmias.

The overall aims of symptom management in angina are: to dilate coronary arteries to allow maximal myocardial perfusion; to decrease the heart rate to minimize oxygen demands of the myocardium, and lengthen diastole when cardiac perfusion occurs; and to prevent platelets from aggregating and forming platelet plugs. In addition to this, reversible risk factors need to be addressed to limit the progression of the disease.

Circulation

Control of vascular tone
Alpha-adrenoceptor activation

Alpha-adrenoceptor activation (Fig. 7.12) causes contraction of vascular smooth muscle through the activation of phospholipase C (PLC). The resulting increased level of IP_3 causes the release of calcium from the endoplasmic reticulum, thus increasing the calcium level. Calcium then binds to calmodulin, thus activating myosin light-chain kinase (MLCK) and allowing contraction.

Beta$_2$-adrenoceptor activation

Beta$_2$-adrenoceptor activation (Fig. 7.12) causes relaxation of vascular smooth muscle through the activation of adenylyl cyclase. The resulting increased level of cAMP activates protein kinase A, which phosphorylates and inactivates MLCK.

M$_3$ receptor activation

M$_3$ receptor activation causes relaxation of vascular smooth muscle through the release of endothelium-derived relaxing factor (EDRF), which is believed to be nitric oxide (NO; Fig. 7.12). Guanylyl cyclase is

activated by NO, thus increasing the levels of cGMP and activating protein kinase G. Protein kinase G inhibits contraction by phosphorylating contractile proteins.

Renin–angiotensin system

A decrease in plasma volume results in the activation of the renin–angiotensin system (RAS), which is summarized in Fig. 7.13 (see also Ch. 9).

Angiotensin-converting enzyme (ACE) catalyses the production of angiotensin II. Angiotensin II causes:

- Potent vasoconstriction (40 times as potent as noradrenaline).
- Release of noradrenaline.
- Stimulation of the secretion of aldosterone.

ACE also catalyses the inactivation of bradykinin, which is an endogenous vasodilator.

Aldosterone is a steroid that induces the synthesis of sodium channels and Na$^+$/K$^+$ ATPase pumps in the luminal membrane of the cortical collecting ducts. This results in a greater amount of sodium and, consequently, water being reabsorbed, thus increasing the blood volume and pressure.

Certain renal diseases and renal artery occlusion will cause activation of the RAS and result in the development of hypertension.

Hypertension

Normal blood pressure is generally regarded as 120/80 mmHg (systolic pressure/diastolic pressure). Hypertension is defined as a diastolic arterial pressure greater than 90 mmHg, or a systolic arterial pressure greater than 140 mmHg. The condition can be fatal if left untreated, as it greatly increases the risk of thrombosis, stroke, and renal failure.

Three factors determine blood pressure. These are blood volume, cardiac output, and peripheral vascular resistance.

'Primary' or 'essential' hypertension accounts for 90–95% of all cases of hypertension. This has no known cause, but it is associated with:

- Age (40+).
- Obesity.
- Physical inactivity.
- Smoking and alcohol consumption.
- Genetic predisposition.

'Secondary hypertension' accounts for the remaining 5–10% of cases of hypertension. The cause is usually one of the following:

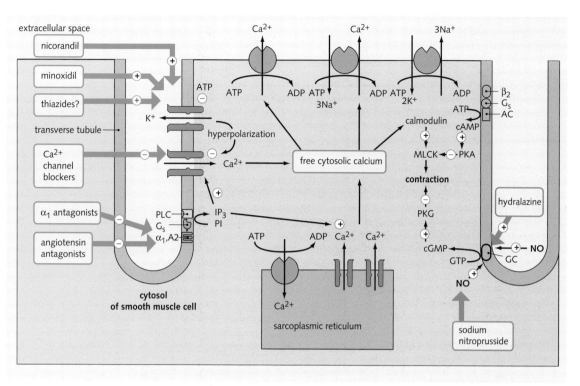

Fig. 7.12 Drugs affecting vascular tone. (AC, adenyl cyclase; α_1, α_1-adrenoceptor; A2, angiotensin II; β_2, β_2-adrenoceptor; GC, guanylyl cyclase; GS, stimulatory G-protein; IP_3, inositol triphosphate; MLCK, myosin light-chain kinase; NO, nitric oxide; PLC, phospholipase C; PI, phosphatidylinositol; PKA, protein kinase A; PKG, protein kinase G.)

- Renal disease, which activates the RAS.
- Endocrine disease, e.g. phaeochromocytoma, steroid-secreting tumour of the adrenal cortex, adrenaline-secreting tumour of the adrenal medulla.

Treatment of hypertension
The treatment of hypertension is aimed at various targets; these are summarized in Fig. 7.14.

Vasodilators
Angiotensin-converting enzyme inhibitors
Captopril, enalapril, lisinopril, and ramipril are examples of ACE inhibitors.
Mechanism of action: ACE inhibitors cause inhibition of ACE with consequent reduced angiotensin II and aldosterone levels (Fig. 7.13), and increased bradykinin levels. This causes vasodilatation with a consequent reduction in peripheral resistance, little change in heart rate and cardiac output, and reduced sodium retention.
Route of administration: Oral.
Indications: Hypertension, heart failure, and renal dysfunction (especially in diabetic patients to slow progression of diabetic or reduced renal functional nephropathy).
Contraindications: Pregnancy, renovascular disease, aortic stenosis.
Adverse effects: Characteristic cough, hypotension, dizziness and headache, diarrhoea, and muscle cramps.
Therapeutic notes: First dose hypotension is relatively common, and so these drugs should ideally be given just before bed.

Angiotensin-II receptor antagonists
Losartan and valsartan are examples of angiotensin-II receptor antagonists.
Mechanism of action: Angiotensin-II receptor antagonists cause inhibition at the angiotensin II receptor (Fig. 7.12), resulting in vasodilatation with a consequent reduction in peripheral resistance.
Route of administration: Oral.
Indications: Hypertension.
Contraindications: Pregnancy, breastfeeding. Caution in renal artery stenosis and aortic stenosis.
Adverse effects: Cough (less common than with ACE inhibitors), orthostatic hypotension, dizziness, headache and fatigue, hyperkalaemia, and rash.

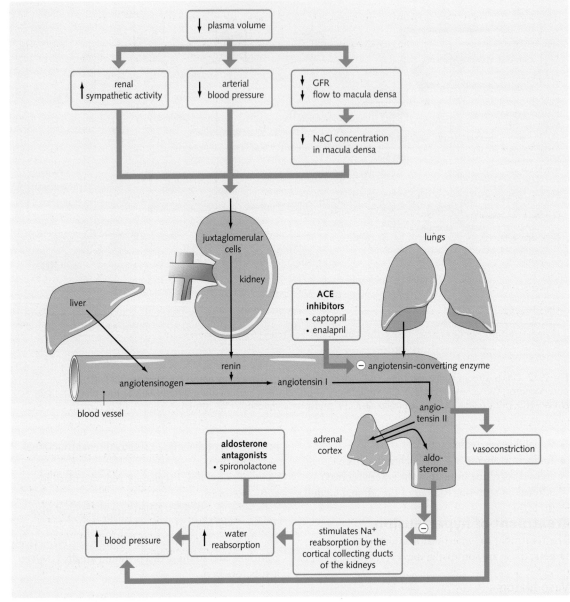

Fig. 7.13 Renin–angiotensin system and angiotensin-converting enzyme (ACE) inhibitors. (GFR, glomerular filtration rate.)

Calcium antagonists

Nifedipine has more effect upon vascular tone than diltiazem or verapamil, which are more cardio-selective (Fig. 7.12, p. 135).

Alpha₁-adrenoceptor antagonists

Prazosin and doxazosin are examples of α_1-adrenoceptor antagonists.

Mechanism of action: α_1-adrenoceptor antagonists cause inhibition of α_1-adrenoceptor-mediated vasoconstriction—consequently reducing peripheral resistance and venous pressure (Fig. 7.12). They also

lower plasma low-density lipoprotein (LDL) cholesterol levels, very-low-density lipoprotein (VLDL) levels, and triglyceride (TGA) levels, and increase high-density lipoprotein (HDL) cholesterol levels—thus reducing the risk of coronary artery disease.

Route of administration: Oral.

Indications: Hypertension (especially in patients with CCF), prostate hyperplasia (reduced bladder and prostate resistance), and coronary artery disease.

Contraindications: Prazocin should not be given to people with CCF due to aortic stenosis.

Advantages and disadvantages of drugs used in hypertension with respect to associated conditions

	Diuretic	β-Blocker	ACE inhibitor/angiotensin II receptor antagonist	Calcium channel blockers	α-Blocker
Diabetes	Care[a]	Care[a]	Yes	Yes	Yes
Gout	No	Yes	Yes	Yes	Yes
Dyslipidaemia	Care[b]	Care[b]	Yes	Yes	Yes
Ischaemic heart disease	Yes	Yes	Yes	Yes	Yes
Heart failure	Yes	Care[c]	Yes	Care[d]	Yes
Asthma	Yes	No	Yes	Yes	Yes
Peripheral vascular disease	Yes	Care	Care[e]	Yes	Yes
Renal artery stenosis	Yes	Care	No	Yes	Yes
Pregnancy	Caution	Not in late pregnancy	No	No	Caution

[a] Diuretics may aggravate diabetes: β-blockers worsen glucose intolerance and mask symptoms of hypoglycaemia.

[b] Both diuretics and β-blockers disturb the lipid profile.

[c] There is some evidence for beneficial effects of some β-blockers when used cautiously in heart failure.

[d] Verapamil and diltiazem may exacerbate heart failure, although amlodipine appears to be safe.

[e] Patients with peripheral vascular disease may also have renal artery stenosis; therefore ACE inhibitors should be used cautiously.

Fig. 7.14 Advantages and disadvantages of drugs used in hypertension with respect to associated conditions. (Reproduced from *Clinical Medicine,* 4th edn, by P Kumar and M Clark, 1998. By permission of WB Saunders.)

Adverse effects: Postural hypotension, dizziness, headache and fatigue, weakness, palpitations, and nausea.

Hydralazine

Hydralazine is a second- or third-line drug for the treatment of mild to moderate hypertension.
Mechanism of action: Hydralazine effects are unclear, though it appears to interfere with the action of IP_3 in vascular smooth muscle, thereby reducing peripheral resistance and blood pressure (Fig. 7.12).
Route of administration: Oral, intravenous.
Indications: Moderate to severe hypertension. Also used in conjunction with β-blockers and thiazides in hypertensive emergencies, and in hypertensive pregnant women.
Contraindications: Idiopathic systemic lupus erythematosus, severe tachycardia.
Adverse effects: Tachycardia, fluid retention, nausea and vomiting, and headache.

Minoxidil

Owing to its adverse effects, minoxidil is the drug of last resort in the long-term treatment of hypertension.

Mechanism of action: Minoxidil activates of vascular smooth muscle ATP-sensitive potassium channels, resulting in hyperpolarization of the cell membrane and consequent reduced calcium entry through L-type channels (Fig. 7.12). The overall effect is inhibition of smooth muscle contraction, and subsequent vasodilatation.
Route of administration: Oral for hypertension; topical cream for baldness.
Indications: Severe hypertension. Baldness.
Contraindications: Phaeochromocytoma or porphyria.
Adverse effects: Hirsutism (limits use in women), sodium and water retention, tachycardia, and cardiotoxicity.
Therapeutic notes: Though unrelated chemically, the drug diazoxide acts in a similar fashion to minoxidil, and activates potassium channels, resulting in vasodilatation.

Sodium nitroprusside

Mechanism of action: Sodium nitroprusside is a prodrug that spontaneously decomposes into NO inside smooth muscle cells. NO activates guanylyl cyclase, thus increasing intracellular cGMP levels, and causing vasodilatation (Fig. 7.12).

Route of administration: Intravenous.

Indications: Sodium nitroprusside is given in hypertensive crises, for controlled hypotension in surgery, and in heart failure.

Contraindications: Sodium nitroprusside should not be given to patients with severe hepatic impairment, vitamin B_{12} deficiency, or Leber's optic atrophy.

Adverse effects: Headache and dizziness, nausea, abdominal pain, palpitations, and retrosternal discomfort.

Therapeutic notes: Sodium nitroprusside is broken down in the body to thiocyanate, which has a half-life of only a few minutes, though prolonged exposure to nitroprusside and thiocyanate can result in thiocyanate toxicity (weakness, nausea, and inhibition of thyroid function).

The more common adverse effects of the vasodilating drugs are hypotension and headache, both of which directly result from reducing peripheral vascular resistance.

Diuretic drugs

Diuretics used in hypertension include thiazides, loop diuretics, and potassium-sparing diuretics.

See Chapter 9 for details of each of these drugs.

Mechanism of action: The antihypertensive action of diuretic drugs does not seem to correlate with their diuretic activity: loop diuretics are powerful diuretics but only moderate antihypertensives; thiazides are moderate diuretics but powerful antihypertensives.

It has recently been suggested that the antihypertensive effects of diuretics (especially the thiazides) are not necessarily a result of their diuretic effect, but rather may be due to activation of ATP-regulated potassium channels in resistance arterioles, with a mechanism of action similar to that of nicorandil and minoxidil. This causes hyperpolarization, and consequently, inhibition of calcium entry into vascular smooth muscle cells with consequent vasodilatation and reduced peripheral vascular resistance (Fig. 7.12).

Centrally acting antihypertensive drugs

Clonidine, methyldopa and moxonidine are examples of centrally acting antihypertensive drugs. These agents are second- or third-line drugs in the treatment of hypertension.

Mechanism of action: Centrally acting antihypertensive drugs are α_2-adrenoceptor agonists. The activation of presynaptic α_2-adrenoceptors causes inhibition of noradrenaline release and consequent vasodilatation. The activation of postsynaptic α_2-adrenoceptors causes vasoconstriction, although presynaptic effects dominate.

Centrally acting antihypertensive drugs reduce the activity of the vasomotor centre in the brain, causing reduced sympathetic activity and subsequent vasodilatation. They also reduce heart rate and cardiac output.

Route of administration: Oral. Clonidine can be given by intravenous infusion.

Indications: Hypertensive patients when first-line antihypertensive agents are ineffective or contraindicated. Methyldopa is safe for hypertension in pregnancy, asthmatic patients, and those with heart failure.

Contraindications: Methyldopa should not be given to people with depression, liver disease, or phaeochromocytoma.

Adverse effects: Dry mouth, sedation, orthostatic hypotension, male sexual dysfunction, and galactorrhoea. Methyldopa can cause diffuse parenchymal liver injury, fever, and, rarely, haemolytic anaemia. Clonidine can cause a withdrawal hypertensive crisis on stopping treatment.

Phaeochromocytoma

Phaeochromocytoma is a rare endocrine tumour, most commonly of the adrenal gland. These tumours can secrete adrenaline and various intermediates in its biosynthesis. These vasoactive compounds result in the clinical signs and symptoms of phaeochromocytomas, which include facial flushing, sweating, breathlessness, anxiety, tachycardia, and paroxysmal hypertension.

Medical management of phaeochromocytoma-induced hypertension relies on the powerful α-adrenoceptor antagonist phenoxybenzamine. Alpha-adrenoceptor blockade reduces peripheral vascular resistance and lowers blood pressure. The use of β-adrenoceptor antagonists is dangerous, as tumour-secreted sympathomimetics act unopposed on α-adrenoceptors, increasing both peripheral vascular resistance and blood pressure.

Phenoxybenzamine

Mechanism of action: Phenoxybenzamine antagonizes α-adrenoceptors in the vascular smooth muscles, resulting in vasodilatation.

Route of administration: Oral, intravenous.

Indications: Hypertensives episodes in phaeochromocytoma.

Contraindications: History of cerebrovascular events, post-myocardial infarction.

Adverse effects: Postural hypotension, tachycardia, nasal congestion.

Therapeutic notes: Phentolamine is another powerful α-adrenoceptor antagonist that can be used in phaeochromocytoma, though has a much shorter half-life, and is commonly used prior to, and during surgery to excise the tumour.

Vasoconstrictors and the management of shock
Shock

Shock is a state of circulatory collapse, characterized by an arterial blood pressure unable to maintain adequate tissue perfusion. Shock is a life-threatening condition.

The body responds inappropriately to shock, releasing mediators such as histamine, prostaglandins, bradykinin, and 5-hydroxytryptamine (5-HT, serotonin), which cause capillary dilatation and increased capillary permeability. This further reduces blood pressure and cardiac output.

Signs of shock include:
- Very low arterial blood pressure.
- A weak, rapid pulse.
- Cold, pale, sweaty skin.
- Rapid breathing.
- Dry mouth.
- Reduced urine output.
- Anxiousness.

Causes of shock include:
- Haemorrhage.
- Burns.
- Dehydration.
- Severe vomiting or diarrhoea.
- Bacterial septicaemia.
- Myocardial infarction.
- Pulmonary embolism.

Types of shock include:
- Hypovolaemic, which is caused by a reduction in the circulating blood volume.
- Cardiogenic, reduced cardiac output due to 'pump failure'.
- Septic, which is caused by massive vasodilatation.
- Anaphylactic, a severe allergic reaction, in which there is a massive generalized release of vasodilating mediators.
- Spinal, disruption of neuronal control upon vascular tone, and cardiac output.

Management of shock

The medical management of shock ultimately depends upon its underlying cause, e.g. if a child is shocked due to chronic diarrhoea and vomiting, fluid and electrolyte replacement is most appropriate management.

The following drugs are useful in restoring blood pressure and tissue perfusion, but on the whole they do not address the underlying cause of the different types of shock.

Sympathomimetic amines

Examples of sympathomimetic amines include adrenaline, noradrenaline, phenylephrine, and ephedrine.

Sympathomimetic amines raise blood pressure at the expense of vital organs such as the kidneys, and they raise peripheral resistance, which is already high in patients with shock.

Mechanism of action: Adrenaline and noradrenaline are agonists at both α- and β-adrenoceptor, and phenylephrine an α_1-adrenoceptor agonist. Ephedrine is a β-adrenoceptor agonist and causes noradrenaline release. These drugs work either by activating alpha-adrenoceptors which then activate phospholipase C, causing vasoconstriction and a consequent increase in arterial blood pressure, or by activating β-adrenoceptors which then activate adenylyl cyclase, causing an increased heart rate, increased cardiac contractility, and vasodilatation.

Route of administration: Parenterally, commonly intravenously.

Indications: Shock, acute hypotension, and reversal of hypotension caused by spinal or epidural anaesthesia. Adrenaline is used in cardiac arrest and anaphylaxis.

Contraindications: Sympathomimetic amines should not be given to people who are pregnant or have hypertension.

Adverse effects: Tachycardia, anxiety, insomnia, arrhythmias, dry mouth, and cold extremities.

Therapeutic notes: In a cardiac arrest, adrenaline is used at a concentration of 1 mg per 10 mL (1 : 10 000) intravenously, whereas in anaphylaxis, adrenaline is used at a concentration of 1 mg per 1 mL (1 : 1000) intramuscularly.

Dopamine and dobutamine

Mechanism of action: Dopamine is a precursor of noradrenaline. It activates dopamine receptors and α- and β-adrenoceptors. When administered by intravenous infusion, dopamine acts on:

- Dopamine receptors, causing vasodilatation in the kidneys at low doses.
- Alpha$_1$-adrenoceptors, causing vasoconstriction in other vasculature.
- Beta$_1$-adrenoceptors, causing positive inotropic and chronotropic effects.

Dobutamine has no effect upon dopaminergic receptors, but does activate β$_1$-adrenoceptors.

If renal perfusion is not impaired, dobutamine and dopamine are a more appropriate means of treating shock than α-adrenoceptor agonists. This form of treatment maintains renal perfusion, and inhibits the activation of the RAS.

Route of administration: Intravenous.
Indications: CCF (emergencies only), cardiogenic shock, septic shock, hypovolaemic shock, cardiomyopathy, and cardiac surgery.
Contraindications: Tachyarrhythmias; dopamine is contraindicated in people with phaeochromocytoma.
Adverse effects: Tachycardia and hypertension; dopamine causes nausea and vomiting, and hypotension.
Therapeutic notes: Although low doses of dopamine cause vasodilatation, high doses cause vasoconstriction and may exacerbate heart failure.

Vasopressin and desmopressin

Vasopressin (antidiuretic hormone; ADH), and desmopressin are examples of antidiuretic peptides.

Vasopressin is short acting ($t_{1/2}$ = 10 minutes) while desmopressin is longer acting ($t_{1/2}$ = 75 minutes).

Mechanism of action: Antidiuretic peptides activate V$_1$ receptors on smooth muscle cells, which stimulate phospholipase C, causing contraction. They also activate V$_2$ receptors on the tubular cells of the kidneys, which stimulate adenylyl cyclase and thereby increase the permeability of these cells to water, and reduce sodium and water excretion.

Vasopressin has a much greater affinity for V$_2$ receptors than V$_1$ receptors; desmopressin is selective for V$_1$ receptors.

Route of administration: Oral, intravenous, intranasal.
Indications: Pituitary diabetes insipidus. The antidiuretic peptides are no longer used in the management of shock, though their pharmacology is both academically interesting, and a potential target for future drugs.
Contraindications: Vascular disease, chronic nephritis.
Adverse effects: Fluid retention, nausea, pallor, abdominal cramps, and belching. They may induce anginal attacks (due to coronary vasoconstriction).

Corticosteroids

The use of corticosteroids in septic shock remains controversial, though they are also given by intravenous injection in the treatment of anaphylactic shock as an adjunct to adrenaline (Ch. 11).

It is possible to distinguish between the types of shock clinically:

- Hypovolaemic—low JVP, cool, clammy peripheries, confusion/restlessness.
- Cardiogenic—raised JVP, cool, clammy peripheries, anxiousness/agitation.
- Septic—warm, sweaty peripheries, pyrexia, nausea.
- Anaphylactic—warm peripheries, urticaria, nausea.
- Spinal—history of trauma or spinal anaesthesia.

Tachycardia, hypotension and tachypnoea will feature in all types of shock.

Lipoprotein circulation and atherosclerosis

Lipoproteins provide a means of transporting lipids (cholesterol, triglycerides, and phospholipids), which are insoluble in the blood, around the body.

Four classes of lipoproteins exist. These differ in size, density, constituent lipids, and type of surface protein (apoprotein). They are:

- High-density lipoproteins (HDL).
- Low-density lipoproteins (LDL).
- Very-low-density lipoproteins (VLDL).
- Chylomicrons.

Lipid transport in the blood is via two pathways, exogenous and endogenous, which are summarized in Fig. 7.15.

In the exogenous pathway (numbers refer to those in Fig. 7.15):

1. Diet-derived lipid breakdown leads to the formation of chylomicrons.
2. Lipoprotein lipase (LPL), found in the endothelium of extrahepatic tissues, hydrolyses the triglycerides in chylomicrons to glycerol and free fatty acids (FFAs), for use by the tissues.

3. The chylomicron remnant is taken up by the liver.
4. The liver secretes cholesterol and bile acids into the gut, creating an enterohepatic circulation.

In the endogenous pathway (numbers refer to those in Fig. 7.15):

1. The liver secretes VLDLs, the components of which may be derived either endogenously or from the diet.
2. Lipoprotein lipase (LPL), found in the endothelium of extrahepatic tissues, hydrolyses triglycerides in the VLDLs to glycerol and FFAs, for use by the tissues, and leaves LDL.
3. LDL is then taken up by the liver and extrahepatic tissues.

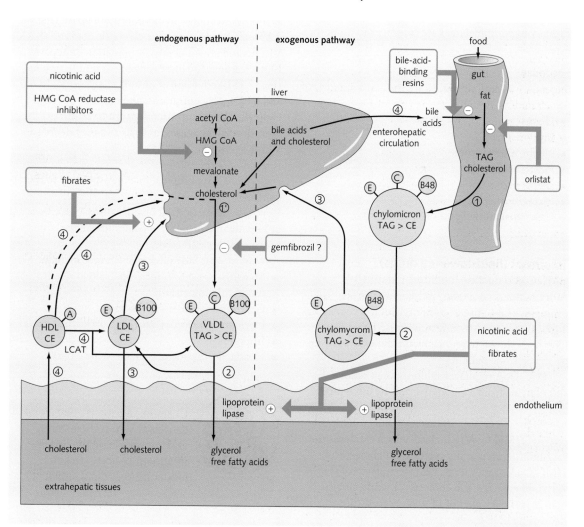

Fig. 7.15 Endogenous and exogenous pathways of lipid transport. (CE, cholesterol ester; HDL, high-density lipoprotein; LCAT, lecithin cholesterol acyltransferase; TAG, triacylglycerol; VLDL, very-low-density lipoproteins; numbers refer to steps in pathways, see text.)

4. HDL is secreted by the liver into the plasma, where it is modified by lecithin cholesterol acyltransferase (LCAT) and uptake of cholesterol from the tissues. Lecithin cholesterol acyltransferase (LCAT) transfers cholesterol esters to LDLs and VLDLs.

Hyperlipidaemias

Hyperlipidaemias are characterized by markedly elevated plasma triglycerides, cholesterol, and lipoprotein concentrations. Cholesterol is deposited in various tissues. Deposition in arterial plaques results in atherosclerosis, which leads to heart attacks, strokes, and peripheral vascular disease. Deposition in tendons and skin results in xanthomas.

Primary

Primary hyperlipidaemias are genetic, and numerous types exist.

Secondary

Secondary hyperlipidaemias are the consequences of other conditions such as:

- Diabetes.
- Liver disease.
- Nephrotic syndrome.
- Renal failure.
- Alcoholism.
- Hypothyroidism.
- Oestrogen administration.

Treatment (lipid-lowering drugs)
HMG CoA reductase inhibitors ('statins')

Atorvastatin, pravastatin, and simvastatin are examples of 3-hydroxy-3-methylglutaryl coenzyme A (HMG CoA) reductase inhibitors. These drugs have been shown to reduce blood cholesterol by up to 35% in some patients.

HMG CoA reductase inhibitors can reduce the risk of dying from a coronary event by up to nearly half.

Mechanism of action: Statins reversibly inhibit the enzyme HMG CoA reductase, which catalyses the rate-limiting step in the synthesis of cholesterol: HMG CoA → mevalonic acid → cholesterol (Fig. 7.15). The decrease in cholesterol synthesis also increases the number of LDL receptors, thus decreasing LDL levels.

Route of administration: Oral.

Indications: Hyperlipidaemia resistant to dietary control, as part of secondary prevention in patients

with serum cholesterol greater than 5.5 mmol/L (though this value will vary depending upon local policy).

Contraindications: Pregnancy, breastfeeding, liver disease.

Adverse effects: Reversible myositis (rare); constipation or diarrhoea; abdominal pain and flatulence; nausea and headache; fatigue and insomnia; and rash.

Fibrates

Fibrates include bezafibrate, ciprofibrate and gemfibrozil. These are broad-spectrum lipid-modulating agents that are ineffective in patients with elevated cholesterol but normal triglyceride concentrations.

Mechanism of action: Fibrates work in several ways, as follows: stimulation of lipoprotein lipase (Fig. 7.15), thus reducing the triglyceride content of VLDLs and chylomicrons; stimulation of hepatic LDL clearance, by increasing hepatic LDL uptake (Fig. 7.15); reduction of plasma triglyceride, LDL, and VLDL concentrations; and increase of HDL-cholesterol concentration (except bezafibrate). Gemfibrozil decreases lipolysis and may decrease VLDL secretion.

Route of administration: Oral.

Indications: Hyperlipidaemia unresponsive to dietary control.

Contraindications: Gall bladder disease, severe renal or hepatic impairment, hypoalbuminaemia, pregnancy, breastfeeding.

Adverse effects: Side effects of fibrates include:

- Myositis-like syndrome (especially if renal function is impaired).
- Gastrointestinal disturbances.
- Dermatitis, pruritus, rash, and urticaria.
- Impotence.
- Headache, dizziness, blurred vision.

 Changing a patient's diet alone can lower serum cholesterol, and this should be the first line treatment option in mild to moderate hyperlipidaemia.

Nicotinic acid

The side effects of nicotinic acid limit its use in the treatment of hyperlipidaemias. Nicotinic acid has

Fig. 7.16 Effects of heparin, vitamin K, and fibrinolytic drugs on the coagulation cascade. (Factor III, factor/tissue thromboplastin.)

been shown to reduce the incidence of coronary artery disease.

Mechanism of action: Nicotinic acid has the following effects: it inhibits cholesterol synthesis (Fig. 7.15), thereby decreasing VLDL and thus LDL production; it stimulates lipoprotein lipase, thus reducing the triglyceride content of VLDLs and chylomicrons; it increases HDL-cholesterol; it increases the levels of tissue plasminogen activator (p. 144); and it decreases the levels of plasma fibrinogen (p. 144).

Route of administration: Oral.

Indications: Hyperlipidaemias unresponsive to other measures.

Contraindications: Pregnancy, breastfeeding.

Adverse effects: Flushing, dizziness, headache, palpitations, nausea and vomiting, and pruritus.

Bile-acid-binding resins

Colestyramine and colestipol have been shown to decrease the rate of mortality from coronary artery disease.

Mechanism of action: Basic anion exchange resins act by binding bile acids in the intestine (Fig. 7.15), thus

preventing their reabsorption and promoting hepatic conversion of cholesterol into bile acids. This increases hepatic LDL receptor activity, thus increasing the breakdown of LDL-cholesterol. Plasma LDL-cholesterol is, therefore, lowered.

Route of administration: Oral.

Indications: Bile-acid-binding resins are especially useful when elevated cholesterol results from a high LDL concentration.

Colestyramine is used in the primary prevention of coronary heart disease in men aged 35–59 years with primary hypercholesterolaemia. It also relieves pruritus associated with partial biliary obstruction and primary biliary cirrhosis.

Contraindications: Complete biliary obstruction.

Adverse effects: Bile-acid-binding resins are not absorbed, and, therefore, they have very few systemic side effects. Side effects include nausea and vomiting, constipation, heartburn, abdominal pain and flatulence, and aggravation of hypertriglyceridaemia. They may interfere with the absorption of fat-soluble vitamins and certain drugs.

Therapeutic regimen: To avoid interference with their absorption, other drugs should not be taken within 1 hour before or 3–4 hours after colestyramine or colestipol administration.

Other lipid-lowering drugs

Fish oils rich in ω-3 marine triglycerides can be useful in the treatment of severe hypertriglyceridaemia, though they may sometimes worsen hypercholesterolaemia. Their role in clinical practice remains to be thoroughly ascertained.

Ispaghula husk is taken orally, and it is presumed to act by binding bile acids, preventing their reabsorption. It is potentially useful in patients with hypercholesterolaemia, but not hypertriglyceridaemia.

Haemostasis and thrombosis

Principles of haemostasis

Haemostasis is the eradication of bleeding from damaged blood vessels.

If haemostasis is defective or unable to cope with blood loss from larger vessels, blood may accumulate in the tissues. This accumulated blood is called a haematoma.

The three stages involved in haemostasis are blood vessel constriction, formation of a platelet plug, and formation of a clot.

Blood vessel constriction

The first response to a severed blood vessel is contraction of the smooth muscle of the vessel. This is mediated by the release of thromboxane A_2 and other substances from platelets.

Blood vessel constriction slows the flow of blood through the vessel, thus reducing the pressure, and pushes opposing surfaces of the vessel together. In very small vessels this results in permanent closure of the vessel, but in most cases blood vessel constriction is insufficient for this to occur.

Platelet plug formation

Exposure to the collagen underlying the vessel endothelium, as occurs during vessel injury, allows platelets to adhere to the collagen by binding to von Willebrand's factors. These factors, secreted by the platelets and endothelium, bind to the exposed collagen; platelets then bind to this complex.

Release of ADP, 5-HT, thromboxane A_2, and other substances by the platelets causes the latter to aggregate, while fibrin acts to bind them together.

The synthesis and release of prostacyclin by the intact endothelium inhibits platelet aggregation, and this acts to limit the extent of the platelet plug.

Intact endothelial cells also produce NO, a potent vasodilator and inhibitor of platelet aggregation.

Clot formation

Blood coagulation is the conversion of liquid blood into a solid gel, known as a clot. A clot consists of a meshwork of fibrin within which blood cells are trapped. It functions to reinforce the platelet plug.

Fibrin is formed from its precursor fibrinogen, through the action of an enzyme called thrombin.

The formation of thrombin occurs via two distinct pathways, the intrinsic and the extrinsic pathways, which together are known as the coagulation cascade. Both pathways involve the conversion of inactive factors into active enzymes, which then go on to catalyse the conversion of other factors into enzymes, and so on (Fig. 7.16).

The extrinsic pathway is so called because the component needed for its initiation is contained outside the blood. Tissue factor binds factor VII on exposure of blood to subendothelial cells, and converts it to its active form, VIIa. This enzyme then catalyses the activation of factors X and IX.

The intrinsic pathway is so called because its components are contained in the blood. It merges with the extrinsic pathway at the step prior to thrombin activation.

The thrombin formed stimulates the activation of factors XI, VIII, and V, and thus acts as a form of positive feedback.

Three naturally occurring anticoagulants limit the extent of clot formation. These are:

- Tissue factor pathway inhibitor, which binds to the tissue factor–VIIa complex, and inhibits its actions.
- Protein C, which is activated by thrombin, and inactivates factors VII and V.
- Antithrombin III, which is activated by heparin, and inactivates thrombin and other factors.

Fibrinolysis

The fibrinolytic or thrombolytic system functions to dissolve a clot once repair of the vessel is under way.

Plasmin digests fibrin. It is formed from plasminogen through the action of plasminogen activators, the best example of which is tissue plasminogen activator (t-PA).

Thrombosis

Thrombosis is the pathological formation of a clot known as a thrombus, which may cause occlusion within blood vessels or the heart, and result in death. Thrombosis causes:

- Arterial occlusion, which may lead to myocardial infarction, stroke, and peripheral ischaemia.
- Venous occlusion, which may lead to deep venous thrombosis and pulmonary embolism.

Arterial thrombi form because of endothelial injury, which is in turn the result of underlying arterial wall pathology, such as atherosclerosis.

Venous and atrial thrombi tend to form as a result of blood stasis, allowing the build-up of platelets and fibrin. People with hypercoagulability, because of a lack of one or more of the naturally occurring anticoagulants, are particularly susceptible.

Arterial thrombi consist mainly of platelets, whereas venous thrombi consist mainly of fibrin.

Management of disorders of haemostasis
Bleeding disorders

Hereditary bleeding disorders are rare. Haemophilia is a genetic disorder in which excessive bleeding occurs, owing to the absence of factor VIII (haemophilia A) or IX (haemophilia B). Von Willebrand's disease is characterized by abnormal bruising and mucosal bleeding.

Acquired bleeding disorders may be due to liver disease, vitamin K deficiency, or anticoagulant drugs.

Caution should be taken when using the following drugs in patients with thromboembolic disease.

Vitamin K

Mechanism of action: Vitamin K is needed for the post-transcriptional γ-carboxylation of glutamic acid residues of prothrombin (factor II) and clotting factors VII, IX, and X by the liver (Fig. 7.17). Vitamin K is also necessary for normal calcification of bone.
Route of administration: Oral, intramuscular, intravenous.
Indications: Vitamin K is used as an antidote to the effects of oral anticoagulants, and in patients with biliary obstruction or liver disease, where Vitamin K deficiency may be a problem. It is also used after prolonged treatment with antibiotics that inhibit the formation of vitamin K by intestinal bacteria, and as prophylaxis against hypoprothrombinaemia in the newborn.

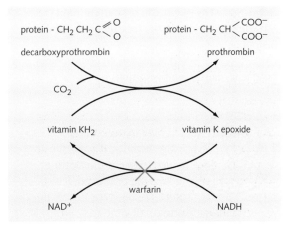

Fig. 7.17 Role of vitamin K in prothrombin formation. Warfarin inhibits the reduction of vitamin K epoxide.

Adverse effects: Side effects of vitamin K include haemolytic anaemia and hyperbilirubinaemia in the newborn.

Protamine

Mechanism of action: Protamine is a strongly basic protein, which forms an inactive complex with heparin, and as such is used in patients in whom heparin treatment has resulted in haemorrhage. High doses of protamine appear to have anticoagulant effects through an unknown mechanism.
Route of administration: Intravenous.
Indications: Haemorrhage secondary to heparinization.
Adverse effects: Nausea, vomiting, flushing, hypotension.

Clotting factors

Deficient clotting factors can be replaced by the administration of fresh plasma. Factors VIII and IX are available as freeze-dried concentrates.
Mechanism of action: All clotting factors are necessary for normal blood coagulation.
Route of administration: Intravenous.
Indications: Haemophilia; antidote to the effects of oral anticoagulants.
Adverse effects: Allergic reactions, including fevers and chills.

Desmopressin

Desmopressin is a synthetic analogue of vasopressin.
Mechanism of action: Desmopressin causes the release of factor VII. Desmopressin is also used in diabetes insipidus, as it has anti-diuretic effects.
Route of administration: Parenteral.

Indications: Desmopressin is given for mild factor VIII deficiency, and in the treatment of diabetes insipidus.

Adverse effects: Fluid retention, hyponatraemia, and headache, nausea, and vomiting.

 The liver is important in coagulation as it is the site at which many of the clotting factors are produced. It also produces bile salts necessary for the absorption of vitamin K, which is needed by the liver to produce prothrombin and clotting factors VII, IX, and X.

Anticoagulants
Vitamin K antagonists
Warfarin, acenocoumarol (nicoumalone), and phenindione are examples of vitamin K antagonists.

Mechanism of action: Vitamin K antagonists block the reduction of vitamin K epoxide, which is necessary for its action as a cofactor in the synthesis of factors II, VII, IX, and X (Fig. 7.16).

Route of administration: Oral.

Indications: Prophylaxis and treatment of deep vein thrombosis and pulmonary embolism; the prophylaxis of embolization in atrial fibrillation and rheumatic disease, and in patients with prosthetic heart valves.

Contraindications: Cerebral thrombosis, peripheral arterial occlusion, peptic ulcers, hypertension, pregnancy.

Adverse effects: Haemorrhage.

Therapeutic notes: The onset of action of vitamin K antagonists takes several hours, owing to the time needed for the degradation of factors that have already been carboxylated ($t_{1/2}$: VII = 6 hours, IX = 24 hours, X = 40 hours, II = 60 hours).

Heparin and the low-molecular weight heparins
Mechanism of action: Heparin activates antithrombin III, which limits blood clotting by inactivating thrombin and factor X. Heparin also inhibits platelet aggregation, possibly as a result of inhibiting thrombin. Low-molecular weight heparins are simply fragments of heparin which exhibit very similar activity to heparin.

Route of administration: Intravenous, subcutaneous.

Indications: Treatment of deep vein thrombosis and pulmonary embolism; prophylaxis against postoperative deep-vein thrombosis and pulmonary embolism in high-risk patients; myocardial infarction.

Contraindications: Heparin should not be given to patients with haemophilia, thrombocytopenia, or peptic ulcers.

Adverse effects: Haemorrhage (treated by stopping therapy or administering a heparin antagonist such as protamine sulphate), skin necrosis, thrombocytopenia, hypersensitivity reactions.

Therapeutic regimen: Heparin is given intravenously by intravenous infusion, or 12 hourly by the subcutaneous route. Low-molecular weight heparins are given as a once daily subcutaneous injection.

Therapeutic notes: Heparin has an immediate onset, and it can, therefore, be used in emergencies.

Hirudins
Mechanism of action: Derived from the medical leech, hirudin, or rather its recombinant derivatives, desirudin and lepirudin, inactivate thrombin.

Route of administration: Subcutaneous, intravenous.

Indications: Desirudin is used in patients with type II (immune) heparin-induced thrombocytopenia. Desirudin is used for prophylaxis of deep-vein thrombosis in patients undergoing hip and knee replacement.

Contraindications: Active bleeding, renal or hepatic impairment.

Adverse effects: Haemorrhage, hypersensitivity reactions.

Antiplatelet agents
Aspirin
Aspirin is acetylsalicylic acid, and originally derived from the willow tree.

Mechanism of action: Aspirin blocks the synthesis of thromboxane A_2 from arachidonic acid in platelets, by acetylating and thus inhibiting the enzyme cyclooxygenase. Thromboxane A_2 stimulates phospholipase C, thus increasing calcium levels and causing platelet aggregation. Aspirin also blocks the synthesis of prostacyclin from endothelial cells, which inhibits platelet aggregation. However, this effect is short lived because endothelial cells, unlike platelets, can synthesize new cyclooxygenase (see Fig. 7.18).

arachidonic acid

aspirin → ⊖ cyclooxygenase

PGG$_2$
PGH$_2$

thromboxanes
e.g. TXA$_2$
platelet

prostaglandins
e.g. PGI$_2$ (prostacyclin)
endothelial cell

Fig. 7.18 Inhibition of cyclooxygenase by aspirin, leading to a reduction in the formation of thromboxane and prostacyclin. (PG, prostaglandin; PGI$_2$, prostacyclin; TXA$_2$, thromboxane A$_2$.)

Route of administration: Oral.
Indications: Prevention and treatment of myocardial infarction and ischaemic stroke. Aspirin is also used as an analgesic and an anti-inflammatory agent (Ch. 4).
Contraindications: Children under 12 years of age; risk of Reye's syndrome. Breastfeeding, haemophilia, peptic ulcers, or known hypersensitivity reactions.
Adverse effects: Bronchospasm, gastrointestinal haemorrhage.
Therapeutic regimen: Aspirin at 150 mg daily after myocardial infarction has been shown to decrease mortality significantly. Given on alternate days, aspirin may reduce the incidence of primary myocardial infarction.

Dipyridamole
Mechanism of action: Dipyridamole causes inhibition of the phosphodiesterase enzyme that hydrolyses cAMP. Increased cAMP levels result in decreased calcium levels and inhibition of platelet aggregation.
Route of administration: Oral.
Indications: Dipyridamole is used in conjunction with warfarin and other oral anticoagulants in the prophylaxis against thrombosis associated with prosthetic heart valves.
Adverse effects: Hypotension, nausea, diarrhoea, and headache.

Clopidogrel
Mechanism of action: Clopidogrel inhibits activation of the glycoprotein IIb/IIIa receptor on the surface of platelets, which is required for aggregation to occur.

Route of administration: Oral.
Indications: Secondary prevention of cardiovascular and cerebrovascular events.
Adverse effects: Haemorrhage, abdominal discomfort, nausea, and vomiting.
Therapeutic notes: If a patient is truly allergic to aspirin, clopidogrel can be used in its place.
　　Ticlopidine acts in a similar fashion to clopidogrel.

Glycoprotein IIb/IIIa inhibitors
Abciximab is the main drug currently in this class.
Mechanism of action: Abciximab is an antibody fragment directed towards the glycoprotein IIb/IIIa (GPIIb/IIIa) receptor of platelets. Binding and inactivation of the GPIIb/IIIa receptor prevents platelet aggregation.
Route of administration: Intravenous.
Indications: Prevention of ischaemic cardiac complications in patients undergoing percutaneous coronary intervention; short-term prevention of myocardial infarction in patients with unstable angina.
Contraindications: Active bleeding.
Adverse effects: Haemorrhage, nausea, vomiting, hypotension.
Therapeutic notes: Tirofiban and eptifibatide also act by inhibiting the GPIIb/IIIa receptor, though are peptide fragments. As peptides, these agents are potentially antigenic, and they should only be used once.

Fibrinolytic agents
Streptokinase
Mechanism of action: Streptokinase forms a complex with, and activates, plasminogen into plasmin, a fibrinolytic enzyme.
Route of administration: Intravenous.
Indications: Life-threatening venous thrombosis, pulmonary embolism, arterial thromboembolism, and acute myocardial infarction.
Contraindications: Recent haemorrhage, trauma, surgery, bleeding diathesis, aortic dissection, coma, history of cerebrovascular disease. Consult BNF for comprehensive list of contraindications.
Adverse effects: Nausea, vomiting, and bleeding.
Therapeutic regimen: Streptokinase is commonly used in conjunction with antiplatelet and anticoagulant drugs.
　　Streptokinase is derived from haemolytic streptococci, and it is therefore antigenic. Repeated administration of streptokinase could result in an anaphylaxis-like reaction. If repeated fibrinolytic

therapy is needed, the non-antigenic tissue-type plasminogen activators should be employed.

Tissue-type plasminogen activators

Alteplase and reteplase are examples of t-PAs.

Mechanism of action: t-PAs are tissue-type plasminogen activators.

Route of administration: Intravenous.

Indications: Myocardial infarction, pulmonary embolism.

Contraindications: As for streptokinase.

Adverse effects: Nausea, vomiting, and bleeding.

 While the administration of a fibrinolytic drug could improve the life expectancy of someone suffering from an acute myocardial infarction, it could also have disastrous effects. There are stringent criteria for administering or not administering fibrinolytic drugs. Learn these from a medical textbook.

Antifibrinolytic agents

Tranexamic acid

Mechanism of action: Tranexamic acid is antifibrinolytic, inhibiting plasminogen activation, and, therefore, preventing fibrinolysis.

Route of administration: Oral, intravenous.

Indications: Tranexamic acid agents is used for gastrointestinal haemorrhage and conditions in which there is haemorrhage or risk of haemorrhage, e.g. haemophilia, menorrhagia, and dental extraction.

Contraindications: Thromboembolic disease.

Adverse effects: Nausea, vomiting, and diarrhoea. Thromboembolic events are rare.

Aprotinin

Mechanism of action: Aprotinin inhibits the proteolytic enzymes plasmin and kallikrein, thus inhibiting fibrinolysis.

Route of administration: Intravenous.

Indications: Aprotinin is used when there is a risk of blood loss after open heart surgery, and for hyperplasminaemia.

Adverse effects: Allergy and localized thrombophlebitis.

Etamsylate

Mechanism of action: Etamsylate corrects abnormal platelet adhesion.

Route of administration: Oral, intravenous.

Indications: Etamsylate is used to reduce capillary bleeding and periventricular haemorrhage in premature infants.

Contraindications: Porphyria.

Adverse effects: Nausea, headache, and rashes.

The blood and fluid replacement

Anaemia

Anaemia is a common problem throughout the world. In the young it is commonly due to nutritional deficiencies (vitamin B12, folate and iron), in fertile women menstrual loss accounts for most cases, and in the elderly, malignancy and renal failure are the more common causes.

Treatment

Iron

Ferrous sulphate, ferrous fumarate and ferrous gluconate are the more common iron salt preparations.

Mechanism of action: Dietary supplementation of iron increases serum iron and stored iron in the liver and bone. Adequate iron is necessary for normal erythropoiesis, as well as for numerous iron-containing proteins.

Route of administration: Oral. Parenteral preparations of iron exist, but they are seldom used.

Indications: Iron-deficiency anaemia.

Contraindications: Caution in pregnancy.

Adverse effects: Gastrointestinal irritation, nausea, epigastric pain, altered bowel habits.

Therapeutic notes: Iron overdose or chronic iron overload can be harmful, and either acquired, or inherited in the form of haemochromatosis. The iron-chelating agent desferrioxamine can be given parenterally, which allows iron to be excreted in the urine.

Vitamin B12

Hydroxocobalamin and cyanocobalamin are vitamin B12 drug preparations.

Mechanism of action: Vitamin B12 is required for DNA synthesis and effective erythropoiesis.

Route of administration: Intramuscular, oral.

Indications: Pernicious anaemia, other macrocytic megaloblastic anaemias.

Contraindications: None.

Adverse effects: Itching, fever, chills, flushing, nausea.

Therapeutic notes: Initial treatment requires regular weekly injections, but once serum vitamin B12 is normalized, injections should be given at 3-monthly intervals.

Folate

Folic acid is the form folate is administered.

Mechanism of action: Folate is required for DNA synthesis and effective erythropoiesis.

Route of administration: Oral.

Indications: Macrocytic megaloblastic anaemias, prevention of neural tube defects in pregnancy.

Contraindications: None.

Adverse effects: None.

Therapeutic notes: Since the introduction of folate acid supplements for pregnant women, the rate of neural tube defects in newborn babies has fallen markedly.

Erythropoietin

Epoetin is a recombinant erythropoietin.

Erythropoietin is synthesized in the kidney in response to a fall in the oxygen tension of the blood passing through it.

Mechanism of action: Erythropoietin acts upon the bone marrow to stimulate stem cells to divide, to produce cells of the red cell lineage.

Route of administration: Parenteral.

Indications: Anaemia of chronic renal failure, anaemia following cancer chemotherapy, prior to autologous blood donation.

Contraindications: Uncontrolled hypertension.

Adverse effects: Dose-dependant increase in blood pressure and platelet count, influenza-like symptoms.

Therapeutic notes: Erythropoietin often features in the news, as an increased haemoglobin concentration most probably improves an athlete's performance, making this drug a potential drug of 'abuse' in sport.

Myeloproliferative disorders

The pharmacological management of the myeloproliferative disorders is outside the remit of this text, though it relies on cytotoxic drugs. Information on these agents should be learnt from a haematology or general medical textbook.

Fluid replacement

Fluid replacement should ideally be achieved orally, though this is often not practical. Intravenous administration of fluids is common-place in hospital.

Intravenous fluids are given for many reasons. In trauma they are used to replace blood loss; in septicaemia they are used to raise blood pressure and tissue perfusion; in the unconscious they are used to replace water and electrolytes lost in the urine and via insensible routes.

There are many types of intravenous fluid. The more common fluids given intravenously are blood, the crystalloids (sodium chloride (normal saline) and dextrose saline), and the colloids (dextrans and gelatin). Each has its role to play in the management of various conditions. Supplements can be added to intravenous fluids to provide the patient with all their requirements.

The art of fluid replacement, and fluid management is best learnt from an anaesthetics or general medical textbook. The names and compositions of the various intravenous fluids can be obtained from the BNF.

- What mechanisms are involved in controlling heart rate?
- What are the differences between nodal and non-nodal cells within the heart?
- What are the more common causes of cardiac failure, and associated signs and symptoms?
- What is meant by the term arrhythmia? What processes may result in arrhythmias?
- What are the principal drugs used in cardiac failure, and their mechanism of action and potential adverse effects?
- How do the anti-arrhythmic drugs act in principle? List the classes of anti-arrhythmics and name an example of each.
- List the more common antianginal drugs, and their mechanism of action, and potential adverse effects.
- What mechanisms are involved in controlling vascular tone?
- Draw a flow diagram of the renin–angiotensin system.
- Indicate on this flow diagram where ACE inhibitors, ATII receptor antagonists and aldosterone antagonists act.
- List the drugs which have vasodilating actions, and summarize their mechanism of action and potential adverse effects.
- Define shock, and outline the main classes of drugs used in its management, and their mechanisms of action.
- List the categories of drugs used in the management of hyperlipidaemia. Summarize their mechanism of action, and adverse effects.
- Outline the steps in haemostasis. List any common disorders of haemostasis.
- Define thrombosis, and name potential complications of this process.
- Name the classes of drugs used in bleeding disorders, their mechanisms of action, and adverse effects.
- List the drugs used to prevent thrombosis, their mechanisms of action, and adverse effects.
- Discuss fibrinolysis, and the agents used today as fibrinolytics, their importance in clinical practice, their mechanisms of action, and potential adverse effects.
- Define anaemia and list its more common causes, and the drugs used to treat these causes.
- Indicate when fluid replacement should be via the intravenous route, rather than the oral route. List some of the intravenous fluids commonly given in hospital.

Reversible airways disease

Asthma

Asthma is a respiratory disease characterized by recurrent reversible obstruction to airflow in the bronchiolar airways. Asthma may be allergic (extrinsic) or non-allergic (intrinsic), though in practice this distinction offers little help.

Allergic asthma

Allergic asthma is the most common form of asthma. Allergic asthma occurs in people sensitive to allergens—antigenic substances in inspired air. Affected individuals have high circulating levels of immunoglobulin E (IgE) and are usually atopic, i.e. genetically prone to allergies. Allergic disorders are discussed in Chapter 4.

Non-allergic asthma

Non-allergic asthma is an intrinsic type of asthma, and it may not be attributable to any allergic reaction. It tends to develop later in life, though on closer questioning a history of childhood asthma-like symptoms often become apparent.

Severe asthma (status asthmaticus)

Severe asthma, or status asthmaticus, is a life-threatening acute deterioration of otherwise stable asthma. It is a potentially fatal condition that must be dealt with as an emergency, and it requires hospital admission. The signs, symptoms, and management of status asthmaticus should be learnt and remembered.

Pathogenesis of asthma

Asthma is characterized by episodes of wheezing and breathlessness caused by bronchospasm, mucosal oedema, and excess mucus formation. In asthma, smooth muscle that surrounds the bronchi is hyperresponsive to stimuli, and underlying inflammatory changes are present in the airways. Asthmatic stimuli include inhaled allergens (e.g. pollen, animal dander), occupational allergens, and drugs or non-specific stimuli such as cold air, exercise, stress, and pollution.

Stimuli cause asthmatic changes through several complex pathways (Fig. 8.1). The possible mechanisms of these pathways include the following:

- Immune reactions (type 1 hypersensitivity) and release of inflammatory mediators: The cross-linking of IgE by allergens causes mast-cell degranulation, and release of histamine and powerful eosinophil and neutrophil chemotactic factors. The eosinophils, neutrophils, and other inflammatory cells release inflammatory mediators that cause a bronchial inflammatory reaction, tissue damage, and an increase in bronchial hyperresponsiveness. Bronchial inflammatory mediators include leukotrienes, prostaglandins, thromboxane, platelet-activating factor, and eosinophilic major basic protein.
- An imbalance in airway smooth muscle tone involving the parasympathetic nerves (vagus), non-adrenergic non-cholinergic (NANC) nerves, and circulating adrenaline that act under normal circumstances to control airway diameter.
- Abnormal calcium flux across cell membranes, increasing smooth muscle contraction, and mast-cell degranulation.
- Leaky tight junctions between bronchial epithelial cells allowing allergen access.

In many patients the asthmatic attack consists of two phases—an immediate-phase response and a late-phase response.

A good understanding of the pathology involved in asthma is imperative to understanding the mechanism of action of the drugs used to treat this common condition.

Immediate-phase response

An immediate-phase response occurs on exposure to the eliciting stimulus. The response consists mainly of bronchospasm. Bronchodilators are effective in this early phase.

Late-phase response

Several hours later, the late-phase response occurs. This consists of bronchospasm, vasodilatation, oedema, and

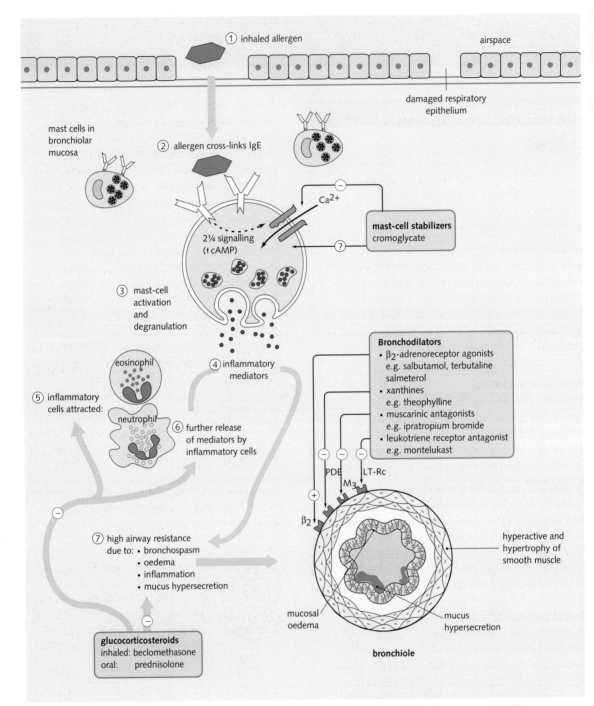

Fig. 8.1 Pathogenesis and drug action in asthma (PDE, phosphodiesterase; LT-Rc, leukotriene receptor). Allergens interact with respiratory mucosa (1), and trigger IgE-mediated mast-cell response (2). Activation of mast cells causes them to degranulate (3) and release various pro-inflammatory mediators (4), which attract and recruit further inflammatory cells (5). These cells also secrete mediators, which amplifies the inflammatory response (6). The over-all effect is narrowing of small airways (7) by bronchospasm, oedema, and increased secretions.

mucus secretion caused by inflammatory mediators released from eosinophils, platelets, and other cells, and neuropeptides released by axon reflexes. Anti-inflammatory drug action is necessary for the prevention and/or treatment of this phase (Fig. 8.1).

Chronic obstructive pulmonary disease

Chronic obstructive pulmonary disease (COPD) occurs mainly in long-standing smokers, and comprises elements of chronic bronchitis and emphysema. Most patients with COPD get some symptom relief from bronchodilators and anti-inflammatory agents in a fashion similar to the asthmatics, yet the response of their airways to these drugs is much less marked, and there are no proven benefits upon life expectancy. Long-term oxygen therapy is also used in patients with COPD.

Management of reversible airways disease

Anti-asthmatic drugs include symptomatic bronchodilators (these are most effective in the immediate-phase response), and prophylactic or anti-inflammatory agents, which prevent and/or resolve the late phase response. The stepwise management of asthma is summarized in Fig. 8.2.

Bronchodilators
Beta$_2$-adrenoceptor agonists
Examples of β_2-adrenoceptor agonists include salbutamol, terbutaline, and salmeterol.

Mechanism of action: Airway smooth muscle does not have a sympathetic nervous supply, but it does contain β_2-adrenoceptors that respond to circulating adrenaline. The stimulation of β_2-adrenoceptors leads to a rise in intracellular cAMP levels and subsequent smooth muscle relaxation and bronchodilation.

Beta$_2$-adrenoceptor agonists may also help prevent the activation of mast cells, as a minor effect.

Modern selective β_2-adrenoceptor agonists are potent bronchodilators and have very few β_1-stimulating properties (i.e. they do not affect the heart).

Route of administration: Inhaled. Oral administration is reserved for children and people unable to use inhalers; intravenous administration for status asthmaticus.

Indications: β_2-adrenoceptor agonists are used to relieve bronchospasm. They may be used alone in mild, occasional asthma, but they are more commonly used in conjunction with other drugs, e.g. corticosteroids.

Contraindications: Caution in hyperthyroidism, cardiovascular disease, and arrhythmias.

Adverse effects: Fine tremor, tachycardia, and hypokalaemia after high doses.

Therapeutic notes: β_2-adrenoceptor agonists treat the symptoms of asthma but not the underlying disease process. Salmeterol is a long-acting drug that can be administered twice daily. It is not suitable for relief of an acute attack.

Anticholinergics
Ipratropium bromide and oxitropium are examples of anticholinergic (antimuscarinic) drugs.

Mechanism of action: Parasympathetic vagal fibres provide a bronchoconstrictor tone to the smooth muscle of the airways. They are activated by reflex on stimulation of sensory (irritant) receptors in the airway walls.

Muscarinic antagonists act by blocking muscarinic receptors, especially the M_3 subtype, which responds to this parasympathetic bronchoconstrictor tone.

Route of administration: Inhaled.

Indications: Anticholinergics are used as adjuncts to β_2-adrenoceptor agonists in the treatment of asthma, and are widely used in the treatment of COPD.

Contraindications: Glaucoma, prostatic hypertrophy, or pregnancy.

Adverse effects: Dry mouth may occur. Systemic anticholinergic effects are very rare.

Xanthines
Theophylline is an example of a xanthine.

Mechanism of action: The xanthines appear to increase cAMP levels in the bronchial smooth muscle cells by inhibiting phosphodiesterase, an enzyme which catalyses the hydrolysis of cAMP to AMP. Increased cAMP relaxes smooth muscle, causing bronchodilation.

Route of administration: Oral. Aminophylline is the intravenous xanthine used in severe asthma attacks.

Indications: Xanthines are used in asthmatic children unable to use inhalers, and adults with predominantly nocturnal symptoms. They are administered intravenously in status asthmaticus.

Contraindications: Cardiac disease, hypertension, hepatic impairment. Xanthines interact with many other drugs and must be prescribed with caution.

Management of asthma (adults and children over 5 years)	
Step 1	Inhaled short-acting β₂-agonist as required
Step 2	Inhaled short-acting β₂-agonist as required *Plus* *Either* regular standard-dose inhaled corticosteroid *Or* regular cromoglicate or nedocromil
Step 3	Inhaled short-acting β₂-agonist as required *Plus* *Either* regular high-dose inhaled corticosteroid *Or* regular standard dose inhaled corticosteroid *plus* regular inhaled long-acting β₂-agonist

Step 4	Inhaled short-acting β₂-agonist as required
	    With
	Regular high-dose inhaled corticosteroid
	    Plus sequential therapeutic trial of one or more of:
	Inhaled long-acting β₂-agonist
	Modified-release oral theophylline
	Inhaled ipratropium or, in adults, oxitropium
	Modified-release oral β₂-agonist
	High-dose inhaled bronchodilators
	Cromoglicate or nedocromil

Step 5	Inhaled short-acting β₂-agonist as required
	    With
	Regular high-dose inhaled corticosteroid *and* one
	or more long-acting bronchodilators
	    Plus
	Regular prednisolone tablets

Stepping down	If control is achieved, stepwise reduction may be possible.

Fig. 8.2 Management of asthma in adults and children over the age of 5 years. Therapy should be started at step 1 and worked upwards until control of symptoms is achieved. Once symptoms have been controlled it may be possible to step down. (Adapted from the *British National Formulary*, 41, March 2001. By permission of the publishers: Royal Pharmaceutical Society of Great Britain and the British Medical Association.)

Adverse effects: Nausea, vomiting, tremor, insomnia, and tachycardia.

Therapeutic notes: Oral xanthines are formulated as sustained-release preparations. Xanthines often cause adverse effects, having a 'narrow therapeutic window', but they are useful as oral drugs in preventing attacks for up to 12 hours.

Leukotriene receptor antagonists

Montelukast and zafirlukast are examples of leukotriene receptor antagonists.

Mechanism of action: The leukotriene receptor antagonists are believed to act at leukotriene receptors in the bronchiolar muscle, antagonizing endogenous leukotrienes, thus causing bronchodilation.

Leukotrienes are though to be partly responsible for airway narrowing that is sometimes observed with the use of non-steroidal anti-inflammatory drugs in asthmatics (NSAIDs; Ch. 4). The NSAIDs inhibit cyclooxygenase, and divert arachidonic acid breakdown via the lipoxygenase pathway, liberating leukotrienes amongst other mediators.

Route of administration: Oral.

Indications: Prophylaxis of asthma.

Contraindications: Elderly, pregnancy, and Churg–Strauss syndrome.

Adverse effects: Gastrointestinal disturbance, dry mouth, and headache.

Therapeutic notes: The leukotriene receptor antagonists are not yet widely used, though their potential as an agent in the combination therapy of asthma is becoming more widely accepted.

In an asthmatic emergency, when thinking what drugs to use, don't forget oxygen.

Prophylactic and anti-inflammatory drugs
Mast-cell stabilizers

Sodium cromoglicate and nedocromil sodium are examples of mast-cell stabilizers.

Mechanism of action: The exact modes of action of mast-cell stabilizers are unclear. These drugs appear to stabilize antigen-sensitized mast cells by reducing calcium influx and subsequent release of inflammatory mediators.

Route of administration: Inhaled.

Indications: Mast-cell stabilizers are useful in young patients (<20 years old) with marked allergic disease and moderate asthma.

Adverse effects: Cough, transient bronchospasm, and throat irritation.

Therapeutic notes: Mast-cell stabilizers have a prophylactic action; they must be taken regularly for several weeks before any beneficial effects are noted. These drugs are, therefore, of no use in acute asthma attacks.

Anti-inflammatory glucocorticoids

Anti-inflammatory glucocorticoids include beclometasone, fluticasone, budesonide, and prednisolone.

Mechanism of action: Corticosteroids depress the inflammatory response in bronchial mucosa and so diminish bronchial hyperresponsiveness. The specific effects include:

- Reduced mucosal oedema and mucus production.
- Decreased local generation of prostaglandins and leukotrienes, with less inflammatory-cell activation.
- Adrenoceptor upregulation.
- Long-term reduced T cell cytokine production, and reduced eosinophil and mast-cell infiltration of bronchial mucosa.

For the intracellular events involved in corticosteroid action see Chapter 11.

Route of administration: Corticosteroids are usually delivered by metered dose inhaler. Oral and intravenous administration is reserved for severe asthma and status asthmaticus.

Indications: Corticosteroids are used in patients with more than minimal symptoms—often in combination with β_2-agonists or drugs that block allergies (Fig. 8.2).

Contraindications: Caution in growing children and in those with systemic and localized respiratory/ENT infections.

Adverse effects: Dysphonia, oral thrush, and systemic penetration in high dosage. If given orally, cushingoid effects may occur (Ch. 11).

Therapeutic notes: The initial treatment of severe or refractory asthma may require oral corticosteroids. If possible, maintenance should be achieved with inhaled corticosteroids via a metered dose, to minimize side effects. Inhaled corticosteroids are usually effective in 3–7 days, but they must be taken regularly.

Use of inhalers, nebulizers, and oxygen

In the treatment of asthma, inhalers and nebulizers are used to deliver drugs directly to the airways. This allows higher drug concentrations to be achieved locally, while minimizing systemic effects. Whatever device is used, less than 15% of the dose is deposited on the bronchial mucosa.

Inhalers

There are several types of inhaler—metered dose, breath-activated spray, and breath-activated powder. They vary in cost, delivery efficiency, and ease of use.

Spacer devices, used in conjunction with inhalers, improve drug delivery, and they are easy to use. Spacers are particularly effective in children.

Nebulizers

Nebulizers convert a solution of drug into an aerosol for inhalation. They are more efficient than inhalers, and they are used to deliver higher doses of drug. They are useful in status asthmaticus and for the acute hospital treatment of severe asthma.

The long-term use of nebulizers is limited by cost, convenience, and the danger of patient over-reliance.

Oxygen

High flow oxygen should be given to any patient in respiratory distress unless they suffer from COPD and have a 'hypoxic drive'. In this situation oxygen can be administered, but at a lower concentration.

Oxygen increases alveolar oxygen tension and decreases the work of breathing necessary to maintain arterial oxygen tension.

Respiratory stimulants and pulmonary surfactants

Respiratory stimulants

Respiratory stimulants, or analeptic drugs, have a very limited place in the treatment of ventilatory failure in patients with chronic obstructive airways disease. They have largely been replaced by the use of ventilatory support.

Doxapram is an example of a respiratory stimulant.
Mechanism of action: Doxapram is used to improve both rate and depth of breathing.

Doxapram is a central stimulant drug that acts on both carotid chemoreceptors and the respiratory centre in the brainstem to increase respiration.
Route of administration: Intravenous.
Indications: Acute respiratory failure.
Adverse effects: Perineal warmth, dizziness, sweating, increase in blood pressure and heart rate.
Therapeutic notes: Apart from naloxone and flumazenil, the respiratory stimulants are seldom employed in clinical practice.

Pulmonary surfactants

Pulmonary surfactants are used in the management of respiratory distress syndrome, which is most common amongst premature babies. Pulmonary surfactants act to decrease the surface tension of the alveoli, and they allow ventilation to occur more easily. They are usually administered via endotracheal tubes directly into the pulmonary tree. Further information on these agents can be obtained from a neonatology text or the BNF.

Antitussives, mucolytics, and decongestants

Antitussives

Antitussives are drugs that inhibit the cough reflex.

Cough is usually a valuable protective reflex mechanism for clearing foreign material and secretions from the airways. In some conditions, however, such as inflammation or neoplasia, the cough reflex may become inappropriately stimulated and, in such cases, antitussive drugs may be used.

Antitussives either reduce sensory receptor activation or work by an ill-defined mechanism, depressing a 'cough centre' in the brainstem.

Drugs that reduce receptor activation
Menthol vapour and topical local anaesthetics
Benzocaine is an example of a topical local anesthetic.
Mechanism of action: Menthol vapour and topical local anaesthetics reduce the sensitivity of peripheral sensory 'cough receptors' in the pharynx and larynx to irritation.
Route of administration: Topical as a spray, lozenge, or vapour.

Indications: Menthol vapour and topical local anaesthetics are used for unwanted cough.

Drugs that reduce the sensitivity of the 'cough centre'
Opioids (Ch. 4)
Opioids reduce the sensitivity of the 'cough centre'. Examples of these drugs include codeine and pholcodine.
Mechanism of action: Although not clearly understood, opioids seem to work via agonist action on opiate receptors, depressing a 'cough centre' in the brainstem.
Route of administration: Oral.
Indications: Opioids are used for inappropriate coughing.
Adverse effects: There are generally few side effects of opioids at antitussive doses. Unlike pholcodine, codeine can cause constipation, and inhibition of mucociliary clearance.

Mucolytics

Mucolytics are drugs that reduce the viscosity of bronchial secretions. They are sometimes used when excess bronchial secretions need to be cleared.

Carbocisteine and mecysteine
Carbocisteine and mecysteine hydrochloride act as mucolytics.
Mechanism of action: Carbocisteine and mecysteine hydrochloride reduce the viscosity of bronchial secretions by cleaving disulphide bonds cross-linking mucus glycoprotein molecules.
Route of administration: Oral.
Indications: Carbocisteine and mecysteine hydrochloride may be of benefit in some chronic obstructive airways disease, although evidence supporting their use does not exist.
Therapeutic notes: A novel drug with 'mucolytic' properties is dornase alfa, a genetically engineered enzyme which cleaves extracellular DNA, and is used in cystic fibrosis, being administered by inhalation.

Decongestants

Nasal decongestion can occur acutely, or be a chronic disorder.

Decongestion relies on administration of agents that ultimately have sympathomimetic effects. This results in vasoconstriction of the mucosal blood vessels of the nose, and a reduction in oedema and secretions.

Ephedrine is the most commonly used decongestant

Mechanism of action: Ephedrine's sympathomimetic activity results in vasoconstriction of nasal blood vessels, limiting oedema and nasal secretions.

Route of administration: Topical or oral.

Indications: Nasal congestion.

Contraindications: Caution in children.

Adverse effects: Local irritation, nausea, headache. Rebound nasal congestion on withdrawal.

Therapeutic notes: Oral preparations are less effective than topical, and they are contraindicated in diabetes, hypertension and hyperthyroidism.

Allergic disorders and drug therapy

Allergic disorders

Allergic reactions occur when the immune system mounts an inappropriate response to an innocuous foreign substance.

Most common allergic disorders are caused by IgE-mediated type I immediate hypersensitivity reactions that occur in a previously sensitized person reexposed to the sensitizing antigen. Type I immediate hypersensitivity reactions are also known as atopic disorders.

Patients with atopic disorders have an inherited predisposition to develop IgE antibodies to allergens that are innocuous and non-antigenic in normal people. These specific IgE antibodies become bound to high-affinity IgE receptors (FcεRI) on the surface of tissue mast cells and blood basophils. The cross-linking of this cell-surface-bound IgE by antigens

(allergens), on subsequent exposure, induces degranulation and release of mediators such as histamine, leukotrienes, and prostaglandins (Fig. 8.3).

The released vasoactive and inflammatory mediators produce many local and systemic effects, including vasodilatation, increased vascular permeability, smooth muscle contraction, oedema, glandular hypersecretion, and inflammatory cell infiltration.

Depending on the site of this reaction and release of mediators, a variety of disorders can result (Fig. 8.4).

Drug therapy of allergic disorders

The most effective therapy in hypersensitivity reactions is avoidance of the offending antigen or environment. When this is not possible, drug therapy can be of use (Fig. 8.5).

Histamine and antihistamines

Histamine is a basic amine that is stored in mast cells (fixed in the tissues) and in circulating basophils; it is also found in the stomach and central nervous system (CNS).

The effects of histamine are mediated by three different receptor types found on target cells (Fig. 8.6).

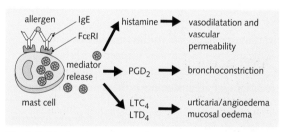

Fig. 8.3 Mechanism of type 1 hypersensitivity (allergic) reaction. (FcεRI, cell surface IgE receptor; LT, leukotriene; PG, prostaglandin.) (Redrawn from Page et al, 2002.)

Fig. 8.4 Type I hypersensitivity/allergic disorders. (GIT, gastrointestinal tract.)

Type I hypersensitivity/allergic disorders			
Disorder	**Site of reaction**	**Response**	**Common allergens**
Anaphylaxis	Circulation	Oedema, circulatory collapse, death	Venoms Drugs
Allergic rhinitis/ hay fever	Nasal passages conjunctiva	Irritation, oedema, mucosal hypersecretion	Pollen Dust
Asthma	Bronchioles	Bronchoconstriction, mucosal secretion, airway inflammation	Pollen Dust
Food allergy	GIT	Vomiting, diarrhoea, urticaria (hives)	Seafood Milk etc.
Wheal and flare	Skin	Vasodilatation and oedema	Insect venom

Fig. 8.5 Drug therapy in allergic disorders.

Drug therapy in allergic disorders			
Disorder	**Drugs used**	**Chapter**	**Mechanism of action**
Anaphylaxis	Adrenaline	5 & 7	Vasoconstriction(α_2) Bronchodilation(β_2)
	Antihistamines	6 & 8	Pro-inflammatory mediator antagonism
	Glucocorticoids	7 & 11	Anti-inflammatory
Allergic rhinitis/ hay fever	Antihistamines	6 & 8	Pro-inflammatory mediator antagonism
	Mast-cell stabilizers	8	Inhibition of mast-cell degranulation
	Glucocorticoids	7 & 11	Anti-inflammatory
	Sympathomimetic vasoconstrictors	5, 7 & 8	Decongestion of nasal mucosa
Asthma	See pp 153–5	8	See pp 153–5
Food allergies	Antihistamines	8	Pro-inflammatory mediator antagonism
Wheal and flare	Antihistamines	8	Pro-inflammatory mediator antagonism

As the major chemical mediator released during an allergic reaction, histamine produces a number of effects, mainly via action on H_1 receptors. Therefore, H_1 antagonists (antihistamines) are of potential benefit in the treatment of allergic disorders.

H_1 Receptor antagonists: antihistamines

There are two types of antihistamines. These are:
- 'Old' sedative types, e.g. chlorphenamine (chlorpheniramine) and promethazine.
- 'New' non-sedative types, e.g. cetirizine and loratadine.

Mechanism of action: Antihistamines work by antagonism of histamine H_1 receptors (Fig. 8.6).

In the periphery, their action can inhibit allergic reactions where histamine is the main mediator involved.

The old-style antihistamines are able to cross the blood–brain barrier where both specific and non-specific actions in the CNS produce sedation and antiemetic effects.

Indications: The main use of antihistamines is in the treatment of seasonal allergic rhinitis ('hay fever'). They are also used for the treatment and prevention of allergic skin reactions such as urticarial rashes, pruritus, and insect bites, and in the emergency treatment of anaphylactic shock.

The old-style antihistamines can also be used as mild hypnotics (Ch. 6), and to suppress nausea in motion sickness, owing to their actions on the CNS.

Route of administration: Orally, topical, transnasal. Intravenous chlorphenamine (chlorpheniramine) can be used in anaphylaxis.

Adverse effects: Old-style antihistamines produce quite pronounced sedation or fatigue, as well as anticholinergic effects such as dry mouth. The newer agents do not do this.

Rare hazardous arrhythmias are associated with the 'new' antihistamines (e.g. terfenadine), especially at high plasma levels or when in combination with imidazole antifungal agents or macrolide antibiotics (Ch. 12).

Hypersensitivity reactions, especially to topically applied antihistamines, may occur.

Mast-cell stabilizers, the anti-inflammatory glucocorticoids, and sympathomimetic decongestants are all used in allergy, and these have already been described.

Remember the allergic reaction can occur locally, systemically, or both.

Histamine receptors	
Histamine receptor	**Effect**
H$_1$	Responsible for most of the actions of histamine in a type I hypersensitivity reaction: • capillary and venous dilatation (producing 'flare' or systemic hypotension) • increased vascular permeability (producing 'wheal' or oedema) • contraction of smooth muscle (producing bronchial and gastrointestinal contraction)
H$_2$	Regulation of gastric acid secretion: • H$_2$-receptors respond to histamine secreted from the enterochromaffin-like cells that are adjacent to the parietal cell (see Chapter 10)
H$_3$	Involved in neurotransmission: • exact physiological role not clear (presynaptic inhibition of neurotransmitter release in the CNS and autonomic nervous system? role in itch and pain perception?)

Fig. 8.6 Effects at histamine receptors.

- What is the definition of asthma?
- Discuss the pathological processes that occur at the cellular level in an asthmatic reaction, and how these produce the signs and symptoms of asthma.
- Describe the broad categories of drugs used to treat reversible airways disease, their mechanism of action, routes of administration, and adverse effects.
- What are the components of the stepwise management of asthma in adults?
- What is chronic obstructive airways disease, and how can it be treated?
- What are the roles and uses of inhalers, nebulizers, and oxygen in the therapy of asthma?
- What drugs might make the symptoms of asthma worse? What are the mechanisms behind this?
- In what clinical setting might a respiratory stimulant be used? Give an example of a respiratory stimulant, and an indication for its use. What are its mechanisms of action and potential adverse effects?
- What is an allergic disorder? Name two examples of allergic disorders, and why they occur.
- What commonly used drugs are employed in the therapy of allergy? What is their route of administration, mechanism of action, and adverse effects?

9. Kidney and Urinary System

Kidney

Principles of renal function

Despite making up only 1% of total body weight, the kidneys receive approximately 25% of the cardiac output.

The volume of plasma filtered by the kidneys is termed the glomerular filtration rate (GFR) and is equal to approximately 180 L/day for a person weighing 70 kg. This means that the entire plasma volume is filtered about 60 times a day.

Functions of the kidney

The kidney has several functions. These include:
- Regulation of body water content.
- Regulation of body mineral content and composition.
- Regulation of body pH.
- Excretion of metabolic waste products, e.g. urea, uric acid, and creatinine.
- Excretion of foreign material, e.g. drugs.
- Secretion of renin, erythropoietin, and 1, 25-dihydroxyvitamin D_3.
- Gluconeogenesis.

The nephron

Each kidney is made up of approximately one million functional units, known as 'nephrons' (Fig. 9.1).

Each nephron consists of:
- A renal corpuscle, which comprises a glomerulus and a Bowman's capsule.
- A tubule, which comprises a proximal tubule, loop of Henle, distal convoluted tubule, and collecting duct system.

Blood supply

Blood reaches each kidney via the renal artery, which divides into numerous branches before forming the afferent arterioles. These afferent arterioles enter the glomerular capillaries (the glomeruli) and leave as the efferent arterioles.

The efferent arteriole leaving most nephrons immediately branches into a set of capillaries known as the 'peritubular capillaries'. These branch extensively and form a network of capillaries surrounding the tubules in the cortex into which

reabsorption from the tubule occurs, and from which various substances are secreted into the tubule.

Glomerular filtration

During glomerular filtration, the fluid fraction of blood in the glomerulus is forced through the capillary endothelium, a basement membrane, and the epithelium of the Bowman's capsule, to enter a fluid-filled space known as the 'Bowman's space'.

Approximately 20% of the plasma entering the glomerulus is filtered. The filtered fluid is known as the glomerular filtrate, and it consists of protein-free plasma.

Tubular function

The tubules are involved in reabsorption and secretion.

Important components of plasma tend to be reabsorbed more or less completely: e.g. sodium and glucose are 99–100% reabsorbed. Waste products are

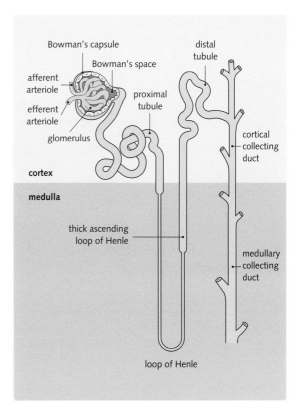

Fig. 9.1 Structure of the juxtaglomerular nephron. (Redrawn from Page et al, 2002.)

only partially reabsorbed: e.g. approximately 45% of urea is reabsorbed.

The tubules secrete hydrogen and potassium ions, as well as organic species such as creatinine, and drugs such as penicillin.

Sodium and water reabsorption

Approximately 99% of filtered water and sodium is reabsorbed, but none is secreted.

Sodium is pumped out of tubular cells into the interstitium by the Na^+/K^+ ATPase in their basolateral membrane. This forms a concentration gradient of sodium: high concentration within the filtrate of the tubule lumen, and low concentration within the cytoplasm of the tubular cells. This gradient forms the basis of most reabsorption and secretion processes that subsequently occur. Sodium reabsorption from the lumen varies according to the section of the tubule (Figs 9.2–9.5).

Water is reabsorbed by passive diffusion, following the movement of sodium ions, and through specific water channels (aquaporins) in the collecting tubules, which greatly increases the reabsorption of water.

Proximal tubule

The Bowman's capsule extends into the proximal tubule, which is made up of an initial convoluted section and a straight section. The proximal tubule is the site into which many drugs are secreted. It is permeable to water and ions.

Approximately two thirds of the filtrate volume is reabsorbed back into the blood in the proximal tubule.

Sodium movement into the cell is coupled with that of glucose and amino acids, whereas chloride movement is by passive diffusion (Fig. 9.2). Reabsorption of bicarbonate also takes place in the proximal tubule.

Loop of Henle

The loop of Henle is shaped like a hairpin; it consists of a descending limb, a thin ascending limb, and a thick ascending limb.

Twenty-five per cent of filtered sodium is reabsorbed in the thick ascending limb (Fig. 9.3), but this portion of the tubule is impermeable to water. Increase in the solute load (sodium) in the interstitium between the ascending loop and the collecting tubules

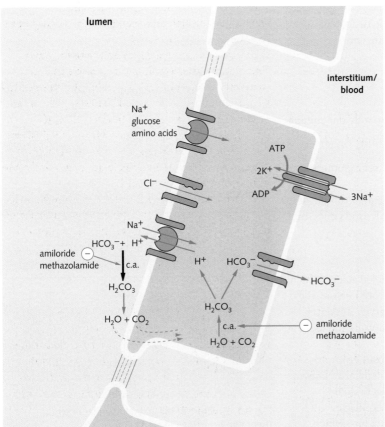

Fig. 9.2 The proximal tubule is one of the sites of bicarbonate (HCO_3^-) reabsorption. Carbonic acid (H_2CO_3) is formed in the cytoplasm from the action of carbonic anhydrase (c.a.) on carbon dioxide (CO_2) and water. H_2CO_3 immediately dissociates into HCO_3^-, which moves down its concentration gradient across the basolateral membrane, and H^+ which is secreted into the lumen in exchange for Na^+. In the lumen, H^+ combines with filtered HCO_3^- to form H_2CO_3 and subsequently CO_2 and water, which are able to diffuse back into the cell.

sets up an osmotic gradient which subsequently permits water reabsorption from the collecting tubules—the countercurrent multiplier system.

Juxtaglomerular apparatus

Where the afferent and efferent arteriole enter the glomerulus, a group of specialized cells, the macula densa, are situated in what is named the juxtaglomerular apparatus. These cells secrete renin, which is fundamental in the renin–angiotensin system. The renin–angiotensin system is involved directly in vascular tone, and in the release of aldosterone (Ch. 7).

Fig. 9.3 Transport mechanism in the thick ascending loop of Henle. Loop diuretics block the $Na^+/K^+/2Cl^-$ co-transporter (1) thereby increasing the excretion of Na^+ and Cl^-. These drugs also decrease the potential difference across the tubule cell, which arises from the recycling of K^+ (2), and this leads to increased excretion of Ca^{2+} and Mg^{2+} by inhibiting paracellular diffusion (3). (Redrawn from Page et al, 2002.)

Distal convoluted tubule and collecting tubule

The distal tubule is continuous with the collecting duct. The collecting duct is the site at which the tubules of many nephrons merge before draining into the renal pelvis. The renal pelvis is continuous with the ureter.

The late distal tubule and collecting duct contain two cell types (Fig. 9.5):

- Principal cells, which incorporate sodium and potassium channels.
- Intercalated cells, which incorporate H^+ ATPases that secrete hydrogen ions.

Sodium movement into the principal cells exceeds potassium movement out, so that a negative potential difference is established. Sodium is transported across the basolateral membrane by Na^+/K^+ ATPase, and potassium is moved into the cell before being forced out by the negative potential.

This part of the tubule is the major site for potassium secretion.

The late distal tubule and collecting duct also contain mineralocorticoid receptors. When aldosterone binds to these, it produces an increase in the synthesis of sodium and potassium channels, Na^+/K^+ ATPase, and ATP, so that sodium reabsorption is increased, and potassium and proton secretion are also increased.

The collecting tubule is also the site for water reabsorption via specific water channels named aquaporins. Fine-tuning the amount of water needed to be reabsorbed is controlled by the hypothalamus, which governs how much antidiuretic hormone (ADH or vasopressin) is released from the pituitary gland. Release of ADH results in more aquaporins being inserted into the luminal membrane, and more water being reabsorbed (Ch. 7).

Atrial natriuretic peptide, derived from the atria of the heart in response to fluid-overload, is believed to act upon the distal nephron causing a water and solute diuresis. This remains a further potential target for future therapeutic manipulation.

Several different sodium channels exist in the renal tubule, which is why the various diuretic drugs act at different sites along its course, and have different molecular actions and clinical side effects.

Oedema

Underlying causes

Oedema occurs when the rate of fluid formation exceeds that of fluid reabsorption from the interstitial fluid into the capillaries.

Oedema has many causes. The more common causes for systemic oedema are congestive cardiac failure and hypoalbuminaemia (including liver failure and the nephrotic syndrome).

Loss of fluid from the intravascular space into the interstitial compartment results in an apparent hypovolaemic state. Poor perfusion of the kidneys activates the renin–angiotensin system, which causes sodium and water retention. This exacerbates the problem of oedema.

Treatment with diuretics

Diuretics are drugs that work on the kidneys to increase urine volume by reducing salt and water reabsorption from the tubules. They are prescribed in the treatment of oedema, where there is an increase in interstitial fluid volume leading to tissue swelling.

Drugs used in the management of renal failure are discussed in Chapter 11.

Loop diuretics

Frusemide (furosemide), bumetanide, and torasemide are examples of loop diuretics.

Loop diuretics cause the excretion of 15–25% of filtered sodium as opposed to the normal 1% or less. This can result in a profound diuresis.
Site of action: Loop diuretics act at the thick ascending segment of the loop of Henle.
Mechanism of action: Loop diuretics inhibit the $Na^+/K^+/2Cl^-$ cotransporter in the luminal membrane (Fig. 9.3). This increases the amount of sodium reaching the collecting duct and, thereby, increases potassium and proton secretion. Calcium and magnesium reabsorption is also inhibited, owing to the decrease in potential difference across the cell normally generated from the recycling of potassium.

Loop diuretics additionally have a venodilator action, which often brings about relief of clinical symptoms prior to the onset of diuresis.
Route of administration: Oral, intravenous or intramuscular. Intravenous route is used in emergencies as therapeutic effect is much quicker (about 30 minutes compared with 4–6 hours for an oral dose).

Indications: Acute pulmonary oedema, oliguria due to acute renal failure, and resistant chronic cardiac failure (CCF) and hypertension.
Contraindications: Loop diuretics should not be given to those with severe renal impairment. They should be given only with extreme caution to patients receiving:

- cardiac glycosides, as the hypokalaemia caused by loop diuretics potentiates the action of cardiac glycosides and consequently increases the risk of cardiac glycoside-induced arrhythmias.
- aminoglycoside antibiotics, as these interact with loop diuretics and increase the risk of ototoxicity and potential hearing loss.

Adverse effects: Hypokalaemia, hyponatraemia, hyperuricaemia, hypotension, and hypovolaemia. Metabolic alkalosis may occur because of increased proton secretion, and consequent excretion. Hypocalcaemia and hypomagnesaemia are also possible.

 Most diuretics drugs block sodium reabsorption from the renal tubule. High solute load in the tubule results in an osmotic diuresis.

Thiazide and related diuretics

Bendroflumethiazide (bendrofluazide), chlortalidone, metolazone, and indapamide are examples of thiazide or related diuretics.

Thiazides produce a moderately potent diuresis, causing the excretion of 5–10% of filtered sodium.
Site of action: Thiazide diuretics act on the early distal tubule.
Mechanism of action: Thiazide diuretics inhibit the Na^+/Cl^- cotransporter in the luminal membrane (Fig. 9.4). Like loop diuretics, they increase the secretion of potassium and protons into the collecting ducts but, in contrast, they decrease calcium excretion by a mechanism possibly involving the stimulation of a sodium/calcium exchange across the basolateral membrane; this is due to reduced tubular cell sodium concentration.
Route of administration: Oral, peak effect at 4–6 hours.
Indications: Hypertension, and oedema secondary to CCF, liver disease, or nephrotic syndrome. Occasionally used for prophylaxis of calcium-containing renal stones.

Fig. 9.4 Transport mechanisms in the early distal tubule. Thiazide diuretics increase the excretion of Na^+ and Cl^- by inhibiting the Na^+/Cl^- cotransporter (1). The reabsorption of Ca^{2+} (2) is increased by these drugs by a mechanism that may involve stimulation of Na^+/Ca^{2+} countertransport (3) due to an increase in the concentration gradient for Na^+ across the basolateral membrane. (Redrawn from Page et al, 2002.)

Contraindications: Hypokalaemia, hyponatraemia, or hypercalcaemia. Caution when prescribing to those taking cardiac glycosides, or to those with diabetes mellitus (thiazides may cause hyperglycaemia).

Adverse effects: Hypokalaemia, hyperuricaemia, hyponatraemia, hypermagnesemia, hypercalcaemia, and metabolic alkalosis.

Potassium-sparing diuretics

Spironolactone, amiloride, and triamterene are all potassium-sparing diuretics.

Potassium-sparing diuretics produce mild diuresis, and they cause the excretion of 2–3% of filtered sodium.

Site of action: Potassium-sparing diuretics work at the late distal tubule and collecting duct.

Mechanism of action: There are two classes of potassium-sparing diuretics (Fig. 9.5):

- Sodium-channel blockers, e.g. amiloride and triamterene. These drugs block sodium reabsorption by the principal cells, thus reducing the potential difference across the cell and reducing potassium secretion. Secretion of proton from the intercalated cells is also decreased.
- Aldosterone antagonists, e.g. spironolactone. Spironolactone is a competitive antagonist at aldosterone receptors, and thus reduces sodium reabsorption and, therefore, potassium and proton secretion. The degree of diuresis depends on aldosterone levels.

Route of administration: Oral.

Indications: In conjunction with other diuretics (thiazides, loop diuretics) in managing heart failure or hypertension, to maintain normal serum potassium levels.

Aldosterone antagonists are used in the treatment of hyperaldosteronism, which can be primary (Conn's syndrome) or secondary (as a result of CCF, liver disease, or nephrotic syndrome).

Contraindications: Potassium-sparing diuretics interact with angiotensin-converting enzyme inhibitors, increasing the risk of hyperkalaemia. They should not be given to patients with renal failure.

Adverse effects: Gastrointestinal disturbances, hyperkalaemia, and hyponatraemia. Aldosterone antagonists have a wide range of adverse effects, including gynaecomastia, menstrual disorders, and male sexual dysfunction.

Therapeutic notes: Low dose spironolactone has beneficial effects in CCF. Several preparations exist which combine a potassium-sparing diuretic with either a thiazide or a loop diuretic, e.g. co-amilofruse, which contains amiloride and frusemide; such drugs are listed in the *British National Formulary*.

Osmotic diuretics

Mannitol is an osmotic diuretic.

Site of action: Osmotic diuretics exert their effects in tubular segments that are water permeable: proximal tubule, descending loop of Henle, and the collecting ducts.

Mechanism of action: Osmotic diuretics are freely filtered at the glomerulus, but only partially, if at all, reabsorbed. Passive water reabsorption is reduce by the presence of this non-reabsorbable solute within

Fig. 9.5 Transport mechanisms in the late distal tubule and collecting duct. Amiloride and triamterene block the luminal Na^+ channels, which reduces the lumen-negative potential difference across the principal cell and decreases the driving force for K^+ secretion from the principal cell and H^+ secretion from the intercalated cell. The net effect is increased Na^+ excretion and decreased K^+ and H^+ excretion. Aldosterone binds to a cytoplasmic mineralocorticoid receptor (MR) stimulating the production of aldosterone-induced proteins (AIP), which (1) activate and increase the synthesis of Na^+ and K^+ channels; (2) increase the synthesis of Na^+/K^+ ATPase, and (3) increase mitochondrial production of adenosine triphosphate (ATP). The effect of aldosterone is to decrease Na^+ excretion and increase K^+ and H^+ excretion in urine, whereas spironolactone, an aldosterone antagonist, has the opposite effects. (Redrawn from Page et al, 2002.)

the tubule lumen. The net effect is increased water loss, with a relatively smaller loss of sodium.

Route of administration: Mannitol is administered intravenously.

Indications: Osmotic diuretics are used mainly for raised intracranial, and, rarely, raised intraocular pressure (glaucoma).

Contraindications: Congestive cardiac failure, pulmonary oedema.

Adverse effects: Chills and fever.

Therapeutic notes: Osmotic diuretics are seldom used in heart failure as expansion of blood volume can be greater than the degree of diuresis produced.

Carbonic anhydrase inhibitors

Carbonic anhydrase inhibitors are no longer used as diuretics, being employed now solely in the management of glaucoma (Ch. 12).

Urinary system

Urinary retention

Acute urinary retention is treated with urethral catheterization. Chronic urinary retention is usually painless, and management depends upon the underlying cause. In men, the most common cause of chronic urinary retention is benign prostatic hyperplasia (BPH). Surgery is the definitive treatment, though many patients can be treated medically. The three classes of drugs that can be employed to treat bladder outflow obstruction secondary to BPH are α-blockers, parasympathomimetics, and antiandrogens.

Alpha-blockers

Doxazosin and prazosin are examples of α-blockers, which act by relaxing the smooth muscle at the urethra opening of the bladder, and so increasing the flow of urine. Since the α-blockers are also used as vasodilators in cardiovascular disease (Ch. 7), hypotension can be a side effect, though they are otherwise well tolerated.

Parasympathomimetics

Carbachol and bethanechol are parasympathomimetics, which act by increasing detrusor muscle contraction. Their effect is most marked when there is bladder outlet obstruction, and they have no role in the relief of acute urinary retention. Side effects include sweating, bradycardia, and intestinal colic. They are now used infrequently, being superseded by catheterization.

Antiandrogens

Finasteride is a specific inhibitor of the enzyme 5α-reductase, which converts testosterone to the more potent androgen dihydrotestosterone. This inhibition loads to a reduction in prostate size, and improvement of urinary flow. The antiandrogens are described in Chapter 11.

Urinary incontinence

Urinary incontinence by definition is the inability to prevent the discharge of urine. The three main types of urinary incontinence are true incontinence, stress incontinence, and urge incontinence.

Urge incontinence is the only type that is practically amenable to pharmacological intervention, mostly with antimuscarinic drugs.

Antimuscarinics

Oxybutynin is the most widely used antimuscarinics for urge incontinence.

Mechanism of action: Oxybutynin relaxes the detrusor muscle of the bladder.

Route of administration: Oral.

Indications: Urinary frequency, urgency, and urge incontinence.

Contraindications: Intestinal obstruction, significant bladder outflow obstruction, and glaucoma.

Adverse effects: Dry mouth, constipation, blurred vision, nausea, and vomiting.

Therapeutic notes: The main side effects are typically the anticholinergic ones, and they are commonly dose-related.

Erectile dysfunction

Erectile dysfunction (impotence) is a very common problem worldwide, and it has numerous causes.

The penis is innervated by autonomic (involuntary) and somatic (voluntary) nerves. Parasympathetic innervation brings about erection, and sympathetic innervation is responsible for ejaculation. Non-adrenergic, non-cholinergic neurotransmission (NANC) also appears to promote erection.

Nitric oxide is believed to be the principal mediator of inducing and sustaining an erection. This highly reactive species activates the guanylyl cyclase enzyme, which subsequently generates cyclic guanosine monophosphate (cGMP).

The synthesis of cGMP in turn activates a protein kinase, which phosphorylates ion channels in the plasma membrane, and causes hyperpolarization of the smooth muscle cell. Intracellular calcium ions are consequently sequestered into the endoplasmic reticulum, and further calcium influx into the cell inhibited by the closure of calcium channels. The overall effect of a fall in intracellular calcium is a relaxation of the smooth muscle, and increased blood flow to the penis.

While nitric oxide has a very short half-life and is molecularly unstable, cGMP is broken down by a specific group of enzymes, the phosphodiesterases, which subsequently results in the penis returning to its flaccid state. Phosphodiesterase type 5 is thought to be the principle species within the penis, and clearly a target for therapeutic manipulation.

Phosphodiesterase inhibitors

Sildenafil is a selective inhibitor of phosphodiesterase type 5.

Mechanism of action: Inhibition of phosphodiesterase-mediated degradation of cGMP. Higher intracellular levels of cGMP result in continual relaxation of penile smooth muscle and maintenance of an erection.

Route of administration: Oral.

Indications: Erectile dysfunction. There are strict guidelines in the United Kingdom as to which groups of patients can be prescribed sildenafil on the National Health Service. These include those patients with: diabetes, multiple sclerosis, Parkinson's disease, poliomyelitis, prostate cancer, severe pelvic injury, single gene neurological disease, spina bifida, or spinal cord injury. For a comprehensive list of criteria, consult the BNF.

Contraindications: Concurrent treatment with nitrates. Conditions in which vasodilatation or sexual activity inadvisable.

Adverse effects: Dyspepsia, headache, flushing, and visual disturbances.

Therapeutic notes: Non-specific inhibition of phosphodiesterase type 6 in the retina is responsible for occasional colour disturbances in some patient's vision. Erection will not occur unless there is sexual stimulation.

Prostaglandin E_1

Alprostadil is a synthetic prostaglandin E_1 analogue, and, like prostaglandin E_1, it has a similar effect to nitric oxide upon penile smooth muscle. Alprostadil can be administered by direct injection into the corpus cavernosum of the penis, or applied into the urethra. The most common and most serious side effect is priapism, and any erection lasting longer than 4 hours should be reported.

Phosphodiesterase enzymes degrade the cyclic nucleotides cAMP and cGMP. Inhibitors of the phosphodiesterases, such as sildenafil, and the less specific xanthines such as theophylline, result in accumulation of these mediators, which brings about the physiological effects of these drugs.

- What fraction of the cardiac output do the kidneys receive, and what is meant by the term glomerular filtration rate?
- List the main functions of the kidney.
- What are the differences between glomerular filtration, tubular secretion and tubular reabsorption? which constituents of blood are filtered, and which are not?
- Describe diuresis, and define a diuretic. Name the classes of diuretic drugs used in clinical practice, and an example of each.
- What is oedema, and what are its more common causes?
- How do loop diuretics work?
- Why should potassium-sparing diuretics be used with caution in renal failure? Explain the pathophysiology.
- What pharmacological treatments are there for the management of urinary outflow obstruction secondary to benign prostatic hyperplasia?
- Antimuscarinic (anticholinergic) drugs are used for urinary incontinence, what are the side effects of anticholinergic drugs?
- What is the mechanism of action of the phosphodiesterase inhibitors in the management of erectile dysfunction? Describe their mechanism of action.

10. Gastrointestinal System

Stomach

Peptic ulceration

The gastric epithelium secretes several substances—hydrochloric acid (HCl) from the parietal cells, digestive enzymes from the peptic cells, and mucus from the mucus-secreting cells. The acid and enzymes convert food into a thick semi-liquid paste called chyme, while mucus protects the stomach from its own corrosive secretions.

Peptic ulceration results from a breach in the mucosa lining the alimentary tract caused by acid and enzyme attack (Fig. 10.1). Unprotected mucosa rapidly undergoes autodigestion leading to a range of damage—inflammation or gastritis, necrosis, haemorrhage, and even perforation as the erosion deepens.

Gastric and duodenal ulcers differ in their location, epidemiology, incidence, and aetiology, but they present with similar symptoms, and are treated on similar principles. Peptic ulcer disease is chronic, recurrent, and common, affecting at least 10% of the population in developed countries. *Helicobacter pylori* plays a role in the pathogenesis of a significant proportion of peptic ulcer disease.

Protective factors

The mucosal defences against acid/enzyme attack consist of:
- The mucus barrier (approximately 500 μm thick), a mucus matrix into which bicarbonate ions are secreted, producing a buffering gradient.
- The surface epithelium, which requires prostaglandins E_2 and I_2, synthesized by the gastric mucosa. These are thought to exert a cytoprotective action by increasing mucosal blood flow.

Acid secretion

The regulation of acid secretion by parietal cells is especially important in peptic ulceration, and it constitutes a major target for drug action (Fig. 10.2). Acid is secreted from gastric parietal cells by a unique proton pump that catalyses the exchange of intracellular protons for extracellular potassium. The secretion of HCl is controlled by the activation of

Weakened mucosal defence	Normal	Increased attack
weakened defences vulnerable to being breached by normal acid/enzyme levels	acid/enzyme attack is adequately balanced by mucosal and other defences	increased attack breaks down the defences that would normally be adequate
e.g. • Helicobacter pylori infection. • loss of normal mucosal defences, e.g. NSAIDs (see Chapter 10)	e.g. • healthy state	e.g. • hyperacidity (Zollinger–Ellison syndrome)

Fig. 10.1 Peptic ulceration. (NSAIDs, non-steroidal anti-inflammatory drugs.) (Adapted from *General and Systematic Pathology*, 2nd edn, by JCE Underwood (ed.), 1996. By permission of Churchill Livingstone.)

Sir Francis Avery–Jones said: 'An ulcer represents the adverse outcome of a conflict between the aggressive forces in the stomach or duodenum (acid/enzymes) and the defence mechanisms (mucus–bicarbonate barrier/surface epithelium)'. This concept can be used as a way to rationalize your thinking of the causes and, therefore, appropriate treatment of peptic ulcers.

three main receptors on the basolateral membrane of the parietal cell. These are:

- Gastrin receptors, which respond to gastrin secreted by the G cells of the stomach antrum.
- Histamine (H_2) receptors, which respond to histamine secreted from the enterochromaffin-like paracrine cells that are adjacent to the parietal cell.
- Muscarinic (M_1, M_3) receptors on the parietal cell, which respond to acetylcholine (ACh) released from neurons innervating the parietal cell.

Although the parietal cells possess muscarinic and gastrin receptors, both ACh and gastrin mainly exert their acid secretory effect indirectly, by stimulating

Fig. 10.2 Acid secretion from parietal cells is reduced by muscarinic antagonists, histamine (H_2) antagonists and the proton pump inhibitors. Gastrin (G) and acetylcholine (Ach) stimulate the parietal cell directly to increase acid secretion and also stimulate enterochromaffin-like cells to secrete histamine, which then acts upon the H_2 receptors of the parietal cell. Antacids raise the luminal pH by neutralizing hydrogen ions. Mucosal strengtheners adhere to and protect ulcer craters, and they may kill *H. pylori*. (Redrawn from Page et al, 2002.)

nearby enterochromaffin-like cells to release histamine. Histamine then acts locally on the parietal cells, where activation of the H_2 receptor results in the stimulation of adenylyl cyclase and the subsequent secretion of acid. Excessive production of gastrin from a rare tumour, a gastrinoma, can result in excess acid production, and in peptic ulceration, a condition known as Zollinger–Ellison syndrome.

Gastro-oesophageal reflux disease

Stomach contents are normally prevented from re-entering the oesophagus by the lower oesophageal sphincter (LOS). Loss of tone of the LOS, or a rise in intra-abdominal pressure are the commonest causes of gastro-oesophageal reflux disease (GORD), of which heartburn, is the major symptom.

Conservative treatment options include weight loss, and raising the head of the patient's bed. Precipitating factors should be avoided, as should excess smoking and alcohol. The drugs used in GORD are the same as for other acid-related disorders (Fig. 10.3).

Prevention and treatment of acid-related disease

Drugs that are effective in the treatment of peptic ulcers either reduce/neutralize gastric acid secretion or increase mucosal resistance to acid-pepsin attack. Peptic ulcers thus treated will heal rapidly, but recurrence is common unless *H. pylori* is eliminated.

Reduction of acid secretion
Proton pump inhibitors

Omeprazole and lansoprazole are examples of proton pump inhibitors (PPIs).

Mechanism of action: PPIs cause irreversible inhibition of H^+/K^+ ATPase that is responsible for proton secretion from parietal cells (Fig. 10.2). They are inactive prodrugs and are converted at acidic pH to sulphonamide, which combines covalently, and therefore irreversibly, with sulphydryl groups on H^+/K^+ ATPase. This inhibition is highly specific and localized.

Route of administration: Oral. Some PPIs can be given intravenously.

Indications: Short-term treatment of peptic ulcers, eradication of *H. pylori*, severe GORD, confirmed oesophagitis, Zollinger–Ellison syndrome.

Contraindications: No important contraindications are reported with PPIs.

Adverse effects: Gastrointestinal upset, nausea, and headaches. There might be a risk of gastric atrophy with long-term treatment.

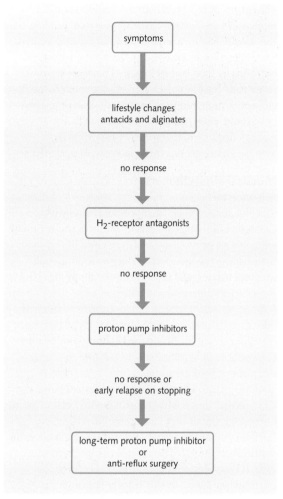

Fig. 10.3 Treatment of gastro-oesophageal reflux disease: a stepwise approach. (Adapted from *Davidson's Principles and Practice of Medicine*, 18th edn, by C Haslett (ed.). By permission of Churchill Livingstone.)

Histamine H_2 receptor antagonists

Examples of H_2 receptor antagonists include cimetidine and ranitidine.

Mechanism of action: H_2 receptor antagonists competitively block the action of histamine on the parietal cell by their antagonism of H_2 receptors (Fig. 10.2).

Route of administration: Oral. Some antihistamines can be given intravenously.

Indications: H_2 receptor antagonists are the first-line treatment of peptic ulcer disease and GORD.

Contraindications: Cimetidine should be avoided by patients stabilized on warfarin, phenytoin, and theophylline.

Adverse effects: Dizziness, fatigue, gynaecomastia, and rash.

Therapeutic notes: H_2 receptor antagonists do not reduce acid production to the same extent as PPIs, but they do relieve the pain of ulcer and promote healing. The drugs are administered at night-time when acid buffering by food is at its lowest. The usual regime is twice daily for 4–8 weeks. Cimetidine inhibits the P_{450} enzyme system, reducing the metabolism of drugs such as warfarin, phenytoin, theophylline, and methylenedioxymethamphetamine (MDMA; 'ecstasy'), potentiating their pharmacological effect.

Mucosal strengtheners
Misoprostol
Mechanism of action: Misoprostol is a synthetic analogue of prostaglandin E. It imitates the action of endogenous prostaglandins (PGE_2 and PGI_2) in maintaining the integrity of the gastroduodenal mucosal barrier, and it promotes healing (Fig. 10.2).
Route of administration: Oral.
Indications: Ulcer healing and ulcer prophylaxis with non-steroidal anti-inflammatory drug (NSAID) use.
Contraindications: Misoprostol should not be given to people with hypotension, or to women who are pregnant or breastfeeding.
Adverse effects: Diarrhoea and abdominal pain.
Therapeutic notes: Misoprostol is most effective at correcting the deficit caused by NSAIDs that inhibit cyclooxygenase-1 and reduce prostaglandin synthesis (Ch. 4). Misoprostol can prevent NSAID-associated ulcers, and, therefore, it is particularly useful in the elderly from whom NSAIDs cannot be withdrawn.

Chelates
Bismuth chelate and sucralfate appear to help protect the gastric mucosa by several means, including inhibiting the action of pepsin, promoting synthesis of protective prostaglandins, and stimulating the secretion of bicarbonate. They are administered orally, and generally well tolerated.

Antacids
Examples of antacids include aluminium hydroxide, magnesium hydroxide, and sodium bicarbonate.
Mechanism of action: Antacids consist of alkaline Al^{3+}, Mg^{2+}, and Na^+ salts that are used to raise the luminal pH of the stomach. They neutralize acid and, as a result, may reduce the damaging effects of pepsin, which is pH dependent (Fig. 10.2). Additionally, Al^{3+} and Mg^{2+} salts bind and inactivate pepsin.
Route of administration: Oral.
Indications: Symptomatic relief of ulcers, non-ulcer dyspepsia, and GORD.

Contraindications: Aluminium hydroxide and magnesium hydroxide should not be given to people with hypophosphataemia. Sodium bicarbonate should be avoided in patients on a salt-restricted diet (in those with heart failure and in hepatic and renal impairment).
Adverse effects: Constipation and diarrhoea.
Therapeutic notes: Antacids are still useful for the relief of symptoms of ulceration; frequent high dosing can promote ulcer healing, but this is rarely practical.

Alginates
Alginate-containing antacids are administered orally, and they form an impenetrable raft that floats on the surface of the gastric contents. This layer prevents gastric acid from refluxing into the oesophagus, and it is, therefore, most useful in GORD. This class of drug is very well tolerated, but it does not have any effect upon acid secretion, or on preventing or healing of peptic ulcers.

Helicobacter pylori eradication regimes
H. pylori plays a significant role in the pathogenesis of peptic ulcer disease. It does not cause ulcers in everyone it infects (50–80% of the population) but, of those who develop ulcers, 90% can be found to have an *H. pylori* infection in their antrum.

Treatment of peptic ulcer disease should include eradication of *H. pylori*. The rate of recurrence of duodenal ulcer after healing can be as high as 80% within 1 year when *H. pylori* eradication is not part of the treatment, but less than 5% when *H. pylori* is eradicated.

The ideal treatment for *H. pylori* eradication is not yet clear. Current regimes under evaluation include:
- The 'classic' triple therapy: 1 or 2 weeks' treatment with omeprazole, metronidazole, and amoxicillin or clarithromycin. This eliminates *H. pylori* in 90% of patients but adverse effects, compliance, and resistance can be problematic.
- Dual therapy: omeprazole is given in combination with a single antibiotic, usually either amoxicillin or clarithromycin; this is less effective at *H. pylori* eradication, and it is not recommended.

 Peptic ulcer disease is very common, and potentially life-threatening. Always check with patients if they have an ulcer, or suffer with ulcer-like symptoms, before prescribing NSAIDs.

Nausea and vomiting

Nausea is an unpleasant feeling in the upper abdomen and throat, which usually precedes vomiting, though for many patients nausea is experienced without vomiting. Nausea alone can be as distressing as the act of vomiting itself. The more common causes of nausea and vomiting are shown in Fig. 10.4. The act of vomiting is coordinated in the vomiting centre within the brainstem. This centre receives neuronal input from several sources, though fibres from the chemoreceptor trigger zone (CTZ) of the fourth ventricle appear fundamental in bringing about emesis. The CTZ lies outside the blood–brain barrier, and it is sensitive to many stimuli, such as drugs and endogenous and potentially exogenous chemical mediators. The CTZ contains numerous dopamine receptors, which partially explains why antiparkinsonian drugs (dopaminergic drugs) often induce nausea and vomiting, while some antidopaminergic drugs are used as antiemetics.

Treatment
Emetic drugs
It is advantageous, occasionally, to induce emesis (vomiting) to empty the stomach of an ingested toxic substance. Ipecacuanha is given as a liquid, and this causes gastric irritation resulting in emesis. There is no evidence to support its use, however, and gastric lavage is the preferred method.

Antiemetic drugs
H₁ receptor antagonists
Cyclizine and cinnarizine are antiemetic antihistamines.
Mechanism of action: These antihistamines have little effect on nausea and vomiting induced by substances acting directly upon the CTZ, though appear effective antiemetics in motion sickness and vestibulocochlear disease.

Causes of nausea and vomiting

- Gastrointestinal irritation
- Motion sickness
- Vestibular disease
- Hormone disturbance
- Drugs and radiation
- Exogenous toxins
- Pain
- Psychogenic factors
- Intracranial pathology

Fig. 10.4 Common causes of nausea and vomiting.

Route of administration: Cyclizine—oral, intramuscular, intravenous. Cinnarizine—oral.
Indications: Motion sickness, vestibular disorders, vertigo.
Adverse effects: Drowsiness, dry mouth, blurred vision.
Therapeutic notes: Antihistamines have significant antimuscarinic activity, and they should be used with caution in prostatic hypertrophy, urinary retention, and glaucoma.

Phenothiazines
Prochlorperazine is the most widely used antiemetic drug in this class, though the phenothiazines are also used for their antipsychotic properties (Ch. 6).
Mechanism of action: Numerous effects. Block dopamine, histamine, and muscarinic receptors.
Route of administration: Oral, rectal, and intramuscular.
Indications: Nausea and vomiting, vertigo, psychosis (Ch. 6).
Contraindications: May exacerbate existing parkinsonian symptoms.
Adverse effects: Sedation, postural hypotension, increased prolactin levels, extrapyramidal effects.

Dopamine antagonists
Domperidone and metoclopramide are examples of the antiemetic dopamine antagonists.
Mechanism of action: Domperidone and metoclopramide block dopamine receptors, and they act on the CTZ. Their central antiemetic effect is enhanced as they also promote gastric emptying and small intestine peristalsis.
Route of administration: Metoclopramide—oral, intramuscular, intravenous. Domperidone—oral, rectal.
Indications: Nausea and vomiting, functional dyspepsia.
Contraindications: Metoclopramide is not routinely given to patients under the age of 20 as there is an increased risk of extrapyramidal side effects in the young.
Adverse effects: Extrapyramidal effects, hyperprolactinaemia.

5-HT₃ receptor antagonists
Ondansetron is an example of a 5-HT₃ receptor antagonist.
Mechanism of action: Antagonism of the 5-HT₃ (serotonin) receptor in the CTZ is believed to be responsible for the antiemetic effects of this class of drugs.

Route of administration: Oral, rectal, intramuscular, intravenous.
Indications: Nausea and vomiting, especially associated with administration of cytotoxic drugs.
Adverse effects: Constipation, headache.

Other antiemetics
The synthetic cannabinoid nabilone has antiemetic properties where there is direct stimulation of the CTZ. Hyoscine is a muscarinic-receptor antagonist, and like the antihistamines it is most effective in the treatment of motion sickness. Betahistine dihydrochloride is used in Ménière's disease, though its prime effects are assumed to be upon the vestibulo-cochlear nerve.

Nausea is one of the most distressing symptoms for the patient, and while antiemetic drugs only control symptoms, prescribing them really does bring about immediate relief.

Intestines

Intestinal motility
Normal motility, or peristalsis, of the intestinal tract acts to mix bowel contents thoroughly and to propel them in a caudal direction. Regulation of normal intestinal motility is under neuronal and hormonal control.

Neuronal control
Two principal intramural plexi form the enteric nervous system. These are:
- The myenteric plexus (Auerbach's plexus), located between the outer longitudinal and middle circular muscle layers.
- The submucous plexus (Meissner's plexus), on the luminal side of the circular muscle layer.

Together, these autonomic ganglionated plexi control the functioning of the gastrointestinal tract through complex local reflex connections between sensory neurons, smooth muscle, mucosa, and blood vessels.

Extrinsic parasympathetic fibres from the vagus are excitatory while extrinsic sympathetic fibres are inhibitory.

The enteric autonomic nervous system is a major target in the pharmacological therapy of gastrointestinal disorders.

Hormonal control
The activity of the gastrointestinal tract is influenced both by endocrine (e.g. gastrin) and paracrine (e.g. histamine, secretin, cholecystokinin, vasoactive intestinal peptide) secretions. Other than in the context of local control of acid secretion in the stomach (p. 169), an understanding of these other hormones is not of immediate relevance to an understanding of the pharmacological therapy of gastrointestinal disorders.

Drugs that affect intestinal motility
Four classes of drug are used clinically for their effects on gastrointestinal motility (Fig. 10.5). These are:
- Motility stimulants.
- Antispasmodics.
- Laxatives (purgatives)
- Antidiarrhoeals.

Motility stimulants
Agents that increase the motility of the gastrointestinal tract without a laxative effect are used for motility disorders such as GORD and gastric stasis (slow stomach emptying), or for diagnostic techniques such as duodenal intubation. Domperidone and metoclopramide, in addition to their antiemetic effects, both act to increase gastric and intestinal motility, though their mechanism of action for the latter remains unclear.

Antispasmodics
The smooth muscle relaxant properties of antispasmodic drugs may be useful as adjunctive treatment in non-ulcer dyspepsia, irritable bowel syndrome, and diverticular disease.

The two classes of antispasmodic drug are antimuscarinics and drugs acting directly on smooth muscle.

Antimuscarinics
Examples of antimuscarinics include atropine, propantheline, and dicycloverine (dicyclomine).
Mechanism of action: Antimuscarinics act by inhibiting parasympathetic activity, causing relaxation of gastrointestinal smooth muscle.
Route of administration: Oral.
Indications: Non-ulcer dyspepsia, irritable bowel syndrome, and diverticular disease.

Contraindications: Antimuscarinics tend to relax the lower oesophageal sphincter and should be avoided in GORD. Other contraindications include angle-closure glaucoma, myasthenia gravis, paralytic ileus, and prostatic enlargement.

Adverse effects: Anticholinergic effects—dry mouth, blurred vision, dry skin, tachycardia, urinary retention.

Drugs acting directly on smooth muscle

Mebeverine, alverine, and peppermint oil are examples of drugs that act directly on smooth muscle.

Mechanism of action: Mebeverine, alverine, and peppermint oil are believed to be direct relaxants of smooth muscle.

Route of administration: Oral.

Indications: Irritable bowel syndrome and diverticular disease.

Contraindications: Paralytic ileus.

Adverse effects: Nausea, headache, and heartburn are occasional problems.

 Irritable bowel syndrome is extremely common in all age groups and in both sexes, and it is often self-limiting over time. Sinister pathology should be excluded, and the patient reassured. Dietary modification and antispasmodics from the mainstay of treatment.

Laxatives

Laxatives are drugs used to hasten transit time in the gut and encourage defecation. Laxatives are used to

Fig. 10.5 Intestinal motility: Control and sites of drug action. (ACh, acetylcholine.)

relieve constipation (an infrequent or difficult passage of stool) and to clear the bowel prior to medical and surgical procedures.

It should be remembered that individual bowel habit can vary considerably—the passage of stools twice a day to once every 3 days is normal.

The frequency and volume of stool are best regulated by diet, but drugs may be necessary. The passage of food through the intestine can be hastened by bulk-forming laxatives, osmotic laxatives, stimulant laxatives, or faecal softeners.

Bulk-forming laxatives
Bran, methylcellulose, and ispaghula husk are examples of bulk-forming laxatives.
Mechanism of action: Bulk-forming laxatives increase the volume of the non-absorbable solid residue in the gut, distending the colon and stimulating peristaltic activity.
Route of administration: Oral.
Indications: Constipation, particularly when small hard stools are present.
Contraindications: Dysphagia, intestinal obstruction, colonic atony, faecal impaction.
Adverse effects: Flatulence, abdominal distension and gastrointestinal obstruction.
Therapeutic notes: Adequate fluid intake should be encouraged, and clinical effects may take several days to develop.

Osmotic laxatives
Examples of osmotic laxatives include lactulose and saline purgatives.
Mechanism of action: Osmotic laxatives are poorly absorbed compounds that increase the water content of the bowel by osmosis. Lactulose is a semi-synthetic disaccharide that is not absorbed from the gastrointestinal tract. Similarly, magnesium and sodium salts are poorly absorbed and osmotically active.
Route of administration: Oral.
Indications: Constipation, hepatic encephalopathy.
Contraindications: Intestinal obstruction.
Adverse effects: Flatulence, cramps, and abdominal discomfort.

Stimulant laxatives
Senna, danthron, bisacodyl, and sodium picosulfate are examples of stimulant laxatives.
Mechanism of action: Stimulant laxatives increase gastrointestinal peristalsis and water and electrolyte secretion by the mucosa possibly by stimulating enteric nerves.

Route of administration: Oral.
Indications: Constipation and bowel evacuation prior to medical/surgical procedures.
Contraindications: Intestinal obstruction.
Adverse effects: In the short term, side effects of stimulant laxatives include intestinal cramp. Prolonged use can lead to damage to the nerve plexi resulting in the deterioration of intestinal function and atonic colon. Danthron is potentially carcinogenic, hence its limited use.
Therapeutic notes: Stimulant laxatives should be given for short periods only, and danthron is indicated for use only in the terminally ill.

Faecal softeners
Liquid paraffin and docusate sodium are examples of faecal softeners.
Mechanism of action: Faecal softeners promote defaecation by softening (e.g. docusate sodium) and/or lubricating (e.g. liquid paraffin) faeces to aid their passage through the gastrointestinal tract.
Route of administration: Oral. Docusate sodium can be administered rectally.
Indications: Constipation, faecal impaction, haemorrhoids, and anal fissures.
Contraindications: Should not be given to children less than 3 years old.
Adverse effects: The prolonged use of liquid paraffin may impair the absorption of fat-soluble vitamins A and D and cause 'paraffinomas'.
Therapeutic notes: The prolonged use of faecal softeners is not recommended.

Antidiarrhoeal drugs
Diarrhoea is the passage of frequent, liquid stools. Causes of diarrhoea include infections, toxins, drugs, chronic disease, and anxiety.

Acute secretory diarrhoea usually results from an infection; it is extremely common, and it causes much preventable mortality, especially in children under 2 years of age in developing countries. The vigour with which diarrhoea should be treated depends very much on the cause and the clinical evaluation of patient risk.

There are four approaches to the treatment of severe acute diarrhoea. These are:
- Maintenance of fluid and electrolyte balance through oral rehydration therapy (ORT).
- Use of antimicrobial drugs.
- Use of opiate-like antimotility drugs.
- Use of stool modifiers/adsorbents.

Oral rehydration therapy

ORT should be the first priority in the treatment of acute diarrhoea of all causes, and it can be lifesaving.

ORT solutions are isotonic or slightly hypotonic; they vary in their composition but a standard formula would contain NaCl, KCl, sodium citrate, and glucose in appropriate concentrations.

Intravenous rehydration therapy is needed if dehydration is severe.

Antimicrobial drugs

Antibiotic treatment of diarrhoea is useful only when a pathogen has been identified or is highly suspected. Acute infectious diarrhoea is usually self-limiting. Antibiotic therapy itself carries certain risks including spreading antibiotic resistance among enteropathogenic bacteria, and destroying normal commensal gut flora, allowing overgrowth of the bacterium *Clostridium difficile*, which can result in pseudomembranous colitis—a potentially fatal condition.

Antibiotic treatment is indicated in:
- Severe cholera or *Salmonella typhimurium* infection—tetracycline.
- *Shigella* species infections—ampicillin.
- *Campylobacter jejuni*—erythromycin or ciprofloxacin.

Antibiotics are discussed in detail in Chapter 3.

Opiate-like antimotility drugs

Examples of opiate-like antimotility drugs include loperamide and codeine.
Mechanism of action: Opiate-like antimotility drugs act on μ-opiate receptors in the myenteric plexus, which increases the tone and rhythmic contraction of the intestine, but lessens propulsive activity. Loperamide and codeine also have an antisecretory action.
Route of administration: Oral.
Indications: Opiate-like antimotility drugs have a limited role as an adjunct to fluid and electrolyte replacement in acute diarrhoea. They are also used as adjunctive therapy in some chronic diarrhoeal conditions.
Contraindications: Opiate-like antimotility drugs should not be given to people with diarrhoeal conditions such as acute ulcerative colitis or antibiotic-associated colitis. They are not recommended for children.
Adverse effects: Nausea, vomiting, abdominal cramps, constipation, and drowsiness.

Therapeutic notes: Loperamide is the most appropriate opioid for local effects on the gut.

Stool modifiers/adsorbents

Examples of stool modifiers/adsorbents include kaolin, chalk, charcoal, and methylcellulose.
Mechanism of action: It has been suggested that stool modifiers/adsorbents act by absorbing toxins or by coating and protecting the intestinal mucosa, though there is no evidence to support this.
Route of administration: Oral.
Indications: There is little evidence to recommend adsorbents at all.
Contraindications: Adsorbents are not recommended for acute diarrhoeas.
Adverse effects: Stool modifiers/adsorbents may reduce the absorption of other drugs.
Therapeutic notes: Adsorbents are popular 'remedies' for the treatment of diarrhoea, although there is little evidence of their benefits.

Diarrhoea can be life-threatening, especially in children. Management in most cases relies on fluid replacement, prior to treating the underlying cause.

Inflammatory bowel disease

The inflammatory bowel diseases fall into two categories that share a number of common features. Symptoms often relapse and remit, and their aetiology remains unclear. Crohn's disease can affect the entire gut, and inflammation occurs throughout the full thickness of the bowel wall, while ulcerative colitis affects only the large bowel, and inflammation is limited to bowel mucosa.

Treatment

Treatment of these conditions is not only pharmacological, but it also depends on psychological support, correction of nutritional deficiencies, and often surgical resection.

Drug treatment is aimed at controlling inflammation and bringing about remission, and the mainstay of drug treatment for these diseases are glucocorticoids, aminosalicylates, immunosuppressives, cytotoxics and antibiotics.

Glucocorticoids

Examples of glucocorticoids include prednisolone, budesonide, and hydrocortisone.

Mechanism of action: Glucocorticoids have an anti-inflammatory effect (Ch. 11).

Route of administration: In localized disease glucocorticoids may be administered rectally as enemas, suppositories, or foams. In extensive or severe disease, oral or intravenous therapy may be required.

Indications: Glucocorticoids are given for acute relapses of inflammatory bowel disease.

Contraindications: Bowel obstruction or perforation, or for prolonged periods.

Adverse effects: Cushingoid side effects may occur with long-term glucocorticoid use (Ch. 11).

Therapeutic notes: Budesonide is locally acting and poorly absorbed, so it has fewer systemic side effects.

Aminosalicylates

Sulfasalazine, mesalazine, and olsalazine are examples of aminosalicylates.

Mechanism of action: Sulfasalazine is broken down in the gut to the active component—5-aminosalicylate (5-ASA)—and sulfapyridine, which acts as a vehicle to transport the drug to the colon. Mesalazine is 5-ASA, and olsalazine is two molecules of 5-ASA. The mechanism of action of the active molecule 5-ASA is unknown, though is postulated to act by scavenging free radicals, or interfering with cytokine networks.

Route of administration: Oral, rectal.

Indications: Maintenance therapy of inflammatory bowel conditions.

Contraindications: Aminosalicylates should not be given to people with salicylate hypersensitivity and renal impairment.

Adverse effects: Sulfapyridine is responsible for the majority of this drug's side effects. Nausea, vomiting, headache, and rashes. Blood disorders and oligospermia have been reported.

Immunosuppressives, cytotoxics, and antibiotics.

When steroids are needed to control symptoms but side effects are troublesome or potentially so, the immunosuppressant azathioprine (Ch. 4) is used as an adjunct to other therapies. In addition, cytotoxic drugs such as methotrexate (Ch. 2), anticytokine antibodies and the antibiotic metronidazole (Ch. 3) have all been employed to modulate the disease process with varying degrees of success.

Obesity

Obesity is becoming increasingly common in the west, and it is associated with many diseases, such as cardiovascular disease, diabetes mellitus, gallstones, and osteoarthritis.

Treatment

Dietary restriction and an exercise programme should be explored prior to surgical or pharmacological intervention. The most widely used anti-obesity drugs act directly upon the gastrointestinal tract.

Drugs acting on the gastrointestinal tract

Orlistat and methylcellulose are examples of such anti-obesity drugs.

Mechanism of action: Orlistat is a pancreatitic lipase inhibitor, which reduces the breakdown and subsequent absorption of fat from the gut. Methylcellulose is believed to act as a bulk-forming agent, and reduce food intake by promoting early satiety (fullness).

Route of administration: Oral.

Adverse effects: Orlistat often results in oily, frequent stools, flatulence, and abdominal and rectal pain. Methylcellulose may produce flatulence and abdominal distention.

Other anti-obesity drugs

The centrally acting appetite suppressant phentermine is licensed, but limitations on its use yield marginal weight loss, so it is seldom prescribed. Numerous other drugs are being evaluated for their anti-obesity properties, including the endogenous mammalian peptide leptin, which appears to induce satiety and counteract the properties of another transmitter, neuropeptide Y, which is believed to promote feeding.

Anal disorders

Haemorrhoids, anal fissures, and pruritus are commonly encountered problems. Bland ointments are the best treatment option, with careful attention to cleanliness. When necessary, topical preparations containing local anaesthetic (Ch. 5) or corticosteroids (Ch. 11) may provide symptomatic relief. Perianal thrush can be treated with nystatin (Ch. 3). Haemorrhoids are often treated by injection with a sclerosant, commonly oily phenol.

Stoma care is simple, though it requires a thoughtful, practical approach, and empathy with the patient. Details of specific stoma care options can be obtained from the *British National Formulary.*

Pancreas and gall bladder

Pancreatic supplements

Pancreatic exocrine secretions contain important enzymes that break down proteins (trypsin, chymotrypsin), starch (amylase), and fats (lipase). These are essential for efficient digestion.

Pancreatin is an extract of pancreas containing protease, lipase, and amylase, that is given by mouth to compensate for reduced or absent exocrine secretions in cystic fibrosis, and following pancreatectomy, total gastrectomy, or chronic pancreatitis. Pancreatin is inactivated by gastric acid and so precautions must be taken to optimize delivery of the pancreatin to the duodenum. Pancreatin preparations are best taken with food; histamine H_2 antagonists (e.g. cimetidine) may be taken an hour before ingestion of the pancreatin in order to reduce gastric acid secretion, though acid-resistant (enterically-coated formulations) are now available.

Even though pancreatin contains peptides, which would normally be degraded in the stomach, these tablets are coated in an acid-resistant layer, and the enzymes and proenzymes within them have endogenous resistance to both acid and proteases, and they become active in the small intestine.

Gall bladder

Bile is secreted by the liver and stored in the gall bladder. Bile contains cholesterol, phospholipids, and bile salts. Bile salts are important for keeping cholesterol in solution. The formation of 'stones' in the bile is relatively common (cholelithiasis), and this can result in blockage of the draining duct, with subsequent infection and inflammation (cholecystitis). Surgical removal of the gall bladder (cholecystectomy) has largely replaced the use of drugs in the management of symptomatic gall stones, though drugs are suitable for patients not treatable by other means.

The dissolution of small cholesterol stones is carried out by prolonged oral administration of the bile acid ursodeoxycholic acid.

Ursodeoxycholic acid

The bile salt ursodeoxycholic acid is administered orally, and handled by the body in the same fashion as endogenous bile salt. It works by decreasing both the secretion of cholesterol into the bile and its absorption from the intestine.

The net effect is a reduced cholesterol concentration in the bile, and a tendency for the dissolution of existing stones.

Colestyramine

This orally administered anion-exchange resin binds bile acids in the gut, preventing their reabsorption and enterohepatic recirculation. It is used in the treatment of pruritus associated with partial biliary obstruction and primary biliary cirrhosis, and in hypercholesterolaemia.

- Describe how the pathophysiology of peptic ulceration involves disturbance of the balance between the aggressive forces (acid/enzymes) and the defence mechanisms (mucus–bicarbonate barrier/surface epithelium) of the stomach and duodenum.
- Describe the factors that control acid production and maintain mucosal defences.
- Relate these first two points to the principles by which the pharmacological treatments work.
- Name examples of each of the different classes of drug.
- Discuss the significance of *Helicobacter pylori* in peptic ulceration.
- Describe the treatment options for the eradication of *Helicobacter pylori*.
- List some common causes for each of nausea and vomiting, and outline the physiology of the two.
- Which are the more common antiemetic drugs, and how do they act?
- Briefly describe the endogenous control of intestinal motility.
- What common diseases affect the intestines that require medical treatments?
- Describe functional bowel disease, and list the classes of drugs use in its management.
- Describe what a laxative drug is, and name the various classes of agents that have laxative properties.
- Outline the immediate therapeutic management of a child presenting with chronic diarrhoea.
- Which infectious agents are likely to result in diarrhoea?
- How do the opiate-like drugs affect diarrhoea, and what are their side effects?
- What are the main groups of drugs used to treat chronic inflammatory bowel disease?
- By what routes of administration can the glucocorticoids be given to treat inflammatory bowel disease, and how do they act?
- List the adverse effects of long-term steroid use.
- Describe the drugs available to treat obesity, and briefly summarize how they act.
- Why is pancreatic supplementation important in cystic fibrosis, and what would be the consequences for the patient if they did not take these?

Thyroid gland

Principles of thyroid function
Production of thyroid hormones

The thyroid gland secretes three hormones, triiodothyronine (T_3), thyroxine (T_4) and calcitonin, though T_3 and T_4 are regarded as the 'true' thyroid hormones and reference to thyroid hormones will relate to these. Calcitonin will be discussed at the end of this chapter.

The principal effects of the thyroid hormones are determination of basal metabolic rate, and influence of growth through stimulation of growth hormone synthesis and action. Other effects are summarized in Fig. 11.1.

The follicular cells of the thyroid gland synthesize and glycosylate thyroglobulin before secreting it into their lumen. Iodination of the tyrosine residues on this molecule is catalysed by thyroid peroxidase, and this results in the formation of monoiodotyrosine (MIT) or diiodotyrosine (DIT). The coupling of MIT with DIT produces T_3, and the coupling of two DIT molecules produces T_4. Coupling is also catalysed by thyroid peroxidase.

The thyroglobulin, now known as colloid, is endocytosed into the follicular cells, where it is broken down to release T_3, T_4, MIT, and DIT. T_3 and T_4 are secreted into the plasma; MIT and DIT are metabolized within the cells and their iodide is recycled (Fig. 11.2).

The iodine required for the synthesis of T_3 and T_4 comes mainly from the diet in the form of iodide. Through the action of a thyrotrophin-dependent pump, iodide is concentrated in the follicular cells, where it is converted into iodine by thyroid peroxidase.

Control of thyroid hormone secretion

The production of thyroid hormones is slow but constant, and control of their plasma levels is determined by varying their rate of secretion (Fig. 11.3).

The hypothalamus contains thyroid hormone receptors that are able to detect and respond to decreased levels of T_3 and T_4 by causing the release of thyrotrophin-releasing hormone (TRH).

TRH reaches the anterior pituitary via the portal circulation, and it stimulates TRH receptors on thyrotroph cells, which in turn secrete thyroid-stimulating hormone (TSH).

TSH reaches the thyroid gland through the systemic circulation, where it stimulates thyroid hormone secretion. Both T_3 and T_4 bind to proteins in the plasma (mostly thyroxine binding globulin), and less than 1% of total thyroid hormones are free. It is the free thyroid hormones that exert their physiological effects. T_3 is about five times more biologically active than T_4, and T_4 is converted in some peripheral tissues to T_3.

T_3 and T_4 exert negative feedback upon the hypothalamus and pituitary.

Most modern laboratory thyroid function tests measure just TSH, though levels of free and total T_3 and T_4 can be measured as well as thyroxine-binding globulin.

Thyroid dysfunction
Hypothyroidism

Hypothyroidism—thyroid insufficiency—is relatively common in adults, and it is associated with tiredness and lethargy, weight gain, intolerance to cold, dry skin, bradycardia, and mental impairment.

Children with hypothyroidism manifest delayed bone growth, whereas a deficiency *in utero* also

---

Physiological effects of thyroid hormones

- Fetal development (physical and cognitive)
- Metabolic rate
- Body temperature
- Cardiac rate and contractility
- Peripheral vasodilatation
- Red cell mass and circulatory volume
- Respiratory drive
- Peripheral nerves (reflexes)
- Hepatic metabolic enzymes
- Bone turnover
- Skin and soft tissue effects

Fig. 11.1 Physiological effects of thyroid hormones. (From Page et al, 2002.)

Fig. 11.2 Synthesis of thyroid hormones and the site of action of some antithyroid drugs. (DIT, diiodotyrosine; MIT, monoiodotyrosine; PTU, propylthiouracil; T_3, triiodothyronine; T_4, thyroxine; TSH, thyroid-stimulating hormone.) (Redrawn from Page et al, 2002.)

results in mentally retarded infants; this condition is known as cretinism.

Hashimoto's thyroiditis is an autoimmune disease resulting in fibrosis of the thyroid gland. It is the most common cause of hypothyroidism and, like most autoimmune diseases, it is more prevalent in women.

Myxoedema is also immunological in origin, and it represents the most severe form of hypothyroidism—sometimes causing coma.

Thyroid hormone resistance and reduced TSH secretion will also produce the symptoms of hypothyroidism.

The causes of hypothyroidism are summarized in Fig. 11.4.

Hyperthyroidism

Hyperthyroidism—thyroid excess—results either from the overproduction of endogenous hormone or exposure to excess exogenous hormone.

Symptoms include increased basal metabolic rate (BMR) with consequent weight loss, increased appetite, increased body temperature, and sweating, as well as nervousness, tremor, tachycardia, and classical ophthalmic signs.

Graves' disease (diffuse toxic goitre) is the most common cause of hyperthyroidism. It is an autoimmune disease caused by the activation of TSH receptors by antibodies. This results in an enlargement of the gland and, therefore, excess hormone production.

Toxic nodular goitre is the second most common cause of hyperthyroidism. It is due to either a single adenoma (hyperfunctioning adenoma) or multiple adenomas (multinodular goitre).

The causes of hyperthyroidism are summarized in Fig. 11.5.

Management of thyroid dysfunction
Hyperthyroidism and antithyroid drugs
Thioureylenes

Carbimazole, methimazole, and propylthiouracil (PTU) are examples of thioureylenes. The thioureylenes are the first-line drugs for treatment of hyperthyroidism.

In the body, carbimazole is rapidly converted to active compound methimazole.

Mechanism of action: The thioureylenes cause inhibition of thyroid peroxidase with a consequent

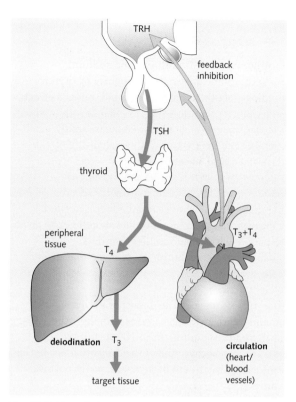

Fig. 11.3 Hypothalamic–pituitary–thyroid axis; control of thyroid hormone synthesis. (T_3, triiodothyronine; T_4, thyroxine; TSH, thyroid-stimulating hormone; TRH, thyrotrophin-releasing hormone.) (Redrawn from Page et al, 2002.)

Causes of hypothyroidism	
Primary	Chronic lymphocytic thyroiditis (Hashimoto's disease)
	Subacute thyroiditis
	Painless thyroiditis (postpartum thyroiditis)
	Radioactive iodine ingestion
	Post thyroidectomy
	Iodine deficiency or excess
	Inborn errors of thyroid hormone synthesis
Secondary	Pituitary disease
Target tissues	Thyroid hormone resistance

Fig. 11.4 Causes of hypothyroidism. (From Page et al, 2002.)

reduction in thyroid hormone synthesis and storage (Fig. 11.2). The effects of PTU may take several weeks to manifest as there are stores of T_3 and T_4. PTU also inhibits the peripheral deiodination of T_4 to T_3.

Causes of hyperthyroidism
• Excess exogenous thyroid hormone
• Diffuse toxic goitre (Graves' disease)
• Hyperfunctioning adenoma (toxic nodule)
• Toxic multinodular goitre
• Painless thyroiditis
• Subacute thyroiditis
• Thyroid stimulating hormone (TSH)-secreting adenoma
• Human chorionic gonadotrophin (hCG)-secreting tumours

Fig. 11.5 Causes of hyperthyroidism. (From Page et al, 2002.)

Route of administration: Oral.

Indications: The thioureylenes are used for hyperthyroidism. Patients sensitive to carbimazole are given PTU.

Contraindications: The thioureylenes should not be given to people with a large goitre. PTU should be given at a reduced dose in patients with renal impairment.

Adverse effects: Nausea and headache; allergic reactions, including rashes; hypothyroidism; and, rarely, hepatotoxicity, bone marrow suppression, and alopecia.

Therapeutic regime: Carbimazole is given at 15–40 mg daily until the patient is euthyroid (4–11 weeks later), then the dose is progressively reduced to a maintenance level of 5–15 mg daily. Treatment is usually given for 18 months. PTU is given at 200–400 mg daily until the patient is euthyroid, then the dose is progressively reduced to a maintenance level of 50–150 mg daily.

Anion inhibitors

Iodine, iodide, and potassium perchlorate are examples of anion inhibitors.

Potassium perchlorate inhibits the uptake of iodine by the thyroid (Fig. 11.2), but it is no longer used, because of the risk of aplastic anaemia.

Iodide is the most rapidly acting treatment against thyrotoxicosis, and it is given in thyrotoxic crisis ('thyroid storm').

Mechanism of action: Iodine and iodide cause inhibition of conversion of T_4 to T_3, of organification, and of hormone secretion. They also reduce the size and vascularity of the gland, which is evident after 10–14 days.

Route of administration: Oral.

Indications: Thyrotoxicosis, and preoperatively.

Contraindications: Iodine and iodide should not be given to breastfeeding women as they cause goitre in infants.

Adverse effects: Iodine and iodide can cause hypersensitivity reactions including rashes, headache, lacrimation, conjunctivitis, laryngitis, and bronchitis. With long-term treatment, depression, insomnia, and impotence can occur.

Therapeutic regime: Iodine and iodide are given 10–14 days before partial thyroidectomy, with either carbimazole or PTU. They should not be given long term as iodine becomes less effective.

Beta-adrenoceptor antagonists

Propranolol and atenolol are examples of β-adrenoceptor antagonists. They are used to attenuate the symptoms of increased thyroid hormone levels, and the effect of increased numbers of adrenoceptors caused by thyroid hormone.

Mechanism of action: β-adrenoceptor antagonists reduce tachycardia, the BMR, nervousness, and tremor.

Route of administration: Oral.

Indications: Thyrotoxic crisis and preoperatively.

Contraindications: β-adrenoceptor antagonists should not be given to people with asthma.

Adverse effects: The side effects of β-adrenoceptor antagonists are given in Chapter 7.

Radioiodine

The use of radioactive iodine to treat hyperthyroidism is not classically considered pharmacology, though the reader should be aware of its place in the management of thyroid disorders; and it is advised to consult a general medical textbook.

Hypothyroidism and thyroid replacement therapy

Levothyroxine

Thyroxine is given as thyroxine sodium in maintenance therapy. It has a half-life of 6 days and a peak onset of 9 days.

Mechanism of action: Thyroxine is converted to T_3 *in vivo*.

Route of administration: Oral.

Indications: Hypothyroidism.

Contraindications: Thyroxine should not be given to people with thyrotoxicosis, and it should be used with caution in those who have cardiovascular disease.

Adverse effects: Arrhythmias, tachycardia, anginal pain, cramps, headache, restlessness, sweating, and weight loss.

Therapeutic regime: The starting dose of thyroxine should be no greater than 100 μg daily (reduce in elderly or those with cardiovascular disease) and increased by 25–50 μg every 4 weeks until a dose of 100–200 μg is reached.

Liothyronine (L-triiodothyronine sodium)

As liothyronine is bound only slightly by thyroid binding globulin, it has a more rapid onset of effects and a shorter duration of action than levothyroxine.

Mechanism of action: Liothyronine is rapidly metabolized *in vivo* to T_3. It has a half-life of 2–5 days and a peak onset of 1–2 days.

Route of administration: Oral, intravenous.

Indications: Liothyronine is given for severe hypothyroidism where a rapid effect is needed.

Contraindications: Liothyronine should not be given to people with cardiovascular disorders.

Adverse effects: Arrhythmias, tachycardia, anginal pain, cramps, headache, restlessness, sweating, and weight loss.

Therapeutic regime: The dosage of liothyronine should be gradually increased as with thyroxine (20 μg liothyronine is equivalent to 100 μg thyroxine). Intravenous liothyronine is the drug of choice in the emergency treatment of myxoedema (hypothyroid) coma.

Endocrine pancreas

Control of plasma glucose

Blood glucose levels are maintained at a concentration of about 5 mmol/L, and usually do not exceed 8 mmol/L. A plasma glucose concentration of 2.2 mmol/L or less may result in hypoglycaemic coma and death due to a lack of energy reaching the brain. A plasma glucose concentration of more than 10 mmol/L exceeds the renal threshold for glucose, which means that glucose will be present in the urine. Osmotic diuresis then occurs.

The islets of Langerhans, located in the pancreas, contain glucose receptors, and they secrete the hormones glucagon and insulin. These hormones are short-term regulators of plasma glucose levels with opposite effects. In addition, their release can be influenced by gastrointestinal hormones and autonomic nerves.

Glucose receptors are also found in the ventromedial nucleus and lateral areas of the hypothalamus. These are able to regulate appetite and feeding, and they also indirectly stimulate the release of a variety of hormones, including adrenaline, growth hormone, and cortisol, all of which affect glucose metabolism.

The hormones involved in blood glucose regulation target the liver, skeletal muscle, and adipose tissue.

Insulin

Insulin is a 51-amino-acid-residue peptide made up of an α- and a β-chain linked by disulphide bonds. It has a half-life of 3–5 minutes and it is metabolized to a large extent by the liver (40–50%), but also by the kidneys and muscles.

In response to high blood glucose levels (as occurs after a meal), as well as to glucosamine, amino acids, fatty acids, ketone bodies, and sulphonylureas (see below), the β-cells of the endocrine pancreas secrete insulin along with a C peptide.

Insulin release is mediated by ATP-dependent potassium channels, located in the membrane of the β-cells. These close in response to elevated cytoplasmic ATP and decreased cytoplasmic ADP levels, resulting in depolarization of the membrane. This triggers calcium entry into the cell through voltage-dependent calcium channels, and subsequent insulin release (Fig. 11.6).

Insulin release is inhibited by low blood glucose levels, growth hormone, glucagon, cortisol, and sympathetic nervous system activation.

The insulin receptor consists of two α- and two β-subunits linked by disulphide bonds. Insulin binds to the extracellular α-subunits, resulting in the internalization of the receptor, and its subsequent breakdown.

The β-subunits display tyrosine kinase activity upon the binding of insulin to the receptor. Autophosphorylation of the β-subunits ensues, resulting in the phosphorylation of phospholipase C with subsequent liberation of diacylglycerol (DAG) and inositol triphosphate (IP_3).

The effects of insulin are summarized in Fig. 11.7.

Diabetes mellitus

Diabetes mellitus involves an inability to regulate plasma glucose within the normal range. It is characterized by an absolute or relative insulin deficiency, leading to hyperglycaemia, glycosuria (glucose in the urine), polyuria (production of large volumes of dilute urine) associated with cellular potassium depletion, and polydipsia (intense thirst).

Effects of insulin on fuel homeostasis	
Carbohydrates	Increase glucose transport Increase glycogen synthesis Increase glycolysis Inhibit gluconeogenesis
Fats	Increase lipoprotein lipase activity Increase fat storage in adipocytes Inhibit lipolysis (hormone-sensitive lipase) Increase hepatic lipoprotein synthesis Inhibit fatty acid oxidation
Proteins	Increase protein synthesis Increase amino acid transport

Fig. 11.7 Metabolic effects of insulin on fuel homeostasis. (From Page et al, 2002.)

Fig. 11.6 Mechanism of insulin secretion from pancreatic β-cells.

There are two forms of diabetes mellitus: insulin-dependent and non-insulin-dependent.

The differences between the two forms are summarized in Fig. 11.8.

The long-term consequences of both types of diabetes are similar, and include increased risk of cardiovascular and cerebrovascular events, peripheral and autonomic neuropathy, nephropathy, and retinopathy.

Insulin-dependent diabetes mellitus (type 1)

In insulin-dependent diabetes mellitus (IDDM), pancreatic β-cells are destroyed by an autoimmune T cell attack. This leads to a complete inability to secrete insulin, and ketoacidosis is a problem. Some untreated IDDM patients have a plasma glucose concentration of up to 100 mmol/L due to insulin deficiency. In this situation, lipolysis is increased, as is the production of ketone bodies from fatty acids. This leads to ketonuria and metabolic acidosis; body fluids become hypertonic, resulting in cellular dehydration, and eventually in hyperosmolar coma.

IDDM is apparent at a young age.

Non-insulin-dependent diabetes mellitus (type 2)

In non-insulin-dependent diabetes mellitus (NIDDM), insulin is often secreted as on average 50% of the β-cells remain active, though there is also peripheral resistance to insulin. Unlike IDDM, this is relatively common in all populations enjoying an affluent life-style. The prevalence of NIDDM increases with age and the degree of obesity.

Ketosis is not a feature of NIDDM as ketone production is suppressed by the small amounts of insulin produced by the pancreas. Hyperosmolar non-ketotic coma is the NIDDM equivalent to ketoacidosis, and it can be fatal if untreated, though it responds rapidly to fluids and insulin.

Secondary diabetes mellitus

Not to be confused with NIDDM, secondary diabetes mellitus accounts for less than 2% of all new cases of diabetes, and it is most commonly due to pancreatic disease (pancreatitis, carcinoma, cystic fibrosis), endocrine disease (Cushing's syndrome, acromegaly), or drug-induced (thiazide diuretics or corticosteroid therapy).

Management of diabetes mellitus
Insulin

The aim of exogenous insulin preparations is to mimic basal levels of endogenous insulin and meal-induced increases in insulin.

Insulin preparations can be human (recombinant), porcine, or bovine in origin, and they are available as short-, intermediate-, and long-acting preparations (Fig. 11.9).

Short-acting insulins are soluble. These preparations most resemble endogenous insulin, and they can be given intravenously in hospital. The rapid-acting insulins aspart and lispro have recently been introduced, which have a faster onset and shorter duration of action than the traditional short-acting insulin.

Intermediate- and long-acting insulins are not as soluble as the short-acting preparations. Their solubility is decreased by precipitating the insulin with zinc or protamine (a basic protein), which prolongs their release into the bloodstream.

The intermediate- and long-acting preparations include:
- Isophane insulin.
- Biphasic isophane insulin.

Features of insulin-dependent and non-insulin-dependent diabetes mellitus

Insulin-dependent diabetes mellitus (IDDM)	Non-insulin-dependent diabetes mellitus (NIDDM)
0.5% prevalence in adults	5% prevalence in adults
Juvenile onset (<30 years)	Maturity onset (>30 years)
Absolute lack of insulin	Relative lack of, or excess, insulin
Not associated with obesity	Often associated with obesity
Insulin therapy	Oral agents (sulphonylureas) usually suffice
Ketoacidosis frequent	Ketoacidosis uncommon
Linked to the presence of islet cell antibody and genetic markers (HLA antigens)	No known autoimmune origin

Fig. 11.8 Features of insulin-dependent and non-insulin-dependent diabetes mellitus.

- Insulin zinc suspension.
- Protamine zinc insulin.

Mechanism of action: Insulin preparations mimic endogenous insulin.

Route of administration: Insulin must always be given parenterally (intravenously, intramuscularly, or subcutaneously), as it is a peptide and, therefore, destroyed in the gastrointestinal tract. Short-acting insulin is given intravenously in emergencies, but administration of the insulin preparations in maintenance treatment is usually subcutaneous.

Indications: IDDM, and NIDDM uncontrolled by other means.

Adverse effects: Local reactions and, in overdose, hypoglycaemia. Protamine can cause allergic reactions. Rarely, there may be immune resistance.

Therapeutic regime: The following regimes are recommended according to the patient:

- Short-acting insulin three times daily (before breakfast, lunch, and dinner) and intermediate-acting insulin at bedtime.
- Short-acting insulin and intermediate-acting insulin mixture twice daily before meals.
- Short-acting insulin and intermediate-acting insulin mixture before breakfast, short-acting insulin before dinner, and intermediate-acting insulin before bedtime.
- Short-acting insulin and intermediate-acting insulin mixture before breakfast is adequate for some NIDDM patients needing insulin.

Therapeutic notes: Preparations are now available that contain mixtures of short- and intermediate- and long-acting insulins, allowing patients to inject themselves only once each time they administer their insulin.

Insulin preparations (subcutaneous)			
Insulin preparation	Action	Peak activity (h)	Duration (h)
Rapid acting insulin	Very rapid	0–2	3–4
Short-acting insulin	Rapid	1–3	3–7
Isophane insulin	Intermediate	2–12	12–22
Insulin zinc suspension	Prolonged	4–24	24–28

Fig. 11.9 Insulin preparations.

Oral hypoglycaemics

The oral hypoglycaemics are administered orally, and, like insulin, they act to lower plasma glucose. The sulphonylureas and the biguanides are the main drugs uses from this class, but newer drugs are also now available.

Sulphonylureas

Gliclazide, tolbutamide, chlorpropamide, and glibenclamide are examples of sulphonylureas.

Mechanism of action: Sulphonylureas block ATP-dependent potassium channels in the membrane of the pancreatic β-cells, causing depolarization, calcium influx, and insulin release.

Route of administration: Oral.

Indications: Sulphonylureas are given for diabetes mellitus, in patients with residual β-cell activity.

Contraindications: Breastfeeding women, or people with ketoacidosis. Long-acting sulphonylureas (chlorpropamide, glibenclamide) should be avoided in the elderly and in those with renal and hepatic insufficiency, as these drugs can induce hypoglycaemia.

Adverse effects: Weight gain; sensitivity reactions, including rashes; gastrointestinal disturbances; headache; and hypoglycaemia.

Therapeutic regime: Tolbutamide is given at 500 mg two or three times daily, and it lasts for 6 hours; chlorpropamide is given at 100–250 mg daily, and it lasts for 12 hours; and glibenclamide is given at 2.5–15 mg daily, and it lasts for 12 hours.

Biguanides

Metformin is the only drug in this class.

Mechanism of action: Metformin increases the peripheral utilization of glucose, by increasing uptake, and decreasing gluconeogenesis. To work, metformin requires the presence of endogenous insulin; therefore, patients must have some functioning β-cells.

Route of administration: Oral.

Indications: NIDDM where dieting and sulphonylureas have proved ineffective.

Contraindications: Metformin should not be given to patients with hepatic or renal impairment (owing to the risk of lactic acidosis) or heart failure.

Adverse effects: Anorexia, headache, nausea and vomiting, lactic acidosis, and decreased vitamin B_{12} absorption.

Therapeutic regime: Metformin is given at 500 mg two or three times daily. It can be used alone or with sulphonylureas. Metformin should be taken with or after food.

Other antidiabetics
Alpha-glucosidase inhibitors
Acarbose is the only available drug in this class.
Mechanism of action: Acarbose inhibits intestinal α-glucosidases, and it delays the absorption of starch and sucrose.
Route of administration: Oral.
Indications: Diabetes mellitus inadequately controlled by diet alone or in combination with other oral hypoglycaemics.
Contraindications: Pregnancy, breastfeeding, bowel disease.
Adverse effects: Flatulence, diarrhoea.
Therapeutic notes: Like metformin, acarbose is particularly useful in the obese diabetic patient.

Thiazolidinediones
Rosiglitazone and pioglitazone belong to the thiazolidinediones.
Mechanism of action: These agents are believed to reduce peripheral insulin resistance, leading to a reduction in plasma glucose.
Route of administration: Oral.
Indications: Uncontrolled NIDDM.
Contraindications: Hepatic impairment, history of heart failure.
Adverse effects: Gastrointestinal disturbance, weight gain. Potentially liver failure.
Therapeutic notes: The thiazolidinediones should only be prescribed by a physician experienced in treating NIDDM, and they are currently only licensed for use in combination with either a sulphonylurea or metformin.

Diet and fluid replacement
Dietary control
Dietary control is important for both IDDM and NIDDM.

The diet should aim to derive its energy from the following constituents, in the following amounts:
- 50% carbohydrate (slowly absorbed forms).
- 35% fat.
- 15% protein.

This regimen aims to reduce total fat intake, increase protein intake, and increase the intake of high fibre foods, which slow the rate of absorption from the gut.

Simple sugars, as found in sweet drinks and cakes, should be avoided.

Meals should be small and regular, thus avoiding large swings in blood glucose levels.

Rehydration therapy
In the acute diabetic patient the fluid deficit can be as high as 7–8 L. Rehydration therapy is essential in order to regain fluid and electrolyte balance, and this takes precedence over the administration of insulin.

The management of the acute diabetic patient is essential to know. Not only is this a very common exam question, you will also encounter it on the wards.

Untreated diabetic patients suffer from hyperkalaemia as potassium requires insulin to enter cells. As soon as insulin is administered, however, potassium follows glucose into cells, and hypokalaemia becomes the danger. The rehydration fluid should, therefore, contain potassium, and plasma potassium concentration should be measured hourly.

Diabetic patients are also at risk of metabolic acidosis due to excessive ketone production. If the acidosis is severe (pH <7.0), bicarbonate can be administered intravenously, though evidence to support this is weak.

Hypoglycaemia
Hypoglycaemia is an uncommon presentation in the untreated diabetic patient, though very common in those taking insulin and sulphonylureas.

The symptoms of hypoglycaemia are driven by the sympathetic nervous system and include:
- Sweating.
- Tremor.
- Anxiety.
- Altered consciousness.

The history may reveal the patient has not eaten as scheduled, exercised, or taken too much insulin.

Management depends upon the consciousness of the patient. If the patient is alert, glucose can be given orally as a syrup, or as simple sugar. If consciousness is altered, oral administration of glucose is dangerous, and there is a risk of the patient aspirating. In this situation, glucose should be administered intravenously, or glucagon can be given by intramuscular or intravenous injection.

Glucose (dextrose monohydrate)

Glucose is administered parenterally as dextrose monohydrate.

Mechanism of action: Dextrose mimics endogenous glucose, and it is utilized by cells.

Route of administration: Intravenous.

Indications: Hypoglycaemia, as part of rehydration therapy.

Contraindications: Hyperglycaemia.

Side effects: Venous irritation and thrombophlebitis. Hypokalaemia may occur.

Therapeutic notes: Glucose is also available in numerous oral preparations, though the patient must be alert and conscious before these are administered as aspiration can occur.

Glucagon

Glucagon is a polypeptide hormone, normally secreted by the pancreatic α-cells.

Mechanism of action: Glucagon acts on the liver to convert glycogen to glucose, and to synthesize glucose from non-carbohydrate precursors (gluconeogenesis). The overall effect is to raise plasma glucose levels.

Route of administration: Parenteral.

Indications: Insulin-induced hypoglycaemia.

Contraindications: Phaeochromocytoma.

Adverse effects: Nausea, vomiting, diarrhoea, and hypokalaemia.

Therapeutic notes: Unlike intravenous glucose, glucagon can be administered easily by non-medical personnel, and it can be carried by the patient as a pre-filled syringe-pen.

In an acute hyperglycaemic attack, it is essential that fluids and soluble insulin are given intravenously to rehydrate the patient rapidly and decrease blood sugar levels.

Adrenal cortex

The adrenal cortex secretes several steroid hormones into the bloodstream. These are categorized by their actions into two main classes—mineralocorticoids and glucocorticoids.

Of the mineralocorticoids, aldosterone is the main endogenous hormone, synthesized in the zona glomerulosa. It affects water and electrolyte balance, and it possesses salt-retaining activity.

Of the glucocorticoids, hydrocortisone (cortisol) and cortisone are the main endogenous hormones, synthesized in the zona fasciculata and zona reticularis. These affect carbohydrate, fat, and protein metabolism, and they suppress inflammatory and immune responses. Cortisol and cortisone also possess some mineralocorticoid activity.

Small quantities of some sex steroids, mainly androgens, are also produced by the adrenal cortex.

Adrenal corticosteroids
Synthesis and release

Adrenal corticosteroids are not preformed; they are synthesized when required from cholesterol.

Glucocorticoids

The release of cortisol is controlled by negative feedback upon the hypothalamo–pituitary–adrenal axis (Fig. 11.10). There is a diurnal pattern of activity with an early morning peak in cortisol release.

A variety of sensorineural inputs regulate the release of corticotrophin-releasing factor (CRF) in the hypothalamus; examples include physiological and psychological 'stress', injury, and infection.

CRF, a 41-amino-acid-residue polypeptide, reaches the anterior pituitary in the hypothalamo-hypophysial portal system, where it stimulates the release of adrenocorticotrophic hormone (ACTH).

ACTH is formed from a larger molecule, pro-opiomelanocortin, and it is released into the circulation, where it stimulates the synthesis and release of cortisol from the adrenal cortex.

Natural and artificial glucocorticoids circulating in the blood exert a negative feedback effect on the production of both CRH and ACTH.

Mineralocorticoids

Aldosterone release is also partially controlled by ACTH, but other factors, especially the renin–angiotensin system (RAS) and plasma potassium levels, are more important.

Mechanism of action of corticosteroids

Endogenous and synthetic corticosteroids act in a similar way (Fig. 11.11). The hormone or drug circulates to peripheral tissues where it enters cells (steroids are lipid soluble) and binds to cytosolic corticosteroid receptors (CR). After hormone binding, these receptors are translocated to the nucleus where they interact with DNA, leading to

189

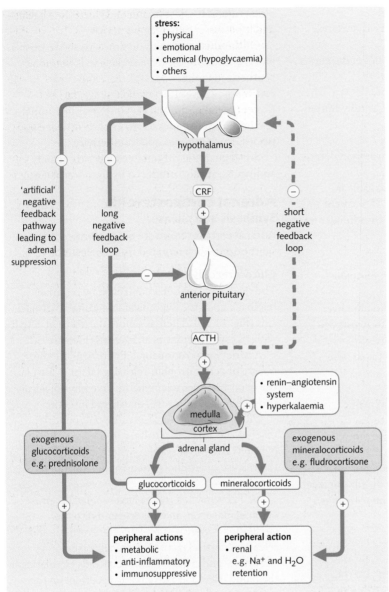

Fig. 11.10 Hypothalamic–pituitary–adrenal axis; control of adrenal corticosteroid synthesis and secretion. (ACTH, adrenocorticotrophin hormone; CRF, corticotrophin-releasing factor.)

the transcription of corticosteroid-responsive genes (CRGs).

The products of these CRGs lead to diverse effects on the target tissues (Fig. 11.12). The actions of corticosteroids are divided into effects on inorganic metabolism (mineralocorticoid effects) and effects on organic metabolism (glucocorticoid effects).

Therapeutic use of corticosteroids

Corticosteroids have wide-ranging and powerful effects on human physiology. There are two main areas where these properties are taken advantage of

in the therapeutic use of corticosteroids—physiological replacement therapy of corticosteroid deficiency, and anti-inflammatory therapy and immunosuppression (Chs 4 and 11).

Exogenous corticosteroids

Both naturally occurring and a number of synthetic corticosteroids are available for clinical use. These vary in their potency, half-life, and the balance between glucocorticoid versus mineralocorticoid activity (Fig. 11.13).

Mechanism of action: Exogenous corticosteroids imitate endogenous corticosteroids.

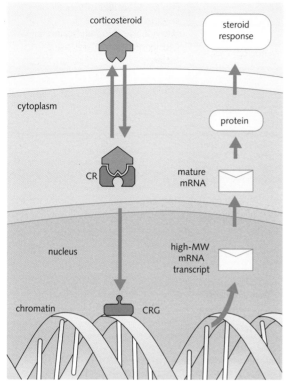

Fig. 11.11 Mechanism of action of corticosteroids at the cellular level. (CR, corticosteroid receptor; CRG, corticosteroid response gene; MW, molecular weight.) (Redrawn from Page et al, 2002.)

Indications: The therapeutic use of corticosteroids falls into the two main categories of physiological replacement therapy, and anti-inflammatory therapy and immunosuppression.

Corticosteroid replacement therapy is necessary when endogenous hormones are deficient, as happens in:

- Primary adrenocortical destruction (Addison's disease).
- Secondary adrenocortical failure due to deficient ACTH from the pituitary, or post adrenalectomy.
- Suppression of the hypothalamo–pituitary– adrenal axis due to prolonged glucocorticoid therapy.

As all the actions of natural corticosteroids are required, a glucocorticoid with mineralocorticoid activity (cortisol) or separate glucocorticoid and mineralocorticoid are given.

The anti-inflammatory and immunosuppressive effects of glucocorticoids are used to treat a wide variety of conditions (Fig. 11.14). In these cases, synthetic glucocorticoids with little mineralocorticoid activity are used (Chs 4 and 11).

Contraindications: Exogenous corticosteroids should not be given to people with systemic infection, unless specific antimicrobial therapy is being given.

Route of administration: Replacement therapy is given orally twice a day at physiological doses to try to mimic, as closely as possible, the level and rhythm of natural corticosteroid secretion.

When used to suppress inflammatory and immune responses, corticosteroids may be given orally or intravenously, but, depending on the condition, the topical administration of glucocorticoids is preferred, if feasible, as it can deliver high concentrations to the target site while minimizing systemic absorption and adverse effects (Fig. 11.14).

At high doses, even topically administered glucocorticoids can achieve systemic penetration.

Adverse effects: Overdosage or prolonged use of corticosteroids may exaggerate some of their normal physiological actions (see earlier), leading to mineralocorticoid and glucocorticoid side effects. Many of these effects are similar to those seen in Cushing's syndrome, a condition caused by excess secretion of endogenous corticosteroids (Fig. 11.15).

The metabolic side effects of glucocorticoids include:

- Central obesity and a 'moon' face, as fat is redistributed.
- Hyperglycaemia, which may lead to clinical diabetes mellitus, due to disturbed carbohydrate metabolism.
- Osteoporosis, due to catabolism of protein matrix in bone.
- Loss of skin structure, with purple striae, and easy bruising, due to altered protein metabolism.
- Muscle weakness and wasting, due to protein catabolism.
- Suppression of growth in children.

Corticosteroid therapy suppresses endogenous secretion of adrenal hormones via negative feedback on the hypothalamo–pituitary–adrenal axis.

Adrenal atrophy can persist for years after withdrawal from prolonged corticosteroid therapy. Replacement corticosteroid therapy is needed to compensate for the lack of sufficient adrenocortical response in times of stress (e.g. illness, surgery).

Steroid therapy must be withdrawn slowly after long-term treatment, as sudden withdrawal can lead to an acute adrenal insufficiency crisis.

With glucocorticoid therapy, the modification of inflammatory and immune reactions leads to an increased susceptibility to infections. This can

Major effects of the corticosteroids	
Glucocorticoids	
Immunological	• decreased production of T and B lymphocytes and macrophages, involution of lymphoid tissue • decreased function of T and B lymphocytes, and reduced responsiveness to cytokines • inhibition of complement system
Anti-inflammatory	• profound generalized inhibitory effects on inflammatory response • reduced production of acute inflammatory mediators, especially the eicosanoids (prostaglandins, leukotrienes, etc.); owing to production of lipocortin, an enzyme that inhibits phospholipase A_2, thus blocking the formation of arachidonic acid and its metabolites—see Chapter 4 • reduced numbers and activity of circulating immunocompetent cells, neutrophils, and macrophages • decreased activity of macrophages and fibroblasts involved in the chronic stages of inflammation, leading to decreased inflammation and decreased healing
Carbohydrate metabolism	• increased gluconeogenesis, decreased cellular uptake and utilization of glucose, increased storage of glycogen in the liver (hyperglycaemic actions)
Fat metabolism	• redistribution of lipid from steroid-sensitive stores (limbs) to steroid-resistant stores (face, neck, trunk)
Protein metabolism	• increased catabolism, decreased anabolism, leading to protein degradation
Cardiovascular	• increased sensitivity of vascular system to catecholamines, reduced capillary permeability leading to raised blood pressure
Central nervous system	• high levels can cause mood changes (euphoria/depression) or psychotic states, perhaps due to electrolyte changes
Anterior hypothalamus and pituitary	• negative feedback effect of CRF and ACTH with the result that endogenous secretion of glucocorticoids is reduced, and may remain so after prolonged glucocorticoid therapy ('adrenal suppression')
Mineralocorticoids	
Kidney	• increases permeability of the apical membrane of cells in the distal renal tubule to sodium • stimulates the Na^+/K^+ ATPase pump leading to reabsorption of Na^+ and loss of K^+ in the urine • water is passively reabsorbed owing to sodium retention; thus extracellular fluid and blood volume are increased (raising blood pressure)

Fig. 11.12 Major effects of corticosteroids. (ACTH, adrenocorticotrophin hormone; CRF, corticotrophin-releasing factor.)

Corticosteroids used therapeutically		
Glucocorticoids		**Mineralocorticoids**
'Natural hormones'	Synthetic	Synthetic
Hydrocortisone (cortisol)	Prednisolone Betamethasone Dexamethasone Beclometasone Triamcinolone	Fludrocortisone Deoxycortone

Fig. 11.13 Examples of therapeutically used corticosteroids.

progress unnoticed because of the suppression of normal indicators of infection, such as inflammation.

Increased susceptibility occurs to normally pathogenic and opportunistic bacterial, viral, and fungal orgnisms. Reactivation of latent infections (e.g. tuberculosis, herpesviruses) can occur.

The effects are most serious when corticosteroids are being used systemically, although topical use can exacerbate superficial skin infections, and inhaled corticosteroids can encourage oropharyngeal thrush, etc.

The other effects of glucocorticoids include mood changes—euphoria and, rarely, psychosis—peptic ulceration due to inhibition of gastrointestinal prostaglandin synthesis, and eye problems such as cataracts and exacerbation of glaucoma.

Conditions in which corticosteroids are used for their anti-inflammatory and immunosuppressive effects		
Systemic uses	Topical uses	
Acute inflammatory conditions e.g. anaphylaxis, status asthmaticus, fibrosing alveolitis, angionecrotic oedema	Asthma	Aerosol
Chronic inflammatory conditions e.g. rheumatoid arthritis, inflammatory bowel disease, systemic lupus erythematosus, glomerulonephritis	Allergic rhinitis	Nasal spray
Neoplastic disease myelomas, lymphomas, lymphatic leukaemias	Eczema	Ointment or cream
Miscellaneous organ transplantation	Inflammatory bowel disease	Foam enema

Fig. 11.14 Examples of conditions in which corticosteroids are used for their anti-inflammatory and immunosuppressive effects.

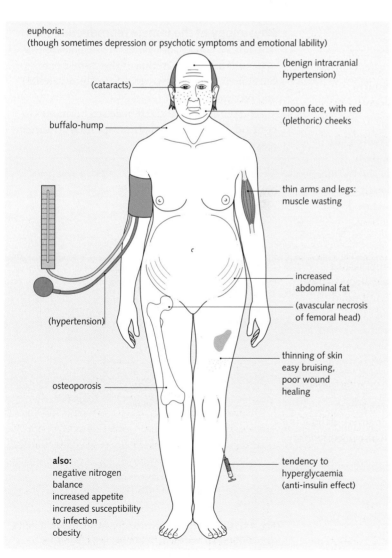

euphoria:
(though sometimes depression or psychotic symptoms and emotional lability)

(cataracts)

(benign intracranial hypertension)

buffalo-hump

moon face, with red (plethoric) cheeks

thin arms and legs: muscle wasting

(hypertension)

increased abdominal fat

(avascular necrosis of femoral head)

thinning of skin easy bruising, poor wound healing

osteoporosis

also:
negative nitrogen balance
increased appetite
increased susceptibility to infection
obesity

tendency to hyperglycaemia (anti-insulin effect)

Fig. 11.15 Effects of prolonged corticosteroid use—the Cushingoid appearance.

193

Fluid retention, hypokalaemia, and hypertension can all be side effects of any corticosteroids that possess significant mineralocorticoid activity.

Therapeutic notes on specific steroid agents
Glucocorticoids

Hydrocortisone (cortisol):
- Is administered orally for adrenal replacement therapy, and possesses mineralocorticoid activity.
- Is administered intravenously in status asthmaticus and anaphylactic shock.
- Is applied topically for eczema, inflammatory bowel conditions, etc.

Prednisolone:
- Is predominantly glucocorticoid in activity.
- Is the oral drug most widely used in allergic and inflammatory diseases.

Deflazacort
- Is derived from prednisolone, with high glucocorticoid activity.
- Is administered orally, and indicated in inflammatory and allergic disorders.

Betamethasone and dexamethasone:
- Have very high glucocorticoid activity with insignificant mineralocorticoid activity.
- Are very potent drugs used orally and by injection to suppress inflammatory and allergic disorders, and to reduce cerebral oedema—they do not possess salt- or water-retaining actions.

Beclometasone:
- Is the dipropionate ester of betamethasone.
- Is a very potent drug with no mineralocorticoid activity that is useful topically, as it is poorly absorbed through membranes and skin.
- Is used as an aerosol in asthma, and as a cream and ointment in eczema to provide high local anti-inflammatory effects with minimal systemic penetration.

Triamcinolone:
- Is a moderately potent drug used in severe asthma.
- Is also administered by intra-articular injection for rheumatoid arthritis.

Mineralocorticoids

Fludrocortisone:
- Has such high mineralocorticoid activity that glucocorticoid activity is insignificant.
- Is administered orally, in combination with a glucocorticoid, in replacement therapy.

Know the adverse effects caused by corticosteroid therapy as they are numerous, common, and a popular exam question. Some of the adverse effects caused by corticosteroids are logical exaggerations of their normal physiological actions, others are more unexpected and must, therefore, be learnt individually.

Reproductive system

Hormonal control of the reproductive system
Physiology of the female reproductive tract

The female gonads, or ovaries, are responsible for oogenesis and the secretion of the steroid sex hormones, namely oestrogens (mainly oestradiol) and progesterone.

The production of the female sex hormones is controlled by the hypothalamic–pituitary–ovarian axis (Fig. 11.16).

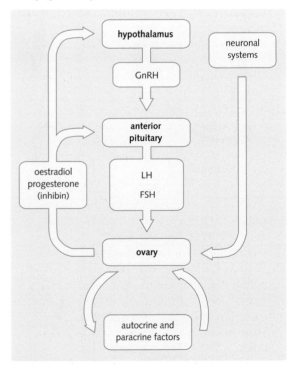

Fig. 11.16 Hypothalamic–pituitary–ovarian axis. (GnRH, gonadotrophin-releasing hormone; LH, luteinizing hormone; FSH, follicle-stimulating hormone.) (Redrawn from Page et al, 2002.)

Gonadotrophin-releasing hormone (GnRH) is secreted by the hypothalamus and stimulates the pulsatile secretion of the gonadotrophins, follicle-stimulating hormone (FSH) and luteinizing hormone (LH) by the anterior pituitary. In turn, these act upon the ovaries to stimulate the release of oestradiol, progesterone, and other ovarian hormones.

The ovarian hormones are able to exert a negative feedback on the hypothalamus and/or the pituitary. Some of these are selective in their inhibition; for example, inhibin selectively inhibits FSH release from the pituitary, activin selectively stimulates FSH release from the pituitary, and gonadotrophin-surge-attenuating factor selectively inhibits LH secretion from the pituitary.

Menstrual cycle

The menstrual cycle is divided into a follicular phase (days 1–14) and a luteal phase (days 14–28). The cycle proceeds as follows (numbers refer to Fig. 11.17):

1. Day 1 is the first day of menstruation, which involves the shedding of the uterine endometrium. Plasma oestrogen levels are low and, therefore, little negative feedback occurs. As a result, the secretion of LH and FSH begins to increase.
2. Ten to twenty-five pre-antral follicles start to enlarge and secrete oestrogen.
3. FSH stimulates the granulosa cells to secrete oestrogen, the levels of which rise.
4. About 1 week into the cycle, one of the follicles becomes dominant, and the others undergo atresia. The dominant follicle secretes increasingly larger amounts of oestrogen.
5. Plasma oestrogen levels rise significantly as a result of increased sensitivity of the granulosa cells to FSH.
6. Elevated oestrogen levels provide negative feedback, and FSH secretion decreases.
7. Plasma oestrogen levels are now so high (>200 pg/mL) that they exert a positive feedback on gonadotrophin secretion. This occurs for about 2 days, during which FSH stimulates the appearance of LH receptors on the granulosa cells.
8. An LH surge occurs. This results in a decrease in oestrogen secretion, an increase in progesterone secretion by the granulosa cells, and the resumption of meiosis in the egg.
9. Oestrogen levels decline after ovulation.
10. The first meiotic division is completed.
11. On day 14, ovulation, the release of the ovum, occurs. This is approximately 18 hours after the LH surge.
12. The granulosa cells are transformed into the corpus luteum, which secretes both oestrogen and progesterone in large quantities.
13. There is a rise in the levels of oestrogen and progesterone. As a result, FSH and LH secretion is suppressed, and their levels fall.
14. If fertilization does not take place, the corpus luteum degenerates after about 10 days.
15. Oestrogen and progesterone levels fall; menstruation is imminent.
16. FSH and LH secretion increase once more, and the 28-day cycle begins again.

Physiology of the male reproductive tract

The male gonads, or testes, are responsible for spermatogenesis and the secretion of the steroid sex hormone testosterone.

Fig. 11.17 The menstrual cycle. (See text for details of numbered stages.) (FSH, follicle-stimulating hormone; LH, luteinizing hormone.)

Spermatogenesis takes place in the lumen of the seminiferous tubules of the testis.

The production of the male sex hormones is controlled by the hypothalamic–pituitary axis (Fig. 11.18).

The Sertoli cells are connected to one another by tight junctions, and they extend from the basement membrane of the seminiferous tubules into the lumen. Under the influence of FSH, these synthesize testosterone receptors and inhibin.

The Leydig cells are found in the connective tissue between the tubules. Under the influence of LH, these synthesize testosterone. Testosterone acts locally to increase sperm production, and also peripherally on the testosterone-sensitive tissues of the body.

Testosterone and inhibin are able to exert negative feedback control over the anterior pituitary, the former decreasing LH secretion and the latter decreasing FSH secretion. In addition, testosterone and inhibin act on the hypothalamus to decrease GnRH secretion.

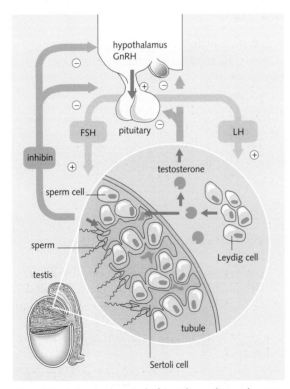

Fig. 11.18 Hormonal control of Sertoli, Leydig, and sperm cell function. (FSH, follicle-stimulating hormone; GnRH, gonadotrophin-releasing hormone; LH, luteinizing hormone.) (Redrawn from Page et al, 2002.)

Drugs that affect the reproductive system
Oral contraceptives
Combined oral contraceptive pill
The combined oral contraceptive pill (COCP) contains both an oestrogen (usually ethinylestradiol, 20–50 µg) and a progestogen (an analogue of progesterone).

COCPs provide a highly effective form of contraception. Their efficacy is reduced by some broad-spectrum antibiotics, which reduce enterohepatic recirculation of oestrogen by killing gut flora.

Mechanism of action: The levels of steroids mimic the luteal phase of the menstrual cycle, and suppress, via negative feedback effects, the secretion of gonadotrophins. As a result, follicular selection and maturation, the oestrogen surge, the LH surge, and consequently ovulation, do not take place.

Route of administration: Oral.

Indications: Contraception and menstrual symptoms.

Contraindications: Pregnancy, breastfeeding, or to those with a history of heart disease or hypertension, hyperlipidaemia or any prothrombotic coagulation abnormality, diabetes mellitus, migraine, breast or genital tract carcinoma, or liver disease.

Adverse effects: Nausea, vomiting and headache, weight gain, breast tenderness, impaired liver function, impaired glucose tolerance in diabetic women, 'spotting' (slight bleeding at the start of the menstrual cycle), thrombosis and hypertension, a slightly increased risk of cervical cancer, and a possibly increased risk of breast cancer.

Therapeutic regime: COCPs are taken for 21 days (starting on the first day of the menstrual cycle) at about the same time each day, with a 7-day break to induce a withdrawal bleed. If the delay in taking the pill is greater than 12 hours, the contraceptive effect may be lost.

Progesterone-only pill (minipill)
The minipill consists of low-dose progestogen; ovulation still takes place and menstruation is normal. The minipill is not as effective as the COCP.

Mechanism of action: The minipill causes thickening of cervical mucus preventing sperm penetration. It also causes suppression of gonadotrophin secretion, and occasionally ovulation, but the latter effect does not occur in the majority of women.

Route of administration: Oral.

Indications: Contraception. It is more suitable for heavy smokers and patients with hypertension or heart disease, diabetes mellitus, and migraine, or in those who have other contraindications for oestrogen therapy.
Contraindications: Pregnancy, arterial disease, liver disease, or breast or genital tract carcinoma.
Adverse effects: Menstrual irregularities, nausea, vomiting and headache, weight gain, and breast tenderness.
Therapeutic regime: The minipill is taken as one tablet daily, at the same time, starting on day 1 of the menstrual cycle and then continuously. If the delay in taking the pill is greater than 3 hours, the contraceptive effect may be lost.

Many female patients forget to mention the oral contraceptive pill when they list their medications, so ensure to ask specifically as there are numerous important drug interactions to consider.

Other contraceptive regimes
Depot-progesterone
Examples of depot-progesterone drugs include medroxyprogesterone acetate and the etonogestrel-releasing implant. These provide contraception that is long term.
Mechanism of action: Depot-progesterone causes thickening of cervical mucus. It also causes suppression of gonadotrophin secretion, and occasionally ovulation, but the latter effect does not occur in the majority of women.
Route of administration: Medroxyprogesterone acetate is administered intramuscularly. The etonogestrel-releasing implant system relies on a hormone rod placed subdermally.
Indications: Contraception.
Contraindications: Pregnancy, arterial disease, liver disease, or breast or genital tract carcinoma.
Adverse effects: Menstrual irregularities, nausea, vomiting and headache, weight gain, and breast tenderness.
Therapeutic notes: Medroxyprogesterone acetate provides protection for about 12 weeks. The etonogestrel-implant system provides protection for 3 years.

Post-coital ('morning-after') pill
The post-coital or 'morning-after' pill provides a form of emergency contraception.
Mechanism of action: High doses of a progestogen alone, or a progestogen with an oestrogen prevent implantation of the fertilized egg. This is 75% effective. Contractions of the smooth muscle are induced, and these accelerate the movement of the fertilized egg into the unprepared uterine endometrium.
Route of administration: Oral.
Indications: The morning-after pill is used for emergency contraception after unprotected intercourse.
Contraindications: Preparations containing oestrogens should not be used in patients who have contraindications to oestrogens (see above).
Adverse effects: Nausea, vomiting and headache, dizziness, and menstrual irregularities.
Therapeutic regime: The morning-after pill regime depends upon the type of pill being taken, but commonly it consist of one or two tablets within 72 hours of intercourse, and one or two subsequent tablets 12 hours later. Consult BNF for details.

Possible contraceptives for males
Male contraceptive drugs remain purely experimental.

Oestrogens and antioestrogens
Oestrogen agonists
The adverse symptoms of the menopause can be attributed to decreased levels of oestrogen that occur as the ovaries being to fail.

Evidence suggests that oestrogen given in low doses to menopausal women will reduce postmenopausal osteoporosis, vaginal atrophy, and the incidence of stroke and myocardial infarction.

A progestogen is co-administered with oestrogen in order to inhibit oestrogen-stimulated endometrial growth and thus reduce the risk of uterine cancer and fibroids.

Examples of oestrogen agonists include oestradiol and oestriol.
Mechanism of action: Oestrogen agonists mimic pre-menopausal endogenous oestrogen levels.
Route of administration: Oral, or by transdermal patches, gels, or subcutaneous implants.

Indications: Oestrogen agonists are used alone for hormone replacement therapy (HRT) in menopausal women who have undergone a hysterectomy, and in conjunction with a progestogen if the patient has a uterus.

Contraindications: Pregnancy, oestrogen-dependent cancer, active or previous thromboembolic disease.

Adverse effects: Increased risk of endometrial cancer and, possibly, an increased risk of breast cancer after many years of treatment.

Therapeutic regime: Oestrogen agonists are given for several years, starting in the perimenopausal period.

Oestrogen antagonists

Examples of oestrogen antagonists include tamoxifen, clomifene, and toremifene.

Mechanism of action: Antioestrogens act at oestrogen receptors in oestrogen-sensitive tissues, such as the breast, bone, endometrium and also feedback to the pituitary, antagonizing endogenous oestrogen.

Route of administration: Tamoxifen is administered orally or by intravenous or subcutaneous injection while clomifene is administered orally.

Indications: Oestrogen antagonists are used to treat female infertility and breast cancer.

Contraindications: Hepatic disease, ovarian cysts, or endometrial carcinoma.

Adverse effects: Multiple pregnancies and hot flushes. Withdrawal causes visual disturbances and ovarian hyperstimulation.

Progestogens and antiprogestogens
Progestogen agonists

Examples of progestogen agonists include progesterone, medroxyprogesterone, dydrogesterone, hydroxyprogesterone, and norethisterone.

Mechanism of action: Progestogen agonists mimic endogenous progesterone.

Route of administration: Oral, or by transdermal patches, gels, or subcutaneous implants.

Indications: Progestogen agonists are given for premenstrual symptoms, severe dysmenorrhoea, menorrhagia, endometriosis, contraception, and as part of HRT.

Contraindications: Pregnancy or to those with arterial disease, liver disease, or breast or genital tract carcinoma.

Adverse effects: Menstrual irregularities, nausea, vomiting and headache, weight gain, and breast tenderness.

Progestogen antagonists

Mifepristone is an example of a progestogen antagonist.

Mechanism of action: Progestogen antagonists bind to progesterone receptors, but they exert no effect. They sensitize the uterus to prostaglandins, and they can, therefore, be used in combination with prostaglandins in the termination of early pregnancy.

Route of administration: Oral.

Indications: Progestogen antagonists are used in the termination of pregnancy.

Contraindications: Progestogen antagonists should not be given to pregnant women (64 days' gestation or more), to women with adrenal failure or haemorrhagic disorders, or to those on anticoagulant or long-term corticosteroid treatment, or to smokers aged 35 years and over.

Adverse effects: Vaginal bleeding, faintness, and nausea and vomiting.

Androgens and antiandrogens
Androgen agonists

Testosterone and mesterolone are examples of androgen agonists.

Mechanism of action: Androgen agonists mimic endogenous androgens.

Route of administration: Oral, intramuscularly, or by implant or cutaneous patch.

Indications: Androgen agonists are given as androgen-replacement therapy in castrated men, for pituitary or testicular disease causing hypogonadism, and for breast cancer.

Contraindications: Androgen agonists should not be given to men with breast or prostate cancer, to people with hypercalcaemia, or to women who are pregnant or breastfeeding.

Adverse effects: Sodium retention causing oedema, hypercalcaemia, suppression of spermatogenesis, virilism in women, and premature closure of epiphyses in prepubertal boys. The incidence of prostate abnormalities and prostate cancer is also increased.

Androgen antagonists

Cyproterone is an androgen antagonist that is a progesterone derivative. Both oestrogens and progestogens have antiandrogenic properties.

Mechanism of action: Androgen antagonists are partial agonists at androgen receptors, and they act on the hypothalamus to reduce the synthesis of gonadotrophins. They inhibit spermatogenesis, causing reversible infertility, but they are not contraceptives.

Route of administration: Oral.

Indications: Androgen antagonists are used for male hypersexuality and sexual deviation, prostate cancer, acne, female hirsutism, and precocious puberty.

Contraindications: Androgen antagonists should not be given to people with hepatic disease or severe diabetes, or to those aged 18 and under as their bones are not fully matured.

Adverse effects: Fatigue and lethargy, and hepatotoxicity.

Therapeutic notes: Finasteride is technically an antiandrogen, though inhibits the enzyme 5α-reductase which metabolizes testosterone to the more potent androgen dihydrotestosterone. Finasteride is indicated in benign prostatic hyperplasia and is administered orally.

Like breast cancer in women, prostate cancer in men is most often hormone-dependent. Exogenous androgens can promote, and antiandrogens suppress tumour growth.

Anabolic steroids

Nandrolone and stanozolol are examples of anabolic steroids.

Mechanism of action: Anabolic steroids are androgenic; they stimulate protein synthesis and promote wound and fracture healing.

Route of administration: Nandrolone is administered by deep intramuscular injection, and stanozolol orally.

Indications: Anabolic steroids can be used for osteoporosis in postmenopausal women, aplastic anaemias, and chronic biliary obstruction.

Contraindications: Hepatic impairment, to men with prostate or breast cancer, or to pregnant women.

Adverse effects: Acne, sodium retention causing oedema, virilization in women, amenorrhoea, inhibition of spermatogenesis, and liver tumours.

Gonadotrophin-releasing hormone agonists and antagonists

Agonists

Goserelin, leuprolide and buserelin are examples of GnRH agonists.

Mechanism of action: GnRH agonists are given intermittently, and mimic endogenous GnRH. Continuous use desensitizes the GnRH receptors on the gonadotrophs and inhibits gonadotrophin synthesis.

Route of administration: Buserelin is administered intranasally; goserelin and leuprolide are administered by subcutaneous injection.

Indications: GnRH agonists are used for ovulation induction in those with GnRH deficiency, endometriosis, precocious puberty, sex-hormone-dependent cancers, and prostate cancer.

Adverse effects: Menopause-like symptoms, including hot flushes, palpitations, decreased libido due to hypo-oestrogenism, and breakthrough bleeding.

Therapeutic regime: Pulsatile administration of GnRH agonists is every 90 minutes for a few minutes. The treatment must not exceed 6 months, and it should not be repeated.

Antagonists

Danazol and gestrinone are examples of a GnRH antagonists.

Mechanism of action: GnRH antagonists inhibit the release of GnRH and the gonadotrophins. They bind to the sex steroid receptors, displaying androgenic, antioestrogenic, and antiprogestogenic effects.

Route of administration: Oral.

Indications: GnRH antagonists are given for endometriosis, menstrual disorders, including menorrhagia, cystic breast disease, and gynaecomastia.

Contraindications: Pregnancy, or to people with hepatic, renal, or cardiac impairment, or those with vascular disease.

Adverse effects: Nausea and vomiting, weight gain, and androgenic effects such as acne and hirsutism.

Therapeutic notes: Cetrorelix and ganirelix are luteinizing hormone releasing hormone antagonists, inhibiting the release of the gonadotrophins. They are administered parenterally, and they are used to treat infertility in specialist centres.

Oxytocic drugs

The oxytocic drugs, oxytocin, ergometrine, prostaglandins E and F [e.g. gemeprost (PGE₁

PGE_1

199

analogue) dinoprostone (PGE_2), and carboprost (15-methyl PGF_{2a})]. All cause uterine contractions.

Oxytocin is a posterior pituitary hormone that acts on uterine muscle to induce powerful contractions. It does this directly and also indirectly by stimulating the muscle to synthesize prostaglandins.

In addition, prostaglandins ripen and soften the cervix, further aiding the expulsion of a uterine mass.

Mechanism of action: Oxytocin acts on oxytocin receptors. The mechanism for ergometrine is not well understood, but it may be via partial agonist action at α-adrenoceptors or 5-hydroxytryptamine receptors. The prostaglandins act at prostaglandin receptors.

Route of administration: Gemeprost and dinoprostone are administered by vaginal pessary; dinoprostone can also be administered extra-amniotically; oxytocin is administered by slow intravenous infusion, and oxytocin and ergometrine together are injected intramuscularly. Prostaglandins can be administered by intravenous infusion.

Indications: Prostaglandins are used to induce abortion. Oxytocin and dinoprostone are used for the induction of labour while oxytocin, ergometrine and carboprost (in those unresponsive to oxytocin and ergometrine) are used for the management of the third stage of labour and prevention and treatment of postpartum haemorrhage.

Contraindications: Oxytocic drugs should not be given to women with vascular diseases; ergometrine should not be used to induce labour.

Adverse effects: Nausea and vomiting, vaginal bleeding, and uterine pain. Oxytocin can cause hypotension and tachycardia.

Bone and calcium

Bone and calcium physiology

Bone is a tissue comprised mainly of calcium, phosphates and a protein meshwork, in addition to the components of the bone-marrow.

Bone functions to provide support, and it enables us to carry out various physiological processes, such as respiration and movement. Bone is also an active tissue and crucial in the homeostasis of calcium and phosphate.

Serum calcium is ultimately controlled by the peptide, parathyroid hormone (PTH) derived from the parathyroid glands. PTH maintains serum calcium by acting on the kidney to reabsorb calcium

from the tubular filtrate, and to stimulate the activation of vitamin D. PTH also acts directly on bone, mobilizing calcium. Activated vitamin D (1,25-dihydroxycholecalciferol) promotes absorption of calcium from the gut. PTH is secreted in response to low serum calcium.

Calcitonin, from the thyroid gland, inhibits calcium mobilization from bone, and decreases reabsorption from the renal tubules.

Disorders of bone and calcium

Osteoporosis is an overall loss of bone mass, and it commonly occurs in women after the menopause, when oestrogens fall, and bone mobilization slowly increases. Other common causes of osteoporosis include thyrotoxicosis, and excessive glucocorticoids (exogenous or endogenous).

Osteodystrophy occurs in renal failure and is driven by secondary hyperparathyroidism.

Rickets (vitamin D deficiency) is now rare in the west, though the adult variant, osteomalacia, is not uncommon.

Hypercalcinemia is a medical emergency, and it is most often due to malignancy.

Rehydration therapy is as important in hypercalcaemia as it is in ketoacidosis (hyperglycaemia), as fluid will be lost in the urine due to osmotic diuresis.

Drugs used in bone and calcium disorders

Bisphosphonates

Disodium etidronate, alendronate, and disodium pamidronate are bisphosphonates.

Mechanism of action: Bisphosphonates inhibit and potentially destroy osteoclasts, which are responsible for mobilizing calcium from bone.

Route of administration: Oral, parenteral.

Indications: Prevention of postmenopausal osteoporosis and corticosteroid-induced osteoporosis, and for the management of hypercalcaemia of malignancy.

Contraindications: Renal impairment, hypocalcaemia.

Adverse effects: Nausea, oesophageal reactions (with oral preparations), hypocalcaemia.

Calcium salts

Calcium gluconate and calcium lactate are calcium salts.

Mechanism of action: Calcium supplementation replace calcium deficiencies.

Route of administration: Oral, intravenous.

Indications: Hypocalcaemia, calcium-deficiency, osteoporosis.

Contraindications: Hypercalcaemia.

Adverse effects: Mild gastrointestinal disturbance, bradycardia, arrhythmias.

Therapeutic notes: If calcium is given parenterally, serum calcium should be repeatedly monitored.

Vitamin D

Vitamin D can be administered in its inactive form as ergocalciferol, or in its active form as calcitriol.

Mechanism of action: Vitamin D acts on the gut to absorb calcium from the diet.

Route of administration: Oral, parenteral.

Indications: Vitamin D deficiency, hypocalcaemia secondary to hypoparathyroidism, renal failure, and postmenopausal osteoporosis.

Contraindications: Hypercalcaemia.

Adverse effects: Symptoms of overdosage include anorexia, lassitude, nausea and vomiting, weight loss, and hypercalcaemia.

Therapeutic notes: Serum calcium should be monitored closely once vitamin D therapy has started, and if symptoms of hypercalcaemia appear.

Calcitonin

Mechanism of action: Calcitonin binds specific receptors on osteoclasts inhibiting their mobilization of bone, and it acts on the kidney to limit calcium reabsorption from the proximal tubules.

Route of administration: Subcutaneous or intramuscular.

Indications: Hypercalcaemia, Paget's disease of bone, bone pain in neoplastic disease.

Contraindications: Caution if history of allergy, or renal impairment.

Adverse effects: Nausea, vomiting, flushing, diarrhoea, tingling of hands.

- How are the thyroid hormones produced and how is the process controlled?
- What are the physiological functions of the thyroid hormones?
- Distinguish between hypothyroidism and hyperthyroidism.
- Describe the classes of drugs used to treat hyperthyroidism and hypothyroidism. Outline their mechanism of action, and potential side effects.
- How are plasma glucose levels controlled?
- Distinguish between type 1 and type 2 diabetes mellitus.
- What are the actions of insulin? Describe the various insulin preparations, their route of administration, and potential adverse effects.
- What other classes of drugs can be used to treat diabetes mellitus? How do these drugs act?
- What is the immediate management of the acute diabetic patient presenting with ketoacidosis?
- What are the clinical features of hypoglycaemia, and what drugs are used in such a situation?
- What are the different types of endogenous steroids produced by the adrenal glands? How do their actions differ?
- Describe the control over endogenous steroid levels in the human body.
- What are the physiological and cellular effects of steroids?
- By what route are exogenous steroids administered to patients, and what are the common side effects of prolonged steroid therapy?
- Name the common sex hormones and regulatory hormones, and indicate their main actions.
- Outline the principles of the female reproductive cycle.
- Describe the agents currently used as contraceptives, and briefly list their mechanism of action, and potential adverse effects.
- What other drugs, aside from those mentioned, affect reproductive function? For each, outline its mode of action.
- Outline the roles and sites of synthesis for vitamin D and parathyroid hormone.
- Describe the drugs used to treat metabolic bone disease, their mechanism of action, and potential adverse effects.

Eyes

Anatomy and physiology

The eyeball is a 25 mm sphere made up of two fluid-filled compartments (the aqueous humour and the vitreous humour) separated by an translucent lens, all encased within four layers of supporting tissue (Fig. 12.1). These four layers consist of:

- The cornea and sclera.
- The uveal tract, comprising the iris, ciliary body, and choroid.
- The pigment epithelium.
- The retina (neural tissue containing photoreceptors).

Light entering the eye is focused by the lens onto the retina, and the signal reaches the brain via the optic nerve.

Control of pupil size
Light

Light levels affect the pupil in two ways (Fig. 12.2):

- High light levels cause pupil constriction, termed miosis.
- Low light levels cause pupil dilation, termed mydriasis.

Autonomic control

The pupils are innervated by the autonomic nervous system, such that:

- Parasympathetic stimulation causes miosis.
- Sympathetic stimulation causes mydriasis.

The dilator pupillae (radial smooth muscle of the iris) is innervated by the sympathetic system, which causes contraction when noradrenaline activates α_1-adrenoceptors. The constrictor pupillae (sphincter

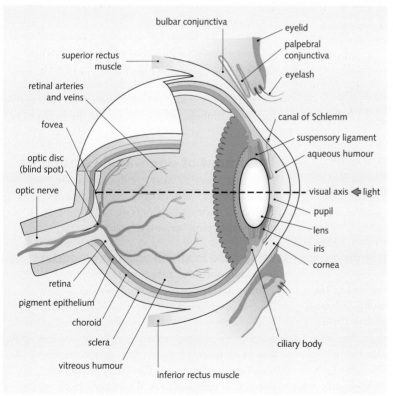

Fig. 12.1 Anatomy of the eye. (Redrawn from Page et al, 2002.)

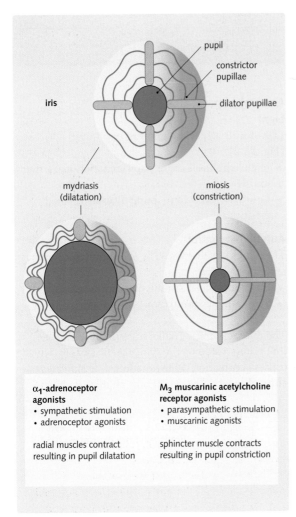

Fig. 12.2 Mechanisms involved in controlling pupil size. (Redrawn from Page et al, 2002.)

Within the figure:

pupil
constrictor pupillae
dilator pupillae
iris

mydriasis (dilatation)

miosis (constriction)

α₁-adrenoceptor agonists
• sympathetic stimulation
• adrenoceptor agonists

radial muscles contract resulting in pupil dilatation

M₃ muscarinic acetylcholine receptor agonists
• parasympathetic stimulation
• muscarinic agonists

sphincter muscle contracts resulting in pupil constriction

Production of aqueous humour

Aqueous humour fills the anterior chamber of the eyeball. It is continuously produced at a rate of 3 mL/day by a special vascular tissue associated with the ciliary body (Fig. 12.3).

The ciliary epithelial cells contain carbonic anhydrase and an ATPase, which transport bicarbonate and sodium.

The aqueous humour flows through the pupil and into the anterior aqueous chamber. Draining fluid leaves the aqueous chamber via the trabecular meshwork and the canal of Schlemm within the surface of the sclera before entering the episcleral veins.

Glaucoma

Glaucoma can be defined as a disorder in which the intraocular pressure (IOP) is raised. This may result in structural changes within the eye, such as cupping of the optic disc, as well as visual field deficits, and potentially blindness.

There are two types of glaucoma: open-angle and closed-angle.

Open-angle glaucoma is the most common type of glaucoma and it may be congenital. It is caused by pathology of the trabecular meshwork that reduces the drainage of the aqueous humour into the canal of Schlemm. Treatment involves either reducing the amount of aqueous humour produced or increasing its drainage.

In closed-angle glaucoma, the angle between the iris and the cornea is very small, and this results in forward ballooning of the iris against the back of the cornea.

smooth muscle of the iris) is innervated by the parasympathetic system, which causes contraction when acetylcholine activates M₃ receptors.

Accommodation

Accommodation is the ability of the eye to change its refractive power. This is determined by the curvature of the lens.

Suspensory ligaments connect the lens to the ciliary muscle. When the ciliary muscle contracts (parasympathetic M₃ receptor activation), the suspensory ligaments relax, resulting in the lens becoming more spherical so that it is able to focus near objects. When the ciliary muscle relaxes, the suspensory ligaments tighten, and the lens becomes elongated and thin, allowing far objects to be focused on the retina.

Treatment of open-angle glaucoma

Most drugs used to treat eye disease can be given topically in the form of drops and ointments. To enable these drugs to penetrate the cornea, they must be lipophilic or uncharged.

Drugs used to inhibit aqueous production
Beta-adrenoceptor antagonists

Timolol and betaxolol are examples of β-adrenoceptor antagonists used in glaucoma.
Mechanism of action: β-adrenoceptor antagonists block β₂-receptors on the ciliary body, and they may also block β-receptors on ciliary blood vessels, resulting in vasoconstriction (they are almost universally referred to as 'β-blockers' in clinical practice) (Fig. 12.3) and reduced aqueous production.

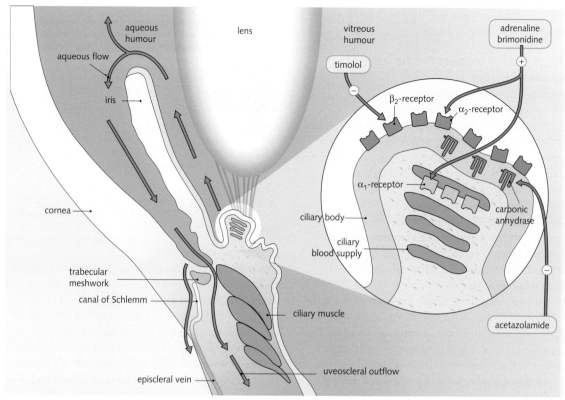

Fig. 12.3 Production and drainage of the aqueous humour. (Redrawn from Page et al, 2002.)

Route of administration: Topical.
Indications: Open-angle glaucoma. β-adrenoceptor antagonists are also used in cardiovascular disease (Ch. 7).
Contraindications: β-adrenoceptor antagonists should not be given to patients with asthma, bradycardia, heart block, or heart failure.
Adverse effects: Systemic side effects include bronchospasm in asthmatic patients, and potentially bradycardia owing to their non-selective action on β-receptors. Other side effects include transitory dry eyes and allergic blepharoconjunctivitis.

Sympathomimetics (adrenoceptor agonists)
Adrenaline, dipivefrine, and brimonidine are commonly used sympathomimetics.
Mechanism of action: Agonism at α-adrenoceptors is thought to be the principle means by which these agents reduce aqueous production from the ciliary body. Adrenaline may also increase drainage of aqueous via the trabecular meshwork (Fig. 12.3).
Route of administration: Topical.
Indications: Open-angle glaucoma. Sympathomimetics are also used in the management of cardiac and anaphylactic emergencies (Ch. 7) and in reversible airways disease (Ch. 8).

Contraindications: Closed-angle glaucoma, hypertension, and heart disease.
Adverse effects: Pain and redness of the eye.
Therapeutic notes: Adrenaline is not very lipophilic and, therefore, it does not penetrate the cornea effectively. This can be overcome by administering dipivefrine hydrochloride, a prodrug that crosses the cornea and that is metabolized to adrenaline once inside the eye.

Carbonic anhydrase inhibitors
Acetazolamide and dorzolamide are carbonic anhydrase inhibitors (CAIs).
Mechanism of action: CAIs inhibit the enzyme carbonic anhydrase, which catalyses the conversion of carbon dioxide and water to carbonic acid, which dissociates into bicarbonate and H^+. Bicarbonate is required by the cells of the ciliary body, and under-production of bicarbonate limits aqueous secretion (Fig. 12.3). CAIs given systemically have a weak diuretic effect (Ch. 9).
Route of administration: Oral, topical, intravenous.
Indications: Open-angle glaucoma.
Contraindications: Hypokalaemia, hyponatraemia, renal impairment. These effects can be reduced if the drug is given in a slow-release form.

205

Adverse effects: Irritation of the eye, nausea, vomiting, diarrhoea, diuresis.

Drugs used to increase the drainage of aqueous humour
Miotics—muscarinic agonists.
Pilocarpine is a muscarinic agonist.

Mechanism of action: Pilocarpine causes contraction of the constrictor pupillae muscles of the iris, constricting the pupil, and allowing aqueous to drain from the anterior chamber into the trabecular meshwork (Fig. 12.3).

Route of administration: Topical.

Indications: Open-angle glaucoma.

Contraindications: Acute iritis, anterior uveitis.

Adverse effects: Eye irritation, headache and browache, blurred vision, hypersalivation. May exacerbate asthma.

The prostaglandin analogue latanoprost is a novel treatment for open-angle glaucoma, and it promotes outflow of aqueous from the anterior chamber. This topically applied drug is indicated in open-angle glaucoma that is resistant to conventional treatment; it may result in a brown pigmentation of the iris.

Glaucoma has a prevalence of approximately 1% in people aged over 40 years.

Treatment of closed-angle glaucoma
Drugs to treat closed-angle glaucoma are used in emergencies as a temporary measure to lower IOP.

Pilocarpine and a carbonic anhydrase inhibitor are often first-line treatments, with mannitol and glycerol being administered systemically and reduce IOP for resistant or more serious cases.

YAG (yttrium–aluminium–garnet) laser surgery provides a permanent cure for closed-angle glaucoma. A hole is made in the iris (iridectomy) to allow increased flow of aqueous humour.

Examining the eye
Mydriatic drugs dilate the pupil, i.e. cause mydriasis, while cycloplegic drugs cause paralysis of the ciliary muscle, i.e. cycloplegia.

Mydriatic and cycloplegic drugs are used in ophthalmoscopy to allow a better view of the interior of the eye.

Effects of commonly used muscarinic antagonists			
Drug	Duration (h)	Mydriatic effect	Cycloplegic effect
Tropicamide	1 – 3	++	+
Cyclopentolate	12 – 24	+++	+++
Atropine	168 – 240	+++	+++

Fig. 12.4 Mydriatics and cycloplegics effects of the commonly used muscarinic antagonists.

Mydriasis and cycloplegia reduce the drainage of the aqueous humour, and they should, therefore, be avoided in patients with closed-angle glaucoma.

Muscarinic antagonists
The most effective mydriatics are the muscarinic antagonists. These block the parasympathetic control of the iris sphincter muscle.

The type of muscarinic antagonist chosen will depend on the length of the procedure and on whether or not cycloplegia is required.

The most commonly used muscarinic antagonists, their duration of action, and their mydriatic and cycloplegic effects are summarized in Fig. 12.4.

Alpha-adrenoceptor agonists
Alpha-adrenoceptor agonists can cause mydriasis by stimulating the sympathetic control of the iris dilator muscle. The sympathetic system does not control the ciliary muscle, however, and, therefore, these drugs do not produce cycloplegia.

The α-agonist most commonly used to produce mydriasis is phenylephrine.

Muscarinic agonists and α-antagonists
A muscarinic agonist such as pilocarpine, or an α-antagonist such as thymoxamine may be used to reverse mydriasis at the end of an ophthalmic examination. This is not usually necessary.

Skin

Anatomy and physiology
The skin is the largest organ in the body, making up on average 16% of the total body weight and covering an area of approximately 1.8 m^2 (Fig. 12.5).

Functions of the skin
The skin has several functions. These include:
- Protection—the skin provides a barrier against chemical, mechanical and thermal stresses,

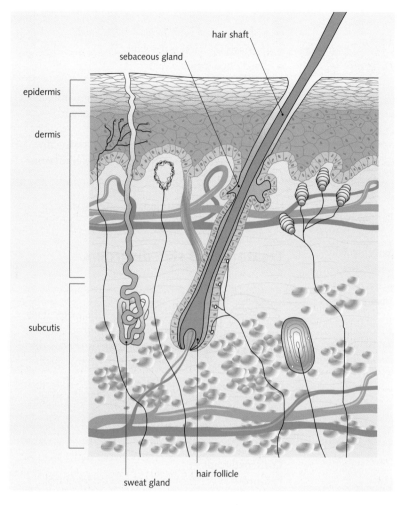

Fig. 12.5 Anatomy of the skin.

hair shaft

sebaceous gland

epidermis

dermis

subcutis

sweat gland

hair follicle

ultraviolet light, dehydration, heat loss, and microorganisms.

- Thermoregulation—hair and subcutaneous fat provide the body with insulation, whereas the sweat glands and increased dermal blood flow allow heat loss.
- Sensation—the skin contains receptors for touch, pressure, temperature, and pain.
- Metabolism—synthesis of vitamin D takes place in the epidermis, and adipose tissue provides a store of energy in the form of triglycerides.

Skin disorders

The most common skin diseases are eczema, acne, psoriasis, skin cancer, viral warts, and urticaria.

Eczema (dermatitis)

Eczema is an inflammatory disease of the skin, defined by the presence of epidermal intercellular oedema or spongiosis.

Eczema can be caused by a number of factors, such as:

- Exogenous irritants and contact allergens.
- Infections.
- Atopy.
- Drugs.
- Certain environmental conditions such as low humidity and ultraviolet light.

Drugs used to treat eczema are summarized in Fig. 12.6.

Acne

Acne affects the pilosebaceous unit and occurs where these are numerous, such as on the face, back, and chest.

Acne is characterized by the presence of keratin plugs in the sebaceous duct openings, known as comedones. Other signs of acne of worsening degrees of severity include inflammatory papules, pustules, nodules, cysts, and scars.

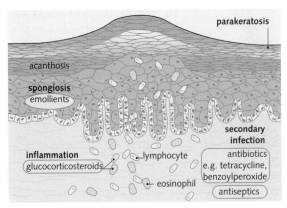

Fig. 12.6 Characteristics of eczema and its drug treatment. (Redrawn from Page et al, 2002.)

Acne is stimulated by androgens, which is why it is related to puberty, and why the antiandrogen cyproterone is often used in females with acne (Ch. 11). The drugs used to treat acne are summarized in Fig. 12.7.

Psoriasis

Psoriasis is a genetic skin disorder that manifests under certain conditions including stress, infection, damage from ultraviolet light, or trauma.

Fig. 12.7 Characteristics of acne and its drug treatment. (Redrawn from Page et al, 2002.)

In psoriasis, the turnover rate of skin is eight times that of normal skin (7 instead of 56 days).

Psoriasis is characterized by:
- Thickened skin plaques.
- Superficial scales.
- Dilated capillaries in the dermis (these might act to initiate psoriasis or as nourishment for hyperproliferating skin).
- An infiltrate of inflammatory cells, especially lymphocytes and neutrophils, in the epidermis and dermis, respectively.

Drugs used to treat psoriasis are summarized in Fig. 12.8.

Treatment of skin disorders

Much is made of the potentially serious effects of steroid therapy, but their usefulness in treating many dermatological conditions should not be ignored. Use steroids with care—but use them!

Corticosteroids

Examples of corticosteroids include clobetasol propionate, betamethasone, clobetasone butyrate, and hydrocortisone (Fig. 12.9).
Mechanism of action: Corticosteroids suppress components of the inflammatory reaction (Ch. 11; Fig. 12.6).
Route of administration: Topically; orally, intradermally or intravenously in severe disease.
Indications: Corticosteroids are used for the relief of symptoms due to inflammatory conditions of the skin other than those due to infection, e.g. in eczema.
Contraindications: Rosacea, or untreated skin infections.
Adverse effects: Most likely to occur with prolonged, or high dose therapy. Local—spread or worsening of infection, thinning of the skin, impaired wound healing, irreversible striae atrophicae. Systemic—immunosuppression, peptic ulceration, osteoporosis, hypertension, cataracts.
Therapeutic notes: Withdrawal of corticosteroids after high doses or prolonged use should be gradual (Ch. 11). Consult *British National Formulary* for up to date guidelines.

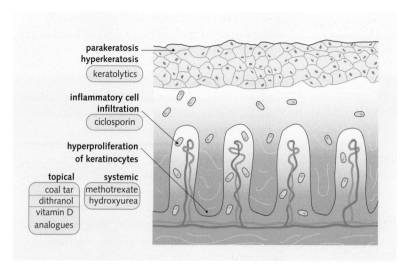

Fig. 12.9 Potency of some topical steroids (UK classification and nomenclature). (Adapted from Graham-Brown et al, *Mosby's Color Atlas and Text of Dermatology*, 1st edn, 1998.)

Potency of some topical steroids (UK classification and nomenclature)		
Group	Approved name	Proprietary name
I (very potent)	Clobetasol propionate	Dermovate®
II (potent)	Betamethasone valerate 0.1%	Betnovate®
	Beclomethasone dipropionate	Propaderm®
	Hydrocortisone 17-butyrate	Locoid®
III (moderately potent)	Clobetasone butyrate	Eumovate®
IV (mild)	Hydrocortisone 1%	Various
	Hydrocortisone 2%	Various

Dithranol

Dithranol is the most potent topical drug for the treatment of psoriasis.

Mechanism of action: Dithranol modifies keratinization, but the mechanism is unclear (Fig. 12.8).

Route of administration: Topical.

Contraindications: Dithranol should not be given to people with hypersensitivity or acute and pustular psoriasis.

Adverse effects: Local skin irritation, staining of skin and hair.

Vitamin D analogues

Calcipotriol and tacalcitol are vitamin D analogue derivatives.

Vitamin D analogues are keratolytics, though also used in vitamin D deficiency related to gastrointestinal/biliary disease and renal failure (Ch. 9).

Mechanism of action: The exact mechanism of action is still unclear, but several effects of vitamin D analogues have been observed. These include inhibition of epidermal proliferation and induction of terminal keratinocyte differentiation (Fig. 12.8).

The anti-inflammatory properties of vitamin D analogues include inhibition of T cell proliferation and of cytokine release, decreased capacity of monocytes to stimulate T cell proliferation and to stimulate lymphokine release from T cells, and inhibition of neutrophil accumulation in psoriatic skin.

Route of administration: Topical.

Indications: Psoriasis.

Contraindications: Vitamin D analogues should not be given to people with disorders of calcium metabolism. They should not be used on the face, as irritation may occur.

Adverse effects: Side effects of vitamin D analogues include local irritation and dermatitis. High doses may affect calcium homoeostasis.

Tar preparations
Coal tar, made up of about 10 000 components, is a keratolytic that is more potent than salicylic acid. It also has anti-inflammatory and antipruritic properties.
Mechanism of action: Coal tar modifies keratinization, but the mechanism is unclear (Fig. 12.8).
Route of administration: Topical.
Indications: Psoriasis and occasionally eczema.
Contraindications: Coal tar should not be given to people with acute or pustular psoriasis or in the presence of an infection. It should not be used on the face, or on broken or inflamed skin.
Adverse effects: Skin irritation and acne-like eruptions, photosensitivity, and staining of the skin and hair.

Salicylates
Salicylic acid is keratolytic at a concentration of 3–6%.
Mechanism of action: Salicylic acid causes desquamation via the solubilization of cell-surface proteins that maintain the integrity of the stratum corneum.
Route of administration: Topical.
Indications: Hyperkeratosis, eczema, psoriasis (combined with coal tar or dithranol preparations), acne, wart and callus eradication.
Contraindications: Sensitivity to the drug, or broken or inflamed skin. High concentrations, such as those needed to treat warts, should not be given to people with diabetes mellitus or peripheral vascular disease, as ulceration may be induced.
Adverse effects: Side effects of salicylic acid include anaphylactic shock in those sensitive to the drug, skin irritation and excessive drying, and systemic effects if used long term.

Emollients
Emollients are used to soothe and hydrate the skin.
A simple preparation is aqueous cream, which is often as effective as more complex drugs.

Most creams are thin emollients, whereas a mixture of equal parts soft white paraffin and liquid paraffin is a thick emollient.

Camphor, menthol, and phenol preparations have antipruritic effects, whereas zinc- and titanium-based emollients have mild astringent (contracting) effects.
Mechanism of action: Emollients hydrate the skin and reduce transepidermal water loss.
Route of administration: Topical. Many emollients can be added to bath water.
Indications: Emollients are used for the long-term treatment of dry scaling disorders.
Contraindications: None.
Adverse effects: Some ingredients, such as lanolin or antibacterials, may induce an allergic reaction.
Therapeutic notes: The use of emollients lessens the need for topical steroids, therefore, limiting potential side effects.

Other drugs used in skin disease
Many other drugs are employed in the management of skin disease. Some of the more common drugs are summarized in Fig. 12.10.

Preparations of drugs for use on skin
Drugs applied to the skin are delivered by a variety of vehicles such as ointments, creams, pastes, powders, aerosols, gels, lotions, and tinctures.

Factors affecting the choice of vehicle include:
- The solubility of the active drug.
- The ability of the drug to penetrate the skin.
- The stability of the drug–vehicle complex.
- The ability of the vehicle to delay evaporation, this being greatest for ointments and least for tinctures.

Factors that affect the absorption of the drug include:
- Body site, in that absorption is greatest from the scrotum and vulva, high from the scalp and face, and lowest from the palms and soles.
- Skin hydration, as occlusive dressings can increase the absorption of a drug tenfold, for example.
- Skin condition, because damage caused by burns and inflammation increases absorption.
- The concentration gradient across the skin (the greater this is, the greater the rate of absorption).

Fig. 12.10 Other drugs used in skin disease, their indications and mechanism of action. (From *Mosby's Color Atlas and Text of Dermatology*, by Graham-Brown et al, 1998. By permission of Mosby.)

Other drugs used in skin disease		
Drug	**Indication**	**Mechanism of action**
Benzoyl peroxide	Acne vulgaris	Antibacterial/keratolytic
Retinoids (vitamin A derivatives)	Psoriasis/acne	Keratolytic/cyto-inhibitory
Psoralen	Psoriasis	Mutates DNA/cytotoxic
Methotrexate	Psoriasis	Cytotoxic
Ciclosporin (cyclosporin)	Psoriasis	Immunosuppressant
Antibacterial, antiviral, antifungal	Skin infections/warts	Antimicrobial
Antiparasite preparations	Skin/hair infestations	Parasite toxins

- How is pupil size controlled?
- Summarize how aqueous humour is produced and drained from the eye.
- What are the differences between open-angle and closed-angle glaucoma?
- Describe the different classes of drugs used to treat glaucoma. For each class, list an example, their mechanism of action, route of administration, and major adverse effects.
- In which situation are mydriatic and cycloplegic drugs used?
- Summarize the common skin disorders and their treatment.
- What are the different classes of drugs used to treat skin disease? For each class list examples, their mechanism of action, route of administration, indications, and major adverse effects.
- Which factors affect the choice of vehicles for drugs used on the skin?
- Which skin diseases may benefit from the use of antibiotic therapy?
- Which factors affect the absorption of drugs used on the skin?

SELF-ASSESSMENT

Multiple-choice Questions

Indicate whether each answer is true or false.

Chapter 1—Introduction to Pharmacology

1. The following are intracellular messengers:

(a) Cyclic adenosine monophosphate.
(b) Diacylglycerol.
(c) Inositol tetraphosphate.
(d) GABA.
(e) Cyclic guanosine monophosphate.

2. A partial agonist:

(a) Brings about the same maximal response as a full agonist.
(b) Can have the same affinity for the receptor as the full agonist.
(c) Can occupy all available receptors.
(d) Always irreversibly binds the receptor.
(e) Has the same efficacy as a full agonist.

3. An antagonist:

(a) Has similar receptor binding affinity to the agonist.
(b) Has similar efficacy to the agonist.
(c) Is always competitive.
(d) With a dose ratio of 10 is a weak antagonist.
(e) Will shift the agonists dose-response curve to the right.

4. Compliance:

(a) Is measured in mmol/L.
(b) Is often high in small children.
(c) Can be enhanced with good communication.
(d) Will be poor if the drug regimen is simple to follow.
(e) Is not important in many diseases.

5. Drugs administered:

(a) Intravenously are subjected to first pass metabolism.
(b) Topically cannot have systemic side effects.
(c) Rectally avoid first pass metabolism.
(d) Orally have the highest possible bioavailability.
(e) Intravenously are more rapidly metabolized than via the oral route.

6. The rate of renal excretion of a drug is usually related to:

(a) The free (not protein-bound) plasma drug concentration.
(b) The total plasma drug concentration.
(c) Tubular reabsorption.
(d) Lipid solubility of the drug.
(e) The volume of distribution of the drug.

7. The volume of distribution:

(a) Of a drug is independent of changes in cardiac output.
(b) Of heparin is approximately 40 litres in a 70 kg man.
(c) Cannot be greater than total body water.
(d) Is dependent on the degree of protein binding.
(e) Is dependent on the pH of the blood.

8. Drugs:

(a) Are commonly excreted by the liver.
(b) That are lipid soluble cannot cross the blood–brain barrier.
(c) Such as paracetamol are directly toxic to the liver.
(d) Can interfere with cytochrome 450 in the liver and alter the metabolism of other drugs.
(e) Are monitored for adverse effects even after being granted a licence for clinical use.

Chapter 2—Cancer

9. Cancer:

(a) Accounts for 25% of deaths in the Western world.
(b) Is always fatal.
(c) Is related to certain viruses.
(d) Chemotherapy relies on structural differences between malignant and non-malignant cells.
(e) Can become resistant to certain drugs.

10. The following are used in cancer chemotherapy:

(a) Bleomycin.
(b) Thalidomide.
(c) Vigabatrin.
(d) Folate agonists.
(e) Polymyxin B sulphate.

11. The following are common adverse effects of chemotherapy:

(a) Bone marrow hyperplasia.
(b) Mouth ulceration.
(c) Impaired wound healing.
(d) Hyperfertility.
(e) Anaemia.

12. Cytotoxic agents include:

(a) Doxazosin.
(b) Alkylating agents.
(c) Mitotic inhibitors.
(d) Antimetabolites.
(e) Cycloplegics.

13. Hormone agonists/antagonists used in cancer therapy include:

(a) Adrenocortical steroids.
(b) Thyroxine.
(c) Oestrogen antagonists.
(d) Prolactin.
(e) Progestogens.

Chapter 3—Infectious Diseases

14. Antibiotics:

(a) Were originally identified from bacteria.
(b) Are commonly classified according to their molecular weight.
(c) Acquire resistance.
(d) Are used as chemotherapy.
(e) Should always be prescribed for sore throats.

15. Antibiotic resistance:

(a) Is only a problem in the Western world.
(b) Can be acquired.
(c) Commonly involves the transfer of nuclear material by viruses.
(d) Is encouraged by indiscreet prescribing of antibiotics.
(e) To penicillin is uncommon.

16. Antibiotics which inhibit bacterial cell-wall synthesis:

(a) Include the penicillins.
(b) Act by forming pores in the bacterial cell wall.
(c) Create cross-linking within the bacterial cell wall.
(d) Include rifampicin.
(e) Can only be given orally.

17. Of the antibiotics which inhibit bacterial protein synthesis:

(a) The aminoglycosides reversibly bind the 30S portion of the bacterial ribosome and inactive it.
(b) Gentamycin can cause deafness.
(c) Tetracyclines are contraindicated in children as they can cause Reye's syndrome.
(d) Chloramphenicol is often used in ophthalmology.
(e) Erythromycin is commonly used in patients who report allergy to penicillins.

18. Infection:

(a) Of the urinary tract is commonly caused by *E. coli*.
(b) With *Clostridium difficile* is commonly precipitated by the use of metronidazole.
(c) Of the central nervous system often requires intrathecal antibiotic therapy.
(d) Of the simple skin wounds is most often treated with flucloxacillin.
(e) With mycobacterial tuberculosis is a notifiable disease.

19. Of the antiviral agents:

(a) Amantadine inhibits viral attachment to host cells.
(b) Aciclovir is used to treat cytomegalovirus.
(c) Zidovudine (AZT) inhibits the viral specific protease.
(d) None have shown clear beneficial effects in HIV management.
(e) Ribavirin is used to treat respiratory syncytial virus in infants.

20. Fungal infections:

(a) Can involve the CNS.
(b) Can never be cured.
(c) Are merely a nuisance in the immunocompromised.
(d) Include *Taenia solium*.
(e) Are always treated systemically.

21. Malaria:

(a) Is caused by the anopheline mosquito.
(b) Can be prevented with chloroquine.
(c) Can be treated with antifolate drugs.
(d) Is seldom resistant to chemotherapy.
(e) Is rare in the United Kingdom.

22. Regarding worm infections:

(a) Therapy is most effective if given intravenously to the patient.
(b) Piperazine results in osmotic lysis of infecting worms.
(c) Immune reactions to dead worms can develop in the host.
(d) Paralysis of infecting worms is ineffective in treating worm infestations.
(e) Like humans, worms rely on GABA at their neuromuscular junctions.

Chapter 4—Inflammation, Pain and Immunosuppression

23. Inflammation/the inflammatory response:

(a) Is an immunologically acquired process.
(b) Relies on endogenous agonist–receptor interactions.
(c) Can be inhibited by opiates.
(d) Relies on the mediators histamine and dopamine.
(e) Involves mast cells.

24. Non-steroidal anti-inflammatory drugs (NSAIDs):

(a) Include paracetamol.
(b) Inhibit the lipoxygenase enzyme.
(c) Inhibit the cyclooxygenase enzyme.
(d) Inhibit the phospholipase A_2 enzyme.
(e) Include clopidogrel.

25. Regarding cyclooxygenase (COX):

(a) Aspirin inhibits COX reversibly.
(b) COX-1 is only expressed during the inflammatory response.
(c) COX converts arachidonic acid to the prostanoids.

(d) COX-2 inhibitors are contraindicated in osteoarthritis.
(e) Inhibition of COX can worsen the symptoms of asthma.

26. Steroidal anti-inflammatory drugs:

(a) Are commonly used to treat aches and sprains.
(b) Are contraindicated in reversible airways disease.
(c) Have a delayed onset of action.
(d) Inhibit lipocortin synthesis.
(e) Can be administered intravenously.

27. Considering rheumatoid arthritis (RA):

(a) RA should not be treated with paracetamol.
(b) RA is an autoimmune disease.
(c) RA does not respond to non-steroidal anti-inflammatory drugs.
(d) Antimalarial drugs, such as chloroquine, are often used in the management of RA.
(e) Treatment with disease-modifying antirheumatic drugs (DMARDs) requires annual screening of the full blood count, and liver and renal function.

28. Regarding gout:

(a) Gout results from pyrophosphate crystals in joints.
(b) Gout is a slowly developing, and seldom presents acutely.
(c) Aspirin should be avoided in its management.
(d) Colchicine inhibits leucocyte migration, and it causes nausea and vomiting in about 80% of patients.
(e) Allopurinol is a methylxanthine.

29. Pain:

(a) Is sensed by nociceptors.
(b) Can be objectively measured.
(c) Usually has a well defined cause.
(d) Can be inhibited by antimalarial drugs.
(e) Perception is only transmitted via nerves.

30. Opiate analgesic drugs:

(a) Can be bought over the counter.
(b) Often cause diarrhoea.
(c) Should not be given intravenously.
(d) Can cause respiratory depression in overdose.
(e) Can cause smooth muscle contraction.

31. Regarding headache:

(a) Headache is a common and non-sinister symptom.
(b) NSAIDs are the first line treatment for headache.
(c) Nausea associated with headache requires hospital admission.
(d) Serotonin (5-HT) agonists are indicated for acute migrainous attacks, constricting cerebral blood vessels.
(e) Antihistamines are indicated for the acute migrainous attack.

32. Which of the following are matched appropriately:

(a) Neuralgic pain may respond to antiepileptics.
(b) Neuralgia commonly occurs due to demyelination.
(c) Amitriptyline is a selective-serotonin reuptake inhibitor.
(d) Ciclosporin is a prodrug.
(e) Azathioprine is cytotoxic to dividing cells.

Chapter 5—Peripheral Nervous System

33. Regarding nerves and nerve conduction:

(a) The resting membrane potential is about +70 mV.
(b) The relative concentrations of sodium and potassium are maintained by the Na^+/K^+ ATPase.
(c) Depolarization occurs when potassium leaves the cell.
(d) Voltage-operated sodium channels are common in all excitable tissues.
(e) The sodium channel contains three gates, m-, h- and n-gates.

34. Local anaesthetics:

(a) Block potassium channels.
(b) Can be given intravenously.
(c) Include cocaine.
(d) Can be given with a vasoconstrictor.
(e) Can be used in heart failure.

35. Anticholinesterases:

(a) Breakdown acetylcholine to choline and acetate.
(b) Increase the amount of acetylcholine in the synaptic cleft.
(c) Include neostigmine.
(d) Are used in the treatment of myasthenia gravis and dementia.
(e) Cross the blood–brain barrier.

36. The autonomic nervous system:

(a) Innervates most smooth and striated muscles.
(b) Relies on acetylcholine released by all postganglion nerve fibres.
(c) Is divided into the sympathetic and parasympathetic nervous systems.
(d) Innervates the adrenal medulla to release glucocorticoids.
(e) Controls heart rate.

37. Regarding adrenoceptors:

(a) α, β and μ are the major divisions of adrenoceptor.
(b) The adrenoceptors are all located in the ganglion.
(c) β_2-adrenoceptors are found only in the lung.
(d) Adrenoceptor agonists include adrenaline and noradrenaline.
(e) Antagonists include atropine.

38. The parasympathetic nervous system:

(a) Relies on acetylcholine released from postganglionic nerve fibres.

(b) Is dependent upon nicotinic and muscarinic receptors in target tissues.
(c) Arises from the thoracolumbar region of the spinal cord.
(d) Increases the rate of contraction of the heart.
(e) Supplies most fibres to the vagus nerve.

Chapter 6—Central Nervous System

39. Parkinsonism:

(a) Is idiopathic.
(b) Is likely to result from excessive dopamine.
(c) Is likely to result from insufficient dopamine.
(d) Can be treated with anticholinergic drugs.
(e) Can be caused by the cardiovascular disease.

40. Treatment for Parkinson's disease:

(a) Usually begins with L-dopa therapy.
(b) Aims to increase dopaminergic activity.
(c) Can be complicated by oculogyric crises.
(d) Can be enhanced by monoamine oxidase inhibitors.
(e) May one day rely on removal of tissue from affected brains.

41. Benzodiazepines:

(a) Are commonly used in the management of depression.
(b) Act at the GABA receptor.
(c) Tend to cause agitation and restlessness.
(d) Can result in dependency.
(e) Should be used with caution for greater than 6 months.

42. Regarding hypnotics and anxiolytics:

(a) Zopiclone has anxiolytic properties, and acts on the GABA receptor.
(b) β-adrenoceptor antagonists act centrally to reduce anxiety.
(c) Barbiturates are non-selective CNS depressants, and cause little sedation.
(d) Chloral hydrate is widely used hypnotic.
(e) Antidepressants are contraindicated in anxiety disorders.

43. Depression:

(a) Is usually bipolar in nature.
(b) Is thought to result from monoamine excess.
(c) Can be treated with monoamine oxidase inhibitors.
(d) Can be treated with antihistamines.
(e) Can be treated with PPIs.

44. Tricyclic antidepressants:

(a) Include lofepramine.
(b) Are safe in overdose.
(c) Act by blocking serotonin (5-HT) and noradrenaline uptake into the presynaptic terminal.
(d) May cause weight loss.
(e) Can be taken with monoamine oxidase inhibitors.

45. The neuroleptics:

(a) Are most useful for treating positive psychotic symptoms.
(b) Can only be given orally.
(c) Act by antagonizing dopamine receptors.
(d) Include metoclopramide.
(e) May cause Parkinson's disease.

46. Considering epilepsy and antiepileptic medication:

(a) Seizures represent abhorrent electrical activity in the brain.
(b) Antiepileptics do not cross the blood–brain barrier.
(c) Phenytoin causes cerebellar signs in overdose.
(d) Carbamazepine is sedating.
(e) Phenytoin is the first line drug in status epilepticus.

47. General anaesthetics:

(a) Are highly specific drugs.
(b) Can be administered intravenously.
(c) Include thiopentone.
(d) Are generally lipid insoluble.
(e) Can cause hypotension.

48. Regarding drug misuse:

(a) Drug misuse is common.
(b) Psychological addiction is easier to break than the physical addiction.
(c) Tolerance develops as the dose of the drug misused increases.
(d) Drug misuse is illegal in the United Kingdom.
(e) Amphetamines are also known as Coke, and Jellies.

Chapter 7—Cardiovascular System

49. Cardiac rate:

(a) Is increased by parasympathetic innervation.
(b) Is slowed by parasympathetic innervation.
(c) Is increased by atropine.
(d) Is increased by salbutamol.
(e) Is elevated in thyrotoxicosis.

50. Considering cardiac failure:

(a) Cardiac glycosides act as negative inotropes.
(b) Diuretics should be avoided in the acute episode.
(c) β-adrenoceptor agonists are indicated for the acute episode.
(d) Angiotensin-converting enzyme inhibitors have proven benefit in the treatment of cardiac failure.
(e) Digoxin can only be given orally.

51. Regarding anti-arrhythmic drugs:

(a) Class I agents block sodium channels.
(b) Adenosine acts to slow the rate of rise of the action potential, and brings about a delay.
(c) Propranolol and sotalol are class II anti-arrhythmics.

(d) Amiodarone acts by blocking potassium channels.
(e) The potassium channel activator nicorandil has anti-arrhythmic properties.

52. Regarding angina:

(a) Angina pain should not be treated with opiates.
(b) Nitrates should be used continuously to prevent angina.
(c) Verapamil and diltiazem predominantly act within the heart.
(d) Warfarin is used in the acute management of unstable angina.
(e) β-adrenoceptor antagonists act by reducing the rate of contraction, and lengthening the duration of diastole.

53. Vascular tone:

(a) Is regulated in part by α- and β-adrenoceptors.
(b) Is increased by nitric oxide.
(c) Is increased by the action of angiotensin II on angiotensin II receptors.
(d) Renal artery stenosis is a cause of essential hypertension.
(e) Angiotensin converting enzyme inhibitors are contraindicated in hyperkalaemia.

54. Regarding shock:

(a) Septic shock is characterized by increased total peripheral resistance.
(b) Corticosteroids will produce an immediate clinical response in a patient with anaphylaxis.
(c) In shock, adrenaline's main action is upon cardiac output.
(d) Oxygen is a first-line drug in the treatment of shock.
(e) Anxiety results from sympathetic activation.

55. The following drugs are used in the treatment of hyperlipidemias:

(a) HMG CoA reductase inhibitors.
(b) Xanthine oxidase inhibitors.
(c) Bezafibrate.
(d) Alfacalcidol.
(e) Cholestyramine.

56. Regarding fibrinolysis:

(a) Heparin is an effective fibrinolytic drug.
(b) Recombinant tissue plasminogen activator commonly stimulates anaphylaxis.
(c) Streptokinase is contraindicated in aortic dissection.
(d) Streptokinase and tissue plasminogen activator are given orally and intravenously.
(e) Streptokinase is indicated in pulmonary embolism.

57. The following drugs are effective antiplatelet agents:

(a) Ibuprofen.
(b) Aspirin.
(c) Clopidogrel.
(d) Dipyridamole.
(e) Heparin.

58. Regarding anaemia:

(a) Vitamin B12 is used in the treatment of pernicious anaemia.
(b) Oral iron preparations often cause dark stools.
(c) Erythropoietin is a first-line drug in iron-deficiency anaemia.
(d) Chronic iron overload can result in cirrhosis of the liver.
(e) Erythropoietin is only effective if the patient has residual renal function.

Chapter 8—Respiratory System

59. Asthma:

(a) Is improved by β-adrenoceptor antagonists.
(b) Is improved by β-adrenoceptor agonists.
(c) Can be made worse by ibuprofen.
(d) Results from irreversible airways narrowing.
(e) Is characterized by stridor.

60. The following drugs have bronchodilating properties:

(a) Beclomethasone.
(b) Theophylline.
(c) Sodium cromoglycate.
(d) Salmeterol.
(e) Ipratropium bromide.

61. The following are common adverse effects of β$_2$-adrenoceptor agonists:

(a) Tremor.
(b) Bradycardia.
(c) Ankle oedema.
(d) Tachycardia.
(e) Oral candida.

62. In asthma:

(a) Salbutamol can be given orally.
(b) Steroids are always given intravenously in the acute attack.
(c) Nebulized bronchodilators are less effective than inhaled bronchodilators.
(d) Oxygen should be restricted to 28% in the acute attack.
(e) The dose of inhaled steroid should not be altered during coexisting respiratory tract infections.

63. The following are correctly paired:

(a) Pulmonary surfactants are indicated in RSV infections.
(b) Naloxone is used in benzodiazepine-induced respiratory depression.
(c) Opiates inhibit the cough reflex.
(d) Ephedrine is a commonly used decongestant.
(e) Naloxone has a very long half-life.

64. Regarding allergy:

(a) IgA is the common mediator in allergic response.
(b) The new antihistamines are non-sedating.

(c) Histamine increases vascular permeability.
(d) Antihistamines are contraindicated in patients with diabetes mellitus.
(e) Histamine causes smooth muscle contraction.

Chapter 9—Kidney and Urinary System

65. The kidney:

(a) Receives 50% of the cardiac output.
(b) Activates vitamin D.
(c) Secretes erythropoietin.
(d) Is sensitive to the antibiotic gentamicin.
(e) Metabolizes most drugs.

66. The following are correctly matched:

(a) Vasopressin is the most potent diuretic.
(b) Loop diuretics act on the thick ascending loop of Henle.
(c) Thiazide diuretics act on the late distal tubule.
(d) Potassium-sparing diuretics act on the late distal tubule.
(e) Mannitol antagonizes aldosterone receptors.

67. Regarding renal failure:

(a) Diuretics should be avoided in acute renal failure.
(b) Hyperkalaemia is common in chronic renal failure.
(c) Hypercalcaemia is common in chronic renal failure.
(d) Metabolic alkalosis is common in chronic renal failure.
(e) NSAIDs are indicated in the management of chronic renal failure.

68. Aldosterone antagonists:

(a) Include sarin.
(b) Promote sodium reabsorption from the late distal tubule.
(c) Include spironolactone.
(d) Have a beneficial effect in treating cardiac failure.
(e) Are used in nephrotic syndrome.

69. Potassium-sparing diuretics:

(a) Include amiodarone.
(b) Include amiloride.
(c) Should only be used with an angiotensin converting enzyme inhibitor.
(d) Can result in hypokalaemia.
(e) May cause gynaecomastia.

70. Loop diuretics:

(a) Can cause hearing loss.
(b) Are only given by the intravenous route.
(c) Have few interactions with β-adrenoceptor antagonists.
(d) Are the most potent of the commonly used diuretics.
(e) Should not be used in acute heart failure.

71. The following are thiazide diuretics:

(a) Metolazone.
(b) Bendrofluazide.
(c) Reboxetine.
(d) Flutamide.
(e) Indapamide.

72. Regarding urinary retention/incontinence:

(a) α-adrenoceptor antagonists relax smooth muscle, increasing the flow or urine.
(b) Parasympathomimetics relax the detrusor muscle, and worsen urinary retention.
(c) In the male, bladder cancer is the commonest cause of urinary retention.
(d) Antimuscarinic drugs relax the detrusor muscle.
(e) Hypotension is a common side effect of α-adrenoceptor blockade.

73. Regarding erectile function/dysfunction:

(a) Nitric oxide is believed to initiate and maintain an erection.
(b) Nitric oxide is broken down by nitric oxide synthase.
(c) Sildenafil inhibits nitric oxide synthase type 5.
(d) Sildenafil inhibits phosphodiesterase type 5.
(e) Sildenafil can be given into the urethra.

Chapter 10—Gastrointestinal System

74. Regarding peptic ulceration:

(a) Ulceration of the gastric and duodenal mucosa is uncommon.
(b) Peptic ulceration is commonly associated with *Helicobacter pylori* infection.
(c) Peptic ulceration is commonly caused by Zollinger–Ellison syndrome.
(d) Gastrin inhibits gastric acid secretion.
(e) Antihistamines by blocking β₁-adrenoceptors.

75. Gastro-oesophageal reflux disease:

(a) Can be exacerbated by smoking, alcohol and obesity.
(b) Should always be referred to a specialist.
(c) Can be treated simply with oral antihistamines.
(d) Can cause metabolic acidosis.
(e) Should not be treated with a proton pump inhibitor.

76. Proton pump inhibitors:

(a) Include the drug fluconazole.
(b) Include the drug lansoprazole.
(c) Inhibit the H^+/K^+ ATPase irreversibly.
(d) Seldom cause side effects.
(e) Are contraindicated in Zollinger–Ellison syndrome.

77. Antacids:

(a) Act to reduce gastric acid secretion from parietal cells.
(b) Include the alginate drugs.
(c) Raise the pH of the stomach.

(d) Are first-line drugs in eradicating *Helicobacter pylori*.
(e) Include aluminium hydroxide.

78. Regarding *Helicobacter pylori*:

(a) *H. pylori* is more common in humans and ferrets than other mammals.
(b) Infection with *H. pylori* will undoubtedly result in peptic ulceration.
(c) *H. pylori* secretes urease, which converts urea to carbon dioxide and water.
(d) *H. pylori* eradication commonly relies on double therapy.
(e) *H. pylori* is not involved in duodenal ulceration.

79. Regarding nausea and vomiting:

(a) Emetic drugs should be used if corrosive agents have been ingested.
(b) The vomiting centre is sensitive to dopamine.
(c) The phenothiazines are useful antiemetics.
(d) Ondansetron is a serotonin (5-HT) receptor antagonist.
(e) Metoclopramide can cause extrapyramidal side effects.

80. Antispasmodics drugs:

(a) Include mebeverine.
(b) Include codeine.
(c) Should not be used in gastro-oesophageal reflux disease.
(d) Can inhibit parasympathetic innervation of the gut.
(e) Are usually given rectally.

81. Regarding laxative drugs:

(a) Lactulose encourages peristalsis.
(b) Senna encourages peristalsis.
(c) Laxatives are indicated in bowel obstruction.
(d) Methylcellulose is a bulk-forming laxative.
(e) Docusate sodium is useful in haemorrhoids.

82. Regarding diarrhoea:

(a) Diarrhoea commonly requires antibiotics in the Western world.
(b) Fluid replacement should always be given intravenously.
(c) Loperamide is given intramuscularly.
(d) Morphine is often administered for diarrhoea.
(e) *Clostridium difficile* is the commonest diarrhoea-causing pathogen in the Western world.

83. Inflammatory bowel disease:

(a) Responds well to laxatives.
(b) Is treated with long-term intravenous steroids.
(c) Can be cured by surgical resection.
(d) Is treated with aspirin derivatives.
(e) Seldom results in nutritional deficiencies.

84. Regarding obesity:

(a) Obesity is associated with diabetes mellitus and osteoarthritis.
(b) Obesity should initially be treated with drugs.
(c) Obesity is often treated with amphetamines.
(d) Orlistat inhibits pancreatic lipase, and subsequent absorption of fat from the gut.
(e) Leptin is used to induce satiety (fullness).

85. The following are correctly paired:

(a) Pancreatic supplementation is indicated in Crohn's disease.
(b) Pancreatin replaces the endocrine function of the pancreas.
(c) Cholestyramine binds bile acids and prevents their reabsorption from the gut.
(d) Ursodeoxycholic acid is used to treat gall stones.
(e) Pancreatin must not be used after total pancreatectomy.

Chapter 11—Endocrine and Reproductive System

86. In hyperthyroidism:

(a) Carbimazole inhibits the action of thyroxine on peripheral tissues.
(b) The thioureylenes inhibit thyroid peroxidase.
(c) Iodine inhibits the conversion of thyroxine to triiodothyronine.
(d) β-adrenoceptor antagonists inhibit thyroxine release.
(e) Symptoms can be reduced by exogenous thyroxine.

87. In hypothyroidism:

(a) Thyroid replacement therapy is given subcutaneously.
(b) Thyroxine is given at standard dose to all patients.
(c) Thyroxine may precipitate cardiac arrhythmias.
(d) In an myxoedema crisis, intravenous thyroxine is administered.
(e) Thyroxine has a half-life of about 6 days.

88. Insulin:

(a) Can be given orally, intramuscularly, intravenously, and subcutaneously.
(b) Acts primarily in the pancreas.
(c) Overdose causes hyperglycaemia.
(d) Should not be used in type 2 diabetes mellitus.
(e) Is used in treating hypercalcaemia.

89. The following are oral hypoglycaemic drugs:

(a) Tolbutamide.
(b) Metformin.
(c) Acarbose.
(d) Rosiglitazone.
(e) Chlorhexidine.

90. Hypoglycaemia:

(a) Is often caused by metformin.
(b) Can present with anxiety.
(c) Should always be treated with intravenous glucose.
(d) Can be reversed by administering intramuscular glycogen.
(e) Can be treated with adrenaline.

91. Regarding the adrenal glands and steroids:

(a) Aldosterone is the principle mineralocorticoid.
(b) Prednisolone is the principle glucocorticoid.
(c) Aldosterone-deficiency can be treated with fludrocortisone.
(d) Cushing's disease is treated with oral hydrocortisone or prednisolone.
(e) Beclomethasone is used topically in skin disease.

92. Side effects of systemic steroid excess include:

(a) Hirsutism.
(b) Pancreatitis.
(c) Bruising.
(d) Sodium and fluid retention.
(e) Hypoglycaemia.

93. The following are indications for oestrogen (or oestrogen and progestogen) therapy:

(a) Contraception.
(b) Menorrhagia.
(c) Breast cancer.
(d) Termination of pregnancy.
(e) Precocious puberty.

94. The following are correct:

(a) Oxytocin relaxes uterine muscle.
(b) Ergometrine is administered orally.
(c) Oxytocin and ergometrine are given together in the third stage of labour.
(d) Ergometrine is used to induce labour.
(e) β-adrenoceptor agonists relax uterine smooth muscle and are used to prevent preterm labour.

95. Regarding the drugs used in disorders of bone and calcium:

(a) Bisphosphonates are contraindicated in hypercalcaemia.
(b) Calcium salts lower serum calcium.
(c) Vitamin D excess causes hypercalcaemia.
(d) Calcitonin inhibits osteoclastic activity.
(e) Hypercalcaemia is treated with vitamin D.

Chapter 12—Eyes and Skin

96. Relating to the eye:

(a) Parasympathetic innervation of the eye causes pupil constriction.
(b) Dilatation of the pupil is mediated by β-adrenoceptor activation.
(c) The ciliary muscle expresses M_2 muscarinic receptors.
(d) Inhibition of parasympathetic innervation of the ciliary muscle makes the lens to become elongated and thin.
(e) Opiate overdose results in pin-point pupils.

97. Glaucoma:

(a) Is defined as raised intracranial pressure.
(b) Treatment is always topical.
(c) Can be treated with miotic drugs.
(d) Is usually painless.
(e) Is a contraindication to selective-serotonin reuptake inhibitor antidepressants.

98. The following are true:

(a) Cycloplegic drugs paralyse the ciliary muscle.
(b) Mydriatic drugs constrict the pupil.
(c) The muscarinic agonist pilocarpine reverses mydriasis.
(d) Once the ciliary muscle is paralysed, the cornea is insensitive to pain.
(e) Steroids should never be applied topically to the eye.

99. Acne:

(a) Is often treated with antiandrogens.
(b) Is made worse by steroids.
(c) Is treated with fibrinolytics.
(d) Is often treated with flucloxacillin.
(e) Can be treated with vitamin A derivatives.

100. The following are true:

(a) Corticosteroids should not be used on undiagnosed skin lesions.
(b) Vitamin D derivatives such as calcipotriol have keratolytic properties.
(c) Coal tar is commonly used in the management of atopic eczema.
(d) Simple emollients may cause hirsutism and hypertension over a prolonged period.
(e) Steroid creams have poor penetration of the skin.

Short-answer Questions

1. Discuss the use of premedication in anaesthesia.

2. Discuss the therapy of hay fever.

3. Describe the classes of drugs used in the treatment of peptic ulcers.

4. What are the main classes of drug used to treat fungal diseases, and what are their mechanisms of action?

5. Which drugs exert their action by modifying γ-aminobutyric acid (GABA) synaptic transmission, and when are they used clinically?

6. Explain the analgesic effect of opioids.

7. Outline the drugs used in the treatment of asthma.

8. Explain the concept of selective toxicity with reference to cytotoxic drugs used in the treatment of cancer.

9. Discuss the different classes of drug used as laxatives.

10. Describe the neurochemical imbalance found in the brains of people suffering from Parkinson's disease, and list the classes of drug used to correct this imbalance.

11. Compare and contrast suxamethonium and atracurium.

12. Explain first pass metabolism.

13. Describe the therapeutic uses of vasoconstrictors.

14. Explain the differences between lidocaine (lignocaine) and amiodarone in their use as anti-arrhythmics.

15. Compare and contrast competitive and non-competitive antagonists.

16. Explain the effects and clinical use of warfarin.

17. Explain how local anaesthetics inhibit nerve conduction.

18. Give an outline of the drug treatment of diabetes mellitus.

19. Explain the clinical use of anticholinesterases and how this is influenced by their duration of action.

20. Explain the role of cAMP as an intracellular messenger in the cardiovascular system.

Essay Questions

1. Drugs are administered by various different routes. Outline the principle routes of administration of drugs using specific examples, with particular reference to the drug absorption, distribution, and metabolism.

2. Discuss the differences between malignant and normal mammalian cells, highlighting the targets available for therapeutic intervention with cytotoxic drugs.

3. Tuberculosis is a reemerging illness worldwide. Outline the nature of this disease, and the current therapeutic approach of its management, with particular emphasis upon the problems of drug-resistance.

4. Rheumatoid arthritis is a disabling and painful disease. Discuss the therapeutic management of this disorder, with particular reference to non-steroidal anti-inflammatory and the disease-modifying antirheumatic drugs.

5. Describe the anatomy and physiology of the autonomic nervous system, with particular reference to the chemical mediators involved in presynaptic and postsynaptic transmission, and the end organ response(s).

6. Discuss the clinical features, biochemical abnormalities and the mechanism of actions of the drugs used in idiopathic Parkinson's disease.

7. Cardiac failure is very common. Discuss the pharmacological strategies that could act to prevent cardiac failure, and the drugs proven to be beneficial in its management.

8. Summarize the clinical features of asthma, and the importance of the drugs used in its management, and in particular their mode of delivery.

9. Erectile dysfunction is common amongst certain groups of the male population. Outline the pathophysiology behind this, and the therapeutic options available to treat it. Consider ethical/social issues regarding state funding for such drugs.

10. Steroids are widely used in clinical practice. Discuss their role and mechanism of action in treating diseases of the skin and gastrointestinal tract, and the complications of long-term use.

1. (a) True—generated by the activation of a G-protein, and adenylyl cyclase.
   (b) True—generated along with IP_3 by activated phospholipase C.
   (c) False—IP_3 is inositol triphosphate.
   (d) False—γ-aminobutyric acid is a neurotransmitter, not an intracellular messenger.
   (e) True—generated by the activation of the guanylyl cyclase enzyme.

2. (a) False—despite the affinity being the same, the partial agonist can never bring about the same response as the full agonist.
   (b) True—see 2a.
   (c) True—though it can still not bring about the same response as the full agonist.
   (d) False—binding is usually reversible, though can be irreversible.
   (e) False—see 2a. Efficacy is the ability of the agonist to bring about a response once bound to the receptor.

3. (a) True—the binding capacity of agonists and antagonists is commonly very similar.
   (b) False—the antagonist will have very little, if any, ability to activate the receptor and bring about a response.
   (c) False—non-competitive antagonists, also known as irreversible antagonists, have a similar effect irrespective of the agonist concentration.
   (d) False—a dose ratio of 10 implies the antagonist is very potent.
   (e) True—higher doses of agonists will be required to bring about the same physiological effect.

4. (a) False—compliance is how well the patient adheres to the drug regimen prescribed by the doctor.
   (b) False—compliance in children depends upon both the child and the parent to cooperate with the drug regimen.
   (c) True—a good doctor–patient relationship improves compliance.
   (d) False—the simpler the regimen, the higher the degree of compliance.
   (e) False—compliance is essential in most diseases, especially infectious diseases such as tuberculosis.

5. (a) False—intravenous drugs bypass first pass metabolism.
   (b) False—high doses of potent steroids can result in systemic effects.
   (c) False—blood draining the rectum is filtered through the liver before entering the systemic circulation.
   (d) False—unpredictable absorption from the gut, and first pass metabolism makes oral drugs less bioavailable.
   (e) True—intravenous drugs will have more rapid speed on onset, and subsequent metabolism than oral drugs.

6. (a) True—the rate of excretion increases with increasing drug concentration.
   (b) False—the free concentration is the determinant.
   (c) True—tubular secretion and tubular reabsorption are important for many drugs.
   (d) False—lipid-soluble drugs are predominantly metabolized in the liver.
   (e) False—the volume of distribution of the drug will influence the plasma half-life but not the rate of renal excretion.

7. (a) False—cardiac output has no effect upon the volume of distribution, as this is a fixed value.
   (b) False—heparin is almost entirely restricted to the intravascular compartment, and has a volume of distribution of 4–5 litres.
   (c) False—some drugs distribute extensively into tissues, and they can have values in excess of total body water.
   (d) True—in the blood or tissues.
   (e) True—in theory, as the degree of ionization of the drug will determine its solubility in the various components of a body.

8. (a) False—drugs are metabolized by the liver, but excreted by the kidneys and in the GI tract.
   (b) False—lipid insoluble drugs cannot cross the blood–brain barrier.
   (c) False—the metabolites of paracetamol are hepatotoxic.
   (d) True—many drugs can either induce or inhibit liver enzymes, altering the metabolism of other drug classes.
   (e) True—the yellow card scheme in the United Kingdom allows drug reactions to be monitored.

9. (a) True—smoking remains the greatest causative agent in the west.
   (b) False—the acute leukaemias in children are now often totally cured.
   (c) True—Epstein–Barr virus, human papilloma virus.
   (d) False—there are few structural differences between cancerous and normal cells; chemotherapy relies on cancer cells dividing more quickly than normal cells.
   (e) True—drug resistance can develop in certain aggressive tumours, as it does in some infectious disease.

10. (a) True—bleomycin is used to treat lymphomas and certain solid tumours.
(b) True—originally designed as an antiemetic but withdrawn due to its teratogenic effects, thalidomide is now used in the treatment of myeloma.
(c) False—vigabatrin is an antiepileptic drug.
(d) False—folate antagonists are used in cancer treatment, and include methotrexate.
(e) False—polymyxin B sulphate is an antifungal drug.

11. (a) False—the bone marrow is commonly suppressed during chemotherapy as its cells are rapidly dividing like malignant cells.
(b) True—the squamous lining of the mouth can become destroyed like the cancer cells.
(c) True—inflammatory responses may be delayed due to non-specific inhibition of diving cells.
(d) False—sterility usually occurs as the stem cells of the gonads are destroyed.
(e) True—bone marrow suppression can lead to pancytopenias, or more commonly anaemia and neutropenia.

12. (a) False—doxazosin is an α-adrenoceptor antagonist used in the treatment of hypertension and urinary outflow obstruction.
(b) True—melphalan is an alkylating agent used in the treatment of myeloma.
(c) True—vincristine is a mitotic inhibitor, and used in the treatment of leukaemias and lymphomas.
(d) True—methotrexate and fluorouracil are antimetabolites, and used to treat leukaemias and solid tumours respectively.
(e) False—cycloplegics are used to paralyse the ciliary muscle of the eye during the ophthalmic examination.

13. (a) True—prednisolone inhibits the growth of cancers of lymphoid origin, and in reducing oedema.
(b) False—thyroxine has no role in cancer therapy, other than in thyroxine-replacement following total thyroidectomy.
(c) True—the oestrogen antagonist tamoxifen is used to treat breast cancers which are oestrogen-dependent.
(d) False—prolactin is not used in cancer therapy.
(e) True—progestogens are used to inhibit endometrial cancers and carcinomas of the breast and prostate.

14. (a) False—antibiotics were originally identified from fungi.
(b) False—antibiotics are usually classified by their site of action, chemical structure or whether they are bactericidal or bacteriostatic.
(c) False—the infective agents (bacteria) acquire resistance, not the antibiotics itself.
(d) True—chemotherapy is simply the term used to denote the use of chemicals (drugs) in treatment of a disease.
(e) False—sore throat does not always mean the infective agent is bacterial; commonly it is viral and unresponsive to antibiotics.

15. (a) False—though more common in the Western world, it is common worldwide.
(b) True—all new cases of antibiotic resistance are now acquired through selection.
(c) False—transfer of resistance genes is by vectors and plasmids, not viruses.
(d) True—resistance is driven by ineffective and indiscriminate use of antibiotics.
(e) False—β-lactamase producing bacteria are very common.

16. (a) True—the penicillins do inhibit bacterial cell-wall synthesis.
(b) False—see 16c.
(c) True—cross-linking inhibits bacterial cell-wall synthesis.
(d) False—rifampicin inhibits bacterial nucleic acid synthesis.
(e) False—most antibiotics can be given enterally and parenterally.

17. (a) False—they bind irreversibly to the 30S portion.
(b) True—in a dose-related fashion.
(c) False—they are contraindicated in children as they are deposited in growing bones and teeth.
(d) True—it has a broad spectrum of activity, and it is useful for superficial bacterial infections of the eye.
(e) True—it has a similar spectrum of activity to the penicillins, but it does not evoke the allergic response.

18. (a) True—*E. coli* is the commonest infective agent in the urinary tract.
(b) False—metronidazole and vancomycin are used to treat *C. difficile* infections.
(c) False—antibiotic penetration of the CSF is usually sufficient.
(d) True—most superficial skin infection is by staphylococcal bacteria.
(e) True—tuberculosis is a notifiable disease.

19. (a) True—by blocking a primitive ion channel in the viral membrane.
(b) False—CMV is resistant to aciclovir.
(c) False—AZT is a reverse transcriptase inhibitor.
(d) False—various antiviral regimens have clear proven benefit in HIV treatment.
(e) True—and is usually delivered by aerosol.

20. (a) True—e.g. *Cryptococcus*, *Candida* and *Aspergillus*.
(b) False—cure is often achieved.
(c) False—can be life threatening.
(d) False—*Taenia* is a worm, *Tinea* is a fungus.
(e) False—many antifungal preparations can be applied locally as creams.

21. (a) False—the mosquito is merely the vector, the infective agents is the *Plasmodium* protozoa.
    (b) True—chloroquine is an effect chemoprophylactic agent, though it does not offer 100% protection.
    (c) True—sulphonamides and dapsone delay parasite replication.
    (d) False—resistance to drugs is becoming more common.
    (e) False—being infected with malaria in the UK is rare, though the disease is not rare in returning travellers.

22. (a) False—most efficient mens of delivering antihelminthic drugs is orally.
    (b) False—piperazine causes a flaccid paralysis of the worm.
    (c) True—this can aid in removing worms and worm fragments.
    (d) False—praziquantel acts in this fashion.
    (e) True—ivermectin paralyses the worm by potentiating the effect of GABA at the NMJ.

23. (a) False—the inflammatory response is an innate mechanism.
    (b) True—numerous endogenous mediators such as histamine act upon specific receptors.
    (c) False—opiates are analgesic drugs, inhibiting the transmission of pain sensation, and they are not anti-inflammatory.
    (d) False—histamine is an inflammatory mediator, dopamine is not.
    (e) True—mast cell degranulation is central in the inflammatory response.

24. (a) False—paracetamol has analgesic and antipyretic properties, but no anti-inflammatory actions.
    (b) False—see 24c.
    (c) True—inhibition of COX is central to NSAIDs actions; lipoxygenase is unaffected by NSAIDs.
    (d) False—the steroid anti-inflammatory drugs inhibit this enzyme.
    (e) False—clopidogrel has antiplatelet properties, but not anti-inflammatory properties.

25. (a) False—aspirin inhibits COX irreversibly.
    (b) False—COX-2 is only expressed during the inflammatory response, COX-1 is the constitutive form.
    (c) True—the prostanoids include the prostaglandins, thromboxane and prostacyclin.
    (d) False—currently COX-2 inhibitors are only licensed in the UK for use in arthritis.
    (e) True—inhibition of COX forces arachidonic acid metabolism down the lipoxygenase pathway, generating bronchoconstricting leukotrienes.

26. (a) False—steroids are usually reserved for more serious inflammatory conditions.
    (b) False—steroids are commonly used in the prophylaxis of asthma.
    (c) True—most steroid actions occur as a result of altered gene expression.
    (d) False—steroids enhance lipocortin synthesis, which itself inhibits phospholipase A_2.
    (e) True—steroids can be administered topically, orally, intravenously, and by inhalation.

27. (a) False—paracetamol is a useful analgesic in RA.
    (b) True—the disease process is mediated by inflammatory cells, which are active against an unknown host target.
    (c) False—NSAIDs form the mainstay of RA treatment.
    (d) True—the antimalarial drugs may inhibit autoimmune leucocytes.
    (e) False—most of the DMARDs require more frequent screening for adverse haematological/biochemical effects.

28. (a) False—gout is monosodium urate, pyrophosphate crystals causes pseudo-gout.
    (b) False—gout nearly always presents very acutely.
    (c) True—aspirin should be avoided, as it inhibits uric acid excretion in the urine.
    (d) True—colchicine appears to inhibit microtubule assembly in inflammatory cells, and it does cause profound nausea and vomiting.
    (e) False—allopurinol inhibits the enzyme xanthine oxidase, which converts purines to urate; methylxanthines include theophylline.

29. (a) True—specialized pain receptors are terms nociceptors.
    (b) False—pain can only be measured subjectively.
    (c) False—many consultations in the community never identify the cause of pain.
    (d) False—antimalarial drugs have no analgesic effects.
    (e) True—there is pure hormonal component to pain.

30. (a) True—weak opiates, such as codeine, can be purchased without prescription.
    (b) False—opiates tend to slow transit time, and result in constipation.
    (c) False—strong opiates are usually given parenterally as they act more quickly, and their bioavailably can be more easily assessed.
    (d) True—opiates can reduce the sensitivity of the respiratory centre to carbon dioxide.
    (e) True—opiates can cause contraction of the sphincter of Oddi and of the ureters.

31. (a) False—Headache is common, but it should never be considered non-sinister until the diagnosis is made.
    (b) True—NSAIDs are effective analgesics, and they may have a role as anti-inflammatories.
    (c) False—Migraine is often accompanied by nausea, though meningitis (meningism) is the concern if nausea is present.
    (d) True—serotonin (5-HT) appears to reverse cerebral blood vessel dilatation.

(e) False—antihistamines are used in migraine prophylaxis to prevent attacks.

32. (a) True—the antiepileptics appear to stabilize neuronal firing.
  (b) False—neuralgia is most commonly caused by nerve or root entrapment.
  (c) False—amitriptyline is a tricyclic antidepressant.
  (d) False—ciclosporin is not a prodrug, azathioprine is.
  (e) True—azathioprine is a fraudulent nucleoside base.

33. (a) False—the resting membrane potential is about −70 mV.
  (b) True—the actual concentrations will also depend upon whether ion channels for sodium and potassium are open or closed.
  (c) False—depolarization is mediated by sodium leaving the cell.
  (d) True—voltage-operated sodium channels are central in electrophysiology.
  (e) False—the sodium channels contain just m- and h-gates.

34. (a) False—local anaesthetics block sodium channels.
  (b) True—intravenous lidocaine (lignocaine) can be used in a Bier's block, though it is now more commonly used to treat cardiac arrhythmias.
  (c) True—cocaine is used in ENT to anaesthetize the nasal septum.
  (d) True—to constrict the vessel and delay the release of the anaesthetic into the systemic circulation.
  (e) False—local anaesthetics, e.g. lidocaine (lignocaine), are used as anti-arrhythmics, but not in heart failure *per se*.

35. (a) False—cholinesterases breakdown acetylcholine.
  (b) True—inhibition of cholinesterases increases the half-life of acetylcholine in the cleft.
  (c) True—neostigmine is an intermediate-acting anticholinesterase.
  (d) True—myasthenia is caused by anti-acetylcholine receptor antibodies, and dementia potentially by depletion of the cholinergic nervous system.
  (e) False—the anticholinesterases do not cross the blood–brain barrier.

36. (a) False—the autonomic nervous system innervates smooth muscle, but not striated muscle.
  (b) False—acetylcholine is used by all preganglionic fibres, but not all postganglionic fibres.
  (c) True—these are the two divisions of the autonomic nervous system.
  (d) False—the autonomic nervous systemic does innervate the adrenal medulla, but to release adrenaline into the systemic circulation.
  (e) True—the vagus nerve carries parasympathetic fibres, and the cardiac nerve sympathetic fibres to the heart.

37. (a) False—α and β are adrenoceptors, μ is an opioid receptor.
  (b) False—α_2-adrenoceptors are preganglionic, but most adrenoceptors are postganglionic in the target tissues.
  (c) False—β_2-adrenoceptors are found in the airways of the lung, but also in vascular smooth muscle, and in the liver.
  (d) True—these are the most potent natural agonists.
  (e) False—atropine is an anticholinergic agent, used to block parasympathetic innervation.

38. (a) True—acetylcholine is released by both the pre- and postganglionic nerve fibres.
  (b) True—mostly muscarinic.
  (c) False—arises from the cranial and sacral regions of the spinal cord.
  (d) False—slows the heart rate.
  (e) True—the vagus is purely a parasympathetic nerve.

39. (a) False—Parkinson's disease is idiopathic, though parkinsonism often has a known cause.
  (b) False—see 39c.
  (c) True—antidopaminergic drugs, or degeneration of the substantia nigra result in low cerebral dopamine.
  (d) True—there is often an imbalance between the dopaminergic and cholinergic systems, and anti-cholinergics aim to rectify this.
  (e) False—parkinsonism can be caused by cerebrovascular disease, but not cardiovascular disease *per se*.

40. (a) False—L-dopa therapy is usually reserved until other treatment options are proving ineffective.
  (b) True—to restore the dopamine deficiency.
  (c) False—oculogyric crises may occur in treatment with the dopamine antagonist metoclopramide.
  (d) True—monoamine oxidase breaks down dopamine, and inhibition of this enzyme helps maintain dopamine activity.
  (e) False—one day transplantation of fetal tissue into affected brains may help Parkinson's patients.

41. (a) False—benzodiazepines are used mainly for anxiety and insomnia and in anaesthetics.
  (b) True—they potentiate the action of GABA on its receptor.
  (c) False—the reverse is true, benzodiazepines are antianxiolytic and sedating.
  (d) True—physical and psychological dependence can occur.
  (e) False—benzodiazepines should not be used for more than 3 weeks as dependency can occur.

42. (a) True—zopiclone has less hang-over effect than some of the benzodiazepines.

(b) False—β-adrenoceptor antagonists act to reduce the symptoms peripherally of anxiety.

(c) False—barbiturates are non-selective depressants of the CNS but are heavily sedating.

(d) False—chloral hydrate is seldom used now in clinical practice, owing to more tolerated drugs on the market.

(e) False—antidepressants can relieve anxiety and insomnia in certain patients.

43. (a) False—depression is commonly unipolar in nature, bipolar disease represent mania.

(b) False—depression is thought to result from monoamine deficiency.

(c) True—monoamine oxidase inhibitors are thought to inhibit monoamine breakdown, restoring the relative deficiency.

(d) False—there is no evidence antihistamines have a role to play in the therapy of depression.

(e) False—PPIs are proton pump inhibitors, and they are indicated in peptic ulcer disease, and in *H. pylori* eradication.

44. (a) True—lofepramine is one of the newer TCAs.

(b) False—TCA in overdose can be fatal.

(c) True—this is their prime mode of action.

(d) False—weight gain is a common side effect.

(e) False—most drugs interact with monoamine oxidase inhibitors.

45. (a) True—negative symptoms are most refractory to drug therapy.

(b) False—many of the neuroleptics can be given by deep intramuscular injection.

(c) True—schizophrenia is proposed to result from dopamine excess.

(d) False—while metoclopramide is a dopamine antagonist, it is not used in the treatment of psychosis.

(e) False—antipsychotic drugs may induce parkinsonism, but Parkinson's disease is idiopathic parkinsonism.

46. (a) True—abhorrent electrical activity in the brain results in the clinical features of epilepsy.

(b) False—the main site of action for the antiepileptics is within the brain.

(c) True—phenytoin can cause cerebellar signs in overdose.

(d) True—a common side effect of carbamazepine is sedation; this is dose-related.

(e) False—benzodiazepines are the first-line drugs in status epilepticus, phenytoin is a second-line drug.

47. (a) False—general anaesthetics are highly non-specific drugs, about whose mechanisms no-one is entirely clear.

(b) True—the induction agents propofol can be used to induce and maintain anaesthesia.

(c) True—thiopentone is a commonly used intravenous agent used for induction.

(d) False—most anaesthetics are highly lipid soluble, and able to penetrate the blood–brain barrier.

(e) True—skeletal and smooth muscle relaxation upon induction can result in hypotension.

48. (a) True—drug misuse also relates to nicotine and alcohol, not just illegal substances.

(b) False—psychological dependence is potentially more difficult to treat than physical dependence.

(c) False—tolerance develops even when the dose of drug taken is constant.

(d) False—not all misused drugs are illegal, e.g. caffeine, nicotine, alcohol.

(e) False—Coke is cocaine, and Jellies is another name for benzodiazepines.

49. (a) False—parasympathetic innervation of the heart via the vagus nerve slows cardiac rate.

(b) True—see 49a.

(c) True—atropine is an anticholinergic, inhibiting parasympathetic inhibition on the heart.

(d) True—salbutamol is a β-adrenoceptor agonist, and as such can increase heart rate.

(e) True—excessive thyroxine increases the basal metabolic rate, and heart rate, and can predispose to arrhythmias (atrial fibrillation).

50. (a) False—cardiac glycosides are positively inotropic, increasing the force of contraction.

(b) False—loop diuretics are first-line drugs in pulmonary oedema.

(c) True—dobutamine and dopamine can be used in CCF emergencies to increase the force of contraction.

(d) True—ACE inhibitors have a clear proven benefit in CCF.

(e) False—digoxin can be given by intravenous infusion in emergencies.

51. (a) True—all class I agents block sodium channels.

(b) True—adenosine causes transient delay in conduction.

(c) False—propranolol is a class II agent, while sotalol is a class III agent.

(d) True—all class III agents block potassium channels.

(e) False—nicorandil is used to prevent angina.

52. (a) False—opiate analgesia is often required in acute angina attacks.

(b) False—patients require a nitrate free period, as they can become insensitive to their effects.

(c) True—verapamil and diltiazem act predominately on the heart to slow the rate and force of contraction; nifedipine acts on the vasculature to cause vasodilatation.

(d) False—anticoagulation in unstable angina is achieved with heparin.

(e) True—β-adrenoceptor antagonists reduce myocardial oxygen demand, and lengthen diastole when myocardial perfusion occurs.

53. (a) True—α- and β-adrenoceptor activation regulate vascular tone.

(b) False—nitric oxide relaxes vascular smooth muscle, reducing vascular tone.
(c) True—angiotensin II is a potent vasoconstrictor.
(d) False—essential hypertension has an unknown cause, renal artery stenosis is a cause of secondary hypertension.
(e) True—ACE inhibitors can themselves cause hyperkalaemia by their inhibitory action on aldosterone.

54. (a) False—septic shock results in nitric oxide release, and vasodilatation.
(b) False—the role of steroids in shock remains unclear, though their action will be delayed as they alter gene expression.
(c) False—adrenaline's main action in shock is to increase vascular tone, and it relaxes smooth muscles of the airways.
(d) True—shock results in hyperfusion and hypoxia of peripheral tissues.
(e) True—sympathetic activation as a result of hypotension drives the symptoms of anxiety.

55. (a) True—HMG CoA reductase inhibitors are also known as statins, and inhibit HMG CoA reductase, which is in the pathway of cholesterol biosynthesis.
(b) False—xanthine oxidase converts purines to uric acid, and xanthine oxidase inhibitors are used in the treatment of gout.
(c) True—bezafibrate is more effective in reducing serum triglycerides than cholesterol.
(d) False—alfacalcidol is a vitamin D derivative used in renal failure.
(e) True—cholestyramine binds bile acids in the gut, preventing their reabsorption, and promoting the breakdown of cholesterol to replace this loss.

56. (a) False—heparin is an anti-coagulant, and has no fibrinolytic properties.
(b) False—rTPa is not commonly antigenic, while streptokinase is derived from bacteria, and is antigenic.
(c) True—fibrinolysis is contraindicated in most active bleeding disorders, and after trauma or surgery.
(d) False—fibrinolytics are given by intravenous infusion only.
(e) True—fibrinolytics are indicated for use in massive pulmonary embolism.

57. (a) False—ibuprofen reversibly inhibits cyclooxygenase, and it has no antiplatelet effects.
(b) True—aspirin irreversibly inhibits cyclooxygenase, preventing the formation of thromboxane A2, which is responsible for platelet aggregation.
(c) True—clopidogrel inhibits the activation of the glycoprotein IIb/IIIa receptor, and is a useful alternative in aspirin sensitive patients.
(d) True—dipyridamole inhibits cAMP degradation, and results in poor platelet aggregation.
(e) False—heparin potentiates the action of anti-thrombin III, and has no effect on platelet aggregation.

58. (a) True—pernicious anaemia is an autoimmune disease resulting in inadequate intrinsic factor, which is responsible for vitamin B12 absorption from the gut.
(b) True—iron in the large bowel is oxidized to dark coloured iron oxides.
(c) False—erythropoietin is ineffective in treating anaemia unless adequate iron stores are present, see 58e.
(d) True—primary and secondary haemochromatosis result in cirrhosis secondary to iron deposition in the liver.
(e) False—erythropoietin is naturally synthesized in the kidney, but acts in the bone marrow. Erythropoietin is used to treat anaemia in renal failure.

59. (a) False—β-adrenoceptor antagonists (β-blockers) may make asthma worse, by inhibiting endogenous β-adrenoceptor activation, which causes smooth muscle relaxation.
(b) True—β-adrenoceptor agonists acts to relax smooth muscle, causing bronchodilatation.
(c) True—ibuprofen and the other NSAIDs inhibit cyclooxygenase, and divert arachidonic acid synthesis down the lipoxygenase pathway, which generates leukotrienes (bronchoconstrictors).
(d) False—asthma is marked by reversible airways narrowing.
(e) False—stridor signifies large airways obstruction, whereas asthma is caused by small airways narrowing, which causes wheeze.

60. (a) False—beclomethasone is a steroid drug, and is used in asthma prophylaxis, and it has no bronchodilating properties.
(b) True—theophylline is a methylxanthine, and inhibits cAMP breakdown. Increased cAMP results in smooth muscle relaxation.
(c) False—sodium cromoglycate is a mast-cell stabilizer, and used in asthma prophylaxis, having no bronchodilating properties.
(d) True—salmeterol is a long acting β_2-adrenoceptor agonist.
(e) True—ipratropium bromide is an antimuscarinic, and inhibits parasympathetic bronchoconstriction.

61. (a) True—this is a commonly reported side effect, and results from skeletal muscle activity.
(b) False—see 61d.
(c) False—ankle oedema is not reported although peripheral vasodilatation may occur.
(d) True—activation of β-adrenoceptors in the heart results in tachycardia.
(e) False—this is, however, a common side effect of inhaled corticosteroids.

62. (a) True—salbutamol may be given by inhalation, nebulized, orally or intravenously.
(b) False—there is debate whether intravenous steroids are any more effective than oral steroids in the acute asthma attack.

(c) False—nebulized drugs are made more available than inhaled drugs.
(d) False—oxygen should be administered at 100%. Oxygen restriction is sometimes indicated in chronic obstructive pulmonary disease.
(e) False—the dose of inhaled steroid is commonly doubled during a respiratory tract infection.

63. (a) False—pulmonary surfactant is used to reduce the surface tension of the alveolus in respiratory distress syndrome (RDS) of neonates.
(b) False—naloxone is used to reverse opiate overdose. Flumazenil is used to reverse benzodiazepine overdose.
(c) True—opiates act in the cough-centre to inhibit the cough reflex.
(d) True—ephedrine causes vasoconstriction, and reduction in oedema and secretions of the nasal mucosa.
(e) False—naloxone has a much shorter half-life than most of the opiates it is used to counteract, and often given repeatedly until the opiate overdosed on is metabolized.

64. (a) False—IgE is the immunoglobulin most strongly related to the allergic response.
(b) True—the old style antihistamines had profound sedating properties as they crossed the blood–brain barrier.
(c) True—histamine increases vascular permeability by opening junctions between endothelial cells.
(d) False—antihistamines are to be used with caution in patients with prostatic hypertrophy, glaucoma, and urinary retention as they have significant antimuscarinic activity.
(e) True—histamine can act directly upon vascular and airways smooth muscle.

65. (a) False—the kidney receives about 25% of the cardiac output.
(b) True—the kidney hydroxylates vitamin D in the 25 position, to generate 1,25 hydroxy-vitamin D.
(c) True—erythropoietin is secreted by the kidney in response to a fall in the oxygen tension of blood flowing through it.
(d) True—gentamicin is nephrotoxic, and ototoxic.
(e) False—most drugs are metabolized by the liver, and subsequently excreted by the kidney.

66. (a) False—vasopressin is an antidiuretic, used to treat diabetes insipidus.
(b) True—loop diuretics including frusemide act to inhibit the $Na^+/K^+/Cl^-$ cotransporter.
(c) False—thiazide diuretics act to inhibit the Na^+/Cl^- cotransporter in the early distal tubule.
(d) True—potassium-sparing diuretics work in the late distal tubule.
(e) False—mannitol's diuretic effect is non-specific, acting as an osmotic diuretic by creating an osmotic load in the tubule lumen.

67. (a) False—diuretics are used in the management of acute renal failure.
(b) True—failing renal function results in potassium accumulating in the body.
(c) False—hypocalcaemia is common, as vitamin D cannot be activated by the kidneys.
(d) False—metabolic acidosis is common, since protons accumulate, and bicarbonate is not synthesized in the kidney.
(e) False—NSAIDs may reduce renal perfusion by inhibiting prostaglandins, which would worsen renal function yet further.

68. (a) False—sarin is a nerve gas, which has anticholinesterase activity.
(b) False—aldosterone antagonists inhibit sodium reabsorption from the late distal tubule.
(c) True—spironolactone is the main aldosterone antagonist.
(d) True—even at doses lower than its diuretic effect, spironolactone improves outcome in cardiac failure.
(e) True—nephrotic syndrome results in secondary hyperaldosteronism, which can be overcome by aldosterone antagonists.

69. (a) False—amiodarone is an anti-arrhythmic drug.
(b) True—amiloride is a commonly used potassium sparing diuretic.
(c) False—caution should be employed when using a potassium sparing diuretics and an ACE inhibitor as both can cause hyperkalaemia.
(d) False—hyperkalaemia is the commonest electrolyte abnormality.
(e) True—spironolactone can cause gynaecomastia, though the other potassium sparing diuretics do not.

70. (a) True—loop diuretics are potentially ototoxic.
(b) False—loop diuretics can be given orally, intravenously or intramuscularly. The intravenous route is used in emergencies.
(c) True—loop diuretics and β-blockers are safe to use together.
(d) True—loop diuretics are termed high-ceiling diuretics and produce the most marked diuresis.
(e) False—acute pulmonary oedema should be treated with intravenous loop diuretics.

71. (a) True—metolazone produces profound diuresis.
(b) True—bendrofluazide is the most widely used thiazide diuretic.
(c) False—reboxetine is a selective noradrenaline retake inhibitor used to treat depression.
(d) False—flutamide is an antiandrogen used in the management of prostatic cancer.
(e) True—indapamide is claimed to lower blood pressure in addition to causing diuresis.

72. (a) True—α-adrenoceptors at the bladder neck cause smooth muscle contraction—antagonism of these relaxes the muscle.

(b) False—parasympathomimetics increase the contraction of the detrusor muscle, aiding urinary flow.

(c) False—prostatic enlargement is the commonest cause of urinary retention in men.

(d) True—antimuscarinic (anticholinergic) drugs relax the detrusor muscle, and result in urinary retention.

(e) True—α-adrenoceptors in the vasculature are activated by systemic α-adrenoceptor blockade, and can decrease total peripheral resistance and blood pressure.

73. (a) True—nitric oxide is believed to increase blood flow into the penis.

(b) False—nitric oxide synthase generates nitric oxide, not degrades it.

(c) False—see 73d.

(d) True—sildenafil is a type 5 specific phosphodiesterase inhibitor.

(e) False—sildenafil can only be given orally. Prostaglandin E_1 can be given into the urethra.

74. (a) False—peptic ulceration is very common amongst patients.

(b) True—H. pylori infection accounts for about 90% of all peptic ulcers.

(c) False—Zollinger–Ellison syndrome is rare, though does itself cause peptic ulceration.

(d) False—gastrin enhances gastric acid release.

(e) False—antihistamines antagonist histamine receptors in the stomach.

75. (a) True—all these factors relax the lower oesophageal sphincter, and exacerbate the symptoms of GORD.

(b) False—most studies suggest dyspepsia only needs referring to a specialist in the over 40s.

(c) True—H_2 antagonists such as cimetidine may be sufficient to overcome the symptoms of GORD.

(d) False—acid hypersecretion into the stomach does not affect the pH of the plasma normally. Repeated vomiting could result in metabolic alkalosis.

(e) False—PPIs are important drugs in the management of acid-related disease.

76. (a) False—fluconazole is an antifungal agent.

(b) True—lansoprazole is a PPI.

(c) True—reversible inhibition of this ATPase would be insufficient in treating peptic ulcer disease.

(d) False—nauseas, vomiting and abdominal discomfort are common adverse reactions.

(e) False—PPIs are first line drugs in the management of Zollinger–Ellison syndrome.

77. (a) False—antacids merely neutralize gastric acid once it is secreted; they have no effect upon acid secretion itself.

(b) False—alginates do not alter stomach pH, merely form an impenetrable raft on top of the gastric contents, preventing reflux into the oesophagus.

(c) True—antacids neutralize gastric acid, making the stomach contents more alkaline.

(d) False—antacids are not first-line drugs in H. pylori eradication regimens.

(e) True—aluminium hydroxide is a clinically used antacid.

78. (a) True.

(b) False—many individuals cary H. pylori in their stomachs, but never develop ulcers.

(c) False—urease converts urea to carbon dioxide and ammonia.

(d) False—triple therapy is more widely used, as it is more effective (PPI, metronidazole and clarithromycin or erythromycin).

(e) False—H. pylori is more strongly associated with gastric ulcers, but it also has a correlation with duodenal ulcers.

79. (a) False—ingested corrosives should be expelled via gastric lavage using a tube, as oesophageal irritation or respiratory aspiration may occur.

(b) True—some dopaminergic drugs result in nausea.

(c) True—the phenothiazines are antidopaminergic .

(d) True—ondansetron is a 5-HT_3 receptor antagonist and believed to act in the chemoreceptor trigger zone.

(e) True—metoclopramide is a dopamine antagonist, and it may produce extrapyramidal side effects.

80. (a) True—mebeverine is a drug acting directly on the smooth muscle of the gut, causing relaxation.

(b) False—codeine slows bowel transit time, but it is not strictly an antispasmodic.

(c) True—antispasmodics may relax the lower oesophageal sphincter, and worsen reflux disease.

(d) True—atropine can be used to block parasympathetic innervation of the gut, which results in smooth muscle relaxation.

(e) False—antispasmodics are usually given orally.

81. (a) False—lactulose is an osmotic laxative, generating an osmotic load in the lumen of the gut.

(b) True—methylcellulose, like bran, simply is an indigestible material, and stimulates peristalsis.

(c) False—laxatives are contraindicated in bowel obstruction.

(d) True—methylcellulose, like bran, simply is an indigestible material, and stimulates peristalsis.

(e) True—docusate sodium is a faecal softener, and used clinically in anal disorders such as haemorrhoids.

82. (a) False—most cases of diarrhoea in the west ar non-infective.

(b) False—fluid replacement should be oral unless dehydration is severe.

(c) False—loperamide is given orally, so it can directly act upon the gut.

(d) False—morphine is not indicated for use in diarrhoea, though it does cause constipation.

(e) False—*C. difficile* causes pseudomembranous colitis, but it is not the commonest infective organism in the west.

83. (a) False—laxatives are not used in the management of IBD.

(b) False—long-term steroids are not used due to their adverse effects, though for the acute episode, steroids should be fully utilized.

(c) True—a total colectomy often completely cures ulcerative colitis.

(d) True—the aminosalicylate sulfasalazine is the main form of treatment for many patients with Crohn's and ulcerative colitis.

(e) False—anaemia, and vitamin deficiencies are common, and these should be addressed.

84. (a) True—obesity is involved in the pathogenesis of several disease processes, including diabetes mellitus, osteoarthritis, cardiovascular disease, and gall stones.

(b) False—diet and exercise are first-line treatment options in the obese.

(c) False—amphetamines were once used to treat obesity, but are no longer used due to their side effects and potential for misuse.

(d) True—orlistat causes steatorrhoea as a result of its mechanism of ation.

(e) False—leptin does induce satiety, but as yet it is not available on the market.

85. (a) False—the pancreas is not involved in Crohn's disease.

(b) False—pancreatin replaces the exocrine function of the pancreas, and contains pancreatic lipase.

(c) True—bile acids are inhibited from re-entering the hepatic circulation, and subsequently lost in stools.

(d) True—while not commonly used, ursodeoxycholic acid decreases the amount of cholesterol in bile, and promotes gall stone dissolution.

(e) False—pancreatin is used to replace the exocrine function of the pancreas.

86. (a) False—carbimazole is a thioureylene, see 86b.

(b) True—thioureylenes inhibit a crucial step in the biosynthesis of thyroxine synthesis within the thyroid gland.

(c) True—iodine is seldom used in practice now due to its adverse effects.

(d) False—β-adrenoceptor antagonists have no effect upon thyroxine release; they merely inhibit the sympathetic symptoms hyperthyroidism can cause.

(e) False—thyroxine therapy is strongly contraindicated in hyperthyroidism, as it will worsen symptoms and sequelae.

87. (a) False—standard replacement therapy is given orally.

(b) False—the dose required is initially calculated, and then altered in response to the patient's thyroid-stimulating hormone levels.

(c) True—thyroxine increases the metabolic rate, and can cause tachycardia and potentially arrhythmias.

(d) False—while intravenous replacement is given in the myxoedema crisis, the drug is T_3 (triiodothyronine) not T_4 (thyroxine).

(e) True—most thyroxine *in vivo* is converted to the more active triiodothyronine.

88. (a) False—insulin is a peptide and cannot be given by the enteral route.

(b) False—insulin acts primarily in the liver, muscle and fat.

(c) False—insulin overdose results in hypoglycaemia as plasma glucose enters the cells.

(d) False—insulin is used in treating type 2 diabetes when other treatments fail.

(e) False—insulin is used to treat hyperkalaemia, as potassium follows glucose into cells from the plasma.

89. (a) True—tolbutamide is a sulphonylurea, and act to stimulate insulin release from residual β-pancreatic cells.

(b) True—metformin is a biguanide, and it increases tissues' sensitivity to insulin.

(c) True—acarbose delays the absorption of sucrose and starch from the gut.

(d) True—rosiglitazone is a thiazolidinedione, and like metformin it is believed to reduce peripheral resistance to insulin.

(e) False—chlorhexidine is a skin disinfectant used in surgical theatres in hospital wards.

90. (a) False—metformin seldom causes hypoglycaemia, the sulphonylureas are more likely to cause hypoglycaemia.

(b) True—hypoglycaemia results in sympathetic activation.

(c) False—if the patient is alert, oral glucose can be administered.

(d) False—hypoglycaemia can be treated with intramuscular glucagon; glycogen is a polymer of glucose stored in the body.

(e) False—adrenaline has no role in the management of simple hypoglycaemia.

91. (a) True—the mineralocorticoids are responsible for water and electrolyte balance, possessing salt-retaining properties.

(b) False—cortisol (hydrocortisone) and cortisone are the principle endogenous glucocorticoids; prednisolone is a synthetic glucocorticoid.

(c) True—fludrocortisone has high mineralocorticoid activity, and little glucocorticoid activity.

233

(d) False—Cushing's disease results from steroid excess; treatment involves removing the adrenal glands, or pituitary gland.

(e) True—though more widely known for its use in asthma, beclomethasone is used in dermatology.

92. (a) True—hirsutism results from increased levels of androgens.
(b) True—steroid excess can result in pancreatitis.
(c) True—steroids can cause thrombocytopenia.
(d) True—steroids act via the aldosterone receptors in the kidney.
(e) False—steroids may cause hyperglycaemia as they antagonize the actions of insulin.

93. (a) True—the combined oral contraceptive pill (COCP) is the most popular form of oral contraceptive, and combines an oestrogen and a progestogen.
(b) True—COCP can be used to treat menorrhagia when any underlying sinister pathology is excluded, as the COCP reduces the severity and duration of the menses.
(c) False—most breast cancers are oestrogen-dependent, and exogenous oestrogens are strongly contraindicated in malignant breast disease.
(d) False—antiprogestogens are used in termination of pregnancy, but not oestrogen or progestogen agonists as these support a pregnancy.
(e) False—precocious puberty is driven by oestrogens in the female, and treatment relies on giving GnRH agonists

94. (a) False—oxytocin causes uterine muscle contraction.
(b) False—ergometrine is a peptide, and must be administered parenterally.
(c) True—'Syntrometrine®' is used in the third stage of labour to deliver the placenta and minimize post-partum bleeding.
(d) False—ergometrine is contraindicated in the first or second stages of labour as the contractions it produced are too forceful.
(e) True—drugs which inhibit preterm delivery are termed tocolytics, and include β-adrenoceptor agonists and ethanol.

95. (a) False—bisphosphonates inhibit osteoclasts, and are used in the management of hypercalcaemia.
(b) False—calcium salts raise serum calcium.
(c) True—vitamin D results in increased absorption of calcium from the gut, and reduced excretion in the urine.
(d) True—calcitonin, like bisphosphonates inhibit osteoclasts.
(e) False—vitamin D raises serum calcium, and is used in hypocalcaemia secondary to vitamin D deficiency.

96. (a) True—parasympathetic activity causes miosis (pupil constriction).
(b) False—dilatation of the pupil is mediated by α_1-adrenoceptor activation.
(c) False—the ciliary muscle contains M_2 muscarinic receptors.
(d) True—anticholinergic drugs have this effect, which results in blurred vision.
(e) True—opiates act centrally on μ- and κ-receptors and cause frank pupil constriction.

97. (a) False—glaucoma is caused by raised intra-ocular pressure.
(b) False—most drugs are given topically, though β-adrenoceptor antagonists and carbonic anhydrase inhibitors can be given systemically.
(c) True—miotic drugs constrict the pupil, allowing aqueous to drain from the posterior to the anterior chambers.
(d) False—acute glaucoma is usually very painful.
(e) False—the tricyclic antidepressants should not be prescribed in glaucoma, as they are anticholinergic, and may worsen glaucoma.

98. (a) True—cycloplegic drugs include tropicamide and are short-acting antimuscarinics.
(b) False—mydriatic drugs dilate the pupil.
(c) True—pilocarpine reverse the antimuscarinic effects of tropicamide.
(d) False—the cornea will remain sensitive to pain unless a local anaesthetic is applied to it.
(e) False—steroids are highly useful drugs in treating inflammatory, not infective, eye disease.

99. (a) True—cyproterone acetate and an oestrogen is used as both a contraceptive pill, and a treatment for acne.
(b) True—steroids probably worsen acne via androgen effects.
(c) False—fibrinolytics break down blood clots; acne is treated with keratolytics, which break down keratin plugs.
(d) False—while many antibiotics are used to treat acne, flucloxacillin is not.
(e) True—the vitamin A derivatives tretinoin and isotretinoin are drugs used in the management of acne.

100. (a) True—infections and some malignancies may become worse if treated with steroids.
(b) True—vitamin D derivatives are both keratolytic and anti-inflammatory.
(c) False—coal tar is most commonly used in psoriasis and occasionally eczema, and never on the face.
(d) False—simple emollient are purely aqueous creams, and do not contain steroids.
(e) False—steroid creams penetrate the skin very well as they are lipid soluble.

1. Premedication is given before the patient is taken to the operating theatre, and it has four component aims. A selection of drugs is used, as no one compound has all the desired effects:
   - Benzodiazepines (give two examples) are used to relieve apprehension and anxiety before anaesthesia, to reduce the amount of anaesthetic required to induce unconsciousness, and, possibly, to sedate postoperatively.
   - Muscarinic antagonists (give two examples) are used to prevent salivation and bronchial secretions, and more importantly to protect the heart from arrhythmias, particularly bradycardia caused by some inhalation agents and neuromuscular blockers.
   - Opioid analgesics (give an example) are often given before an operation as, although the patient is unconscious during surgery, adequate analgesia is important to stop physiological stress reactions to pain, and for the postoperative period.
   - Antiemetic drugs (give an example) can be given to inhibit postoperative emesis. Nausea and vomiting are common after general anaesthesia, often owing to the administration of opioid drugs.

2. Hay fever (seasonal allergic rhinitis) is caused by a type I hypersensitivity reaction to pollen and is characterized by features such as a streaming nose, inflamed eyes, etc.
   Precipitating factors (allergens) should be avoided, but symptomatic relief is often necessary. Antihistamines (H_1 histamine receptor antagonists) are the mainstay of treatment, the initial choice being governed by the degree of sedation required. Older drugs (e.g. chlorpheniramine, trimeprazine) that cross the blood–brain barrier are much more sedative than the newer drugs that don't (e.g. cetirizine, loratadine).
   Other drugs that can be of use are topical nasal formulations of corticosteroids (beclomethasone) and nasal or eye drop preparations of sodium cromoglycate, but these must be used prophylactically. An anticholinergic spray (e.g. ipratropium) can be used for persistent rhinorrhoea.

3. Drugs that are effective in the treatment of peptic ulcers can be classified as follows:
   - Acid secretion inhibitors such as proton pump inhibitors (e.g. omeprazole) irreversibly inhibit the H^+/K^+ ATPase that is responsible for H^+ secretion from parietal cells. Histamine H_2 receptor antagonists (e.g. cimetidine) competitively block the action of histamine on parietal cell H_2 receptors.
   - Mucosal strengtheners such as sucralfate and bismuth chelate polymerize below pH 4 to a gel substance that adheres to and protects ulcer craters.

Bismuth chelate has an additional weak antibacterial effect on *Helicobacter pylori*. Misoprostol is a synthetic analogue of prostaglandin E that imitates the action of endogenous prostaglandins (PGE_2 and PGI_2) in maintaining the integrity of the gastroduodenal mucosal barrier.
   - Antacids such as aluminium hydroxide and sodium bicarbonate are alkaline salts that are used to raise the luminal pH of the stomach.
   - *H. pylori* eradication regimes include the triple therapy (omeprazole, metronidazole, and clarithromycin).

4. The main classes of drug used to treat fungal infections (mycoses) are the polyene macrolides, the imidazoles, and the triazoles, and other antifungal agents.
   - Polyene macrolides (amphotericin B, nystatin) bind to ergosterol in the fungal cell membrane, forming pores through which the cell constituents are lost. This causes fatal damage.
   - Imidazoles and triazoles (clotrimazole, fluconazole) inhibit fungal lipid (especially ergosterol) synthesis in cell membranes, and they also interfere with fungal oxidative enzymes.
   Additionally, three other drugs are increasingly being used:
   - Allylamines (terbinafine) prevents ergosterol synthesis by inhibiting the enzyme squalene oxidase, resulting in squalene accumulation, which leads to membrane disruption and cell death.
   - Flucytosine, which is imported into fungal (but not human) cells, where it is converted into 5-fluorouracil, a potent inhibitor of DNA synthesis.
   - Griseofulvin, the mechanism of action of which is not fully established, but it probably interferes with microtubule formation or nucleic acid synthesis and polymerization.

5. See Fig. SAQ1

6. Opioid analgesic drugs, whether naturally occurring like morphine or chemically synthesized, possess agonist action at opioid receptors. Mu-receptors are thought to be responsible for most of the analgesic effects of opioids, though δ-receptors and κ-receptors are probably important in the periphery and at the spinal level, respectively, and they may also contribute to analgesia.
   Opioids act on these opioid receptors and affect the transmission of pain information from the periphery via the dorsal horn of the spinal cord to higher brain centres.

235

Opioid drugs affect the activity of the dorsal horn relay neurons by several inhibitory inputs. This constitutes the 'gate-control mechanism':

- Opioid receptor agonism (inhibitory) on the dorsal horn relay neurons themselves.
- Activation of descending inhibitory noradrenergic fibres from the locus ceruleus area of the brainstem.
- Activation of descending inhibitory serotonergic fibres from the nucleus raphe magnus and periaqueductal grey areas of the brainstem.

The combined effect of this is to reduce the activity of the dorsal horn relay neurons ('shutting the gate') causing analgesia. Note that the sense of euphoria produced by strong opioids undoubtedly contributes to their analgesic activity by helping to reduce the anxiety and emotive components associated with pain.

7. The two main classes of drugs used in the management of asthma are the bronchodilators, and the prophylactic and anti-inflammatory drugs.

Bronchodilators:

β_2-adrenoceptor agonists act upon β_2-adrenoceptors in the smooth muscle of the airway, causing a rise in cAMP, and subsequent relaxation in the bronchial smooth muscle. The anticholinergics, ipratropium bromide and oxitropium, block muscarinic receptors in the airways, preventing parasympathetic bronchoconstriction. The xanthine, theophylline, inhibits phosphodiesterase breakdown of cAMP, and enhances cAMP's ability to relax smooth muscle. Leukotriene receptor antagonists such as montelukast, are antagonists at leukotriene receptors, and they prevent endogenous agonists (leukotrienes) from bringing about bronchoconstriction.

Prophylactic and anti-inflammatory drugs:

Mast-cell stabilizers, such as sodium cromoglycate, act to prevent pro-inflammatory cells, particularly mast cells, from degranulating, and inhibit their release of

histamine and other bronchoconstricting mediators. Glucocorticoids, including beclomethasone and budesonide, have several potential actions in asthma, including reduction in mucosal oedema, inhibition of pro-inflammatory cytokine synthesis, and adrenoceptor upregulation.

8. Selectively toxic cytotoxic cancer chemotherapy is the use of chemicals or drugs (both natural and synthetic) in an attempt to kill malignant cancer cells preferentially while aiming to cause the minimum of damage to normal host cells. The problem that exists with selective toxicity in the chemotherapy of cancers is that whereas in, e.g., antibacterial chemotherapy, where the target (prokaryote) is of a very different cell type to host (eukaryote), cancer cells are very similar in most ways to normal host cells. This makes identification of targets for selective chemotherapy very difficult.

Cytotoxic drugs are therefore not specifically toxic to cancer cells; the selectivity they show is marginal at best, and they affect all rapidly dividing tissues (both normal and malignant) and thus have a number of general toxic effects: myelosuppression, inhibition of mucosal cell division, alopecia, sterility, etc. Relative selectivity (a higher proportional kill of cancer cells) can be achieved with some cancers because:

- In the malignant tumours, more cells are undergoing proliferation than in normal proliferating tissues.
- Normal cells seem to recover from chemotherapeutic inhibition faster than some cancer cells.
- Synchronized cell cycling may leave discrete periods of vulnerability to cytotoxic drugs.

9. Laxatives are drugs used to increase the motility of the gut and encourage defecation. They are used to relieve constipation (an infrequent or difficult passage of stool) and to clear the gastrointestinal tract before medical or surgical procedures.

Fig. SAQ1

Classes of drug that act by modifying γ-aminobutyric acid (GABA) synaptic transmission		
Drug class & examples	Mechanism of action	Clinical uses
Benzodiazepines *e.g. clonazepam temazepam lorazepam*	Occupation of the benzodiazepine site on the GABA/Cl⁻ channel complex by benzodiazepine receptor agonists enhances the actions of GABA on the Cl⁻ conductance of the neuronal membrane (increase frequency of opening)	Sleep disorders Anxiety disorders Premedication Status epilepticus Alcohol withdrawal
Barbiturates *e.g. thiopentone phenobarbitone*	Occupation of the barbiturate site on the GABA/Cl⁻ channel complex enhances the actions of GABA on the Cl⁻ conductance of the neuronal membrane (increase duration of opening)	Anaesthetic induction Epilepsy
Anticonvulsants *e.g. vigabatrin valproate?*	Irreversible inhibition of GABAγ, increasing brain GABA levels and central GABA release	Epilepsy

Four main classes of laxative are used:

- Bulk laxatives (bran, methylcellulose), which increase the volume of non-absorbable solid residue, distending the colon and stimulating peristaltic activity.
- Osmotic laxatives (lactulose, saline purgatives), which are poorly absorbed compounds that increase the water content of the bowel by osmosis.
- Stimulant laxatives (senna, cascara, sodium picosulphate), which increase gastrointestinal peristalsis by stimulating the mucosa of the gut (probably by irritating local reflexes), the signal arising in the mucosa and being transmitted through the intramural plexi to the smooth muscle of the intestine.
- Faecal softeners (liquid paraffin, docusate sodium), which promote defecation by softening (e.g. docusate sodium) and/or lubricating (e.g. liquid paraffin) the faeces to aid their passage through the gastrointestinal tract.

10. The main pathology in Parkinson's disease is a progressive degeneration of the dopaminergic neurons of the substantia nigra, which project in the nigrostriatal pathway to the corpus striatum (analysis of post-mortem brains of parkinsonian patients shows a substantially reduced concentration of dopamine (less than 10% of normal) in the basal ganglia).

In Parkinson's disease, the inhibitory dopaminergic activity of the nigrostriatal pathway is therefore considerably reduced (20–40%). This results in cholinergic neuron hyperactivity from the corpus striatum, which contributes to the pathological features of parkinsonism. Usually, the activity of this cholinergic neuronal pathway is restrained by inhibition from the dopaminergic pathway that projects from the substantia nigra.

The treatment of parkinsonism is based on correcting the imbalance at the basal ganglia between the dopaminergic and cholinergic systems. Two major groups of drugs are used:

- Drugs that increase dopaminergic activity between the substantia nigra and the corpus striatum. These are dopamine precursors, dopamine agonists, drugs stimulating the release of dopamine, monoamine oxidase B (MAO_B) inhibitors, and catechol-*O*-methyl transferase (COMT) inhibitors.
- Drugs that inhibit striatal cholinergic activity, i.e. anticholinergic drugs.

11. See Fig. SAQ2.

Fig. SAQ2

	Atracurium	Suxamethonium
Block	Non-depolarizing/ competitive	Depolarizing/ non-competitive
Tetanic fade	Present	Absent unless repeatedly or continuously administered
Initial spasms	Absent	Present
Effect of anticholinesterase	Block reversed	Block enhanced unless repeatedly or continuously administered
Effect of competitive antagonist	Block enhanced	Block reduced
Effect of depolarizing agents	Block reversed	Block enhanced
Route of administration	Quaternary ammonium compounds are poorly absorbed orally and must be administered by intravenous injection	Quaternary ammonium compounds are poorly absorbed orally and must be administered by intravenous injection
Rate of onset	Fast	Very fast
Duration	40 minutes	4 minutes
Myasthenia gravis patients	Block enhanced	Block reduced
Side effects	Minimal histamine release Tachycardia	Postoperative muscle pain Bradycardia K^+ release
Clinical use	Neuromuscular blockers for surgery	Neuromuscular blockers for surgery

12. Orally administered drugs, which are usually absorbed in the small intestine, reach the liver via the portal circulation. At this stage, or within the small intestine, they may be extensively metabolized, which is known as firstpass metabolism, and means that considerably less drug reaches the systemic circulation than enters the portal vein. This causes problems because it means that higher doses of drug must be given and, owing to individual variation in the degree of firstpass metabolism, the effects of the drug can be unpredictable. Drugs that are subject to a high degree of firstpass metabolism, such as the local anaesthetic lidocaine (lignocaine), cannot be given orally and so must be administered by some other route.

13. Vasoconstrictors are used in the treatment of shock (a state of circulatory collapse, characterized by an arterial blood pressure unable to maintain adequate tissue perfusion) and hypotension.

   Sympathomimetic amines, including adrenaline, noradrenaline, phenylephrine, and ephedrine, can be administered intravenously. These activate α-receptors, stimulating phospholipase C and causing vasoconstriction and a consequent increase in arterial blood pressure. However, these raise blood pressure at the expense of vital organs such as the kidneys, and raise peripheral resistance, which is already high in patients with shock.

   Dobutamine and dopamine given by intravenous infusion are a more appropriate form of treating shock than α-adrenoceptor agonists, as renal perfusion is not impaired. Dopamine is a precursor of noradrenaline and activates dopamine receptors and α- and β-adrenoceptors.

14. See Fig. SAQ3.

15. See Fig. SAQ4.

16. Warfarin is the most commonly used oral anticoagulant. It is a vitamin K antagonist. Vitamin K is needed for the post-transcriptional γ-carboxylation of glutamic acid residues of prothrombin and clotting factors II, VII, IX, and X by the liver. Warfarin works by blocking the reduction of vitamin K epoxide, a step necessary for its action as a cofactor. It is indicated in the prophylaxis and treatment of deep vein thrombosis and pulmonary embolism, in the prophylaxis of embolization in atrial fibrillation, in patients with prosthetic heart valves, and in rheumatic heart disease.

   Warfarin is well absorbed and can therefore be given orally. The onset of action of this drug takes several hours, owing to the time needed for the degradation of factors that have already been carboxylated. ($t_{1/2}$: II = 60 hours, VII = 6 hours, IX = 24 hours, X = 40 hours).

   Haemorrhage is the main adverse effect, and this can be treated by administering vitamin K.

17. Local anaesthetics are drugs used to inhibit pain by reversibly blocking nerve conduction.
   Small nerve fibres are preferentially blocked, owing to the high surface-area to volume ratio. This results in a differential block whereby the small nociceptive (pain) and autonomic fibres are blocked but not the larger fibres responsible for the mediation of movement and touch.

   Local anaesthetics are weak bases ($pK_a = 8-9$). Only the uncharged form can penetrate lipid membranes; therefore, quaternary ammonium compounds, which are fully protonated, must be injected into the nerve axon if they are to work.

   The majority of local anaesthetics block by two routes—hydrophobic and hydrophilic. The hydrophobic route involves the uncharged form entering the membrane and blocking sodium channels from a site in the protein membrane interface. The hydrophilic route involves the uncharged form crossing the membrane to the inside where the charged form blocks the channel. This latter pathway depends on the channel being open and, therefore, this type of block is use dependent. Use dependency is especially important in the anti-arrhythmic action of local anaesthetics. Blocking sodium channels prevent propagation of a nerve impulse, and results in inhibition of nerve conduction.

   Nerve block occurs when the number of non-inactivated channels is insufficient in order to bring about depolarization to threshold.

   Examples of local anaesthetics include cocaine, procaine, lidocaine (lignocaine), and prilocaine, which vary in their rate of onset, duration, tissue penetration, chemistry, and clinical use.

18. Insulin preparations aim to mimic basal levels of insulin, and meal-induced increases in insulin. They are indicated in insulin-dependent diabetes mellitus. The insulin may be from human, porcine, or bovine sources. The preparations are available as short-, medium- and long-acting agents. The short-acting preparations consist of soluble insulin, and most resemble endogenous insulin. The intermediate-acting preparations are not as soluble, owing to the presence of a buffer such as large insulin crystals or the addition of protamine; examples include protamine zinc insulin and isophane insulin. The long-acting preparations such as insulin zinc suspension consist of insulin zinc crystals. Insulin must always be given parenterally, as it is a peptide and, therefore, destroyed in the gastrointestinal tract. Short-acting insulin is given intravenously in emergencies, but administration of the insulin preparations in maintenance treatment is usually subcutaneous.

   The sulphonylureas are given orally and include gliclazide, chlorpropamide, and glibenclamide. They block the ATP-dependent potassium channels in the membrane of the pancreatic β-cells, causing depolarization, calcium influx, and insulin release.

Fig. SAQ3

	Lidocaine (lignocaine)	Amiodarone
Class	1b	111
Mechanism of action	Blocks voltage-dependent Na^+ channels in their refractory (inactivated) state	K^+ channel blocker which also blocks Na^+ and Ca^{2+} channels, i.e. slows phase 0 and 3, and blocks α and β adrenoceptors
Effect on action potential duration	Decreased	Increased
Effect on effective refractory period	Increased	Increased
Effect on atrioventricular conduction	No effect	Decreased
Route of administration	Intravenously	Oral and intravenous
Indications	Ventricular arrhythmias following myocardial infarction	Ventricular and supraventricular arrhythmias in patients resistant to other drugs
Adverse effects	Hypotension Bradycardia Respiratory depression	Thyroid dysfunction Liver damage Pulmonary disorders Photosensitivity Neuropathy

Fig. SAQ4

	Competitive antagonists	Non-competitive antagonists
Example	Isoprenaline	Nifedipine
Binding to receptor	Reversible	Irreversible
Effect on agonist–receptor interaction	Dilution	Effectively remove receptors from the system
Effect on dose-response curve	Parallel shift to the right	Parallel shift to the right
Effect on maximum response of the agonist dose-response curve	Not depressed—reflects the fact that the block is surmountable by the addition of greater doses of agonist	Depressed, reflecting the fact that the antagonist's effect cannot be overcome by the addition of greater doses of agonist
Other notes	Making the assumption that the competive antagonist is acting in a totally reversible manner, then the pA_2 is equal to the negative logarithm of the K_d for the antagonist	At low concentrations, a parallel shift may occur without a reduced maximum response; since irreversible antagonists effectively remove receptors from the system, this reflects the fact that there must be a number of spare receptors

239

They are indicated in non-insulin-dependent diabetes mellitus, in patients with some β-cell activity.

The biguanides include metformin. They are administered orally and are indicated in non-insulin-dependent diabetes mellitus. They increase the peripheral utilization of glucose and decrease gluconeogenesis, but require the presence of endogenous insulin; therefore, patients must have some functioning β-cells.

Newer oral antidiabetic drugs include the α-glucosidase inhibitor acarbose, which acts in the gut to delay the absorption of starch and sucrose, and the thiazolidinediones, rosiglitazone and pioglitazone, which, like metformin, appear to reduce peripheral insulin resistance.

19. Anticholinesterases inhibit acetylcholinesterase and thus increase the amount of acetylcholine in the synaptic cleft, and enhance cholinergic transmission.

Short-acting anticholinesterases include edrophonium, which is selective for the neuromuscular junction (NMJ) and clinically relevant in the diagnosis of myasthenia gravis. Its duration of action is only 2–10 minutes; it is, therefore, not used therapeutically.

Intermediate-acting anticholinesterases include neostigmine, which is used intravenously to reverse the effects of non-depolarizing blockers. It has a duration of 2–4 hours and is used orally in the treatment of myasthenia gravis. Although neostigmine shows some selectivity for the NMJ, atropine is sometimes co-administered to block the muscarinic effects of the drug. Pyridostigmine has few parasympathetic actions, lasts for 3–6 hours, and is also used orally in myasthenia gravis. Physostigmine shows selectivity for the

postganglionic parasympathetic junction. It is a tertiary amine and its use is therefore associated with central effects such as initial excitation followed by depression and possible respiratory depression and unconsciousness. The central effects can be antagonized by atropine. It is used in the form of eye drops to constrict the pupil and contract the ciliary muscle in the treatment of glaucoma.

Most long-lasting or irreversible anticholinesterases are organophosphorous compounds. Sarin and tabun were developed as nerve gases, and parathion was developed as an insecticide as well as for clinical use. These have many adverse effects, such as bradycardia, hypotension, respiratory problems, depolarizing neuromuscular block, central effects, and possible death from peripheral nerve demyelination.

20. The sympathetic system mediates its effects on the cardiovascular system through activation of β_1-adrenoceptors. These are linked to adenylyl cyclase, an enzyme that catalyses the conversion of ATP to cAMP within the myocardial cells. The cAMP produced causes activation of cAMP-dependent protein kinase A, which phosphorylates serine and threonine residues of voltage-operated calcium channels resulting in their opening. There is a subsequent elevation in intracellular calcium levels, resulting in an increased rate and force of contraction of the heart.

Beta$_1$-adrenoceptor antagonists prevent the activation of adenylyl cyclase and the subsequent rise in cAMP and thus calcium. These are used in the treatment of heart failure and arrhythmias.

Index

Readers are advised to refer to both the individual drugs and their respective drug groups. Cross-references have not been inserted. Drug names are in **bold**.